Canine and Feline Dermatology:

A Systematic Approach

Canine and Feline Dermatology:

A Systematic Approach

GENE H. NESBITT, D.V.M., M.S.

Diplomate, American College of Veterinary Dermatology

Staff Dermatologist, The Animal Medical Center
New York, N.Y.

Assistant Clinical Professor of Dermatology
Department of Dermatology
New York Medical College
Metropolitan Hospital, New York, N.Y.

1983

Lea & Febiger • *Philadelphia*

Lea & Febiger
600 South Washington Square
Philadelphia, PA 19106
U.S.A.

NOTICE

Maximum efforts have been expended by the author and publisher to insure the accuracy of dosage recommendations which are in agreement with standards accepted at the time of publication. Dosage schedules may be changed as new clinical data or more experience with the drug suggest a better protocol. It is urged that reference be made to the manufacturer's recommendations for dosages. Drugs that have been recommended, but are not officially approved for use in a given species should be used only with the knowledge of potential side effects and with caution after the owner is informed of the experimental nature of the drug.

Library of Congress Cataloging in Publication Data

Nesbitt, Gene H.
    Canine and feline dermatology.

    Bibliography: p.
    Includes index.
    1. Veterinary dermatology. 2. Dogs—Diseases.
3. Cats—Diseases. I. Title.
SF901.N47 1983   636.7′08965   82-12747
ISBN 0-8121-0859-0

PRINTED IN THE UNITED STATES OF AMERICA

Print Number: 5 4 3 2 1

Preface

Dermatologic diseases in the dog and cat represent a significant percentage of the cases seen by the small animal practitioner. In many instances the client becomes dissatisfied when the problem cannot be either easily resolved or controlled. When the animal continues to show signs of discomfort or when side effects from the medication start to occur, the veterinarian often becomes frustrated with his failure to know how to approach the problem in a way that will satisfy both the client and himself. The information obtained from the history can be helpful in defining the problem, but can also be time consuming in a busy practice setting. In addition, the physical examination frequently reveals mostly secondary morphologic changes.

This book was written primarily to provide the practitioner and student with a systematic approach to any dermatologic problem by using dermatologic diagnostic and therapeutic keys. These keys can result in a better use of diagnostic tests, a more definitive diagnosis, and improved patient management. The most pertinent historical and clinical data can be obtained quickly and the clinician is directed to the appropriate screening and definitive diagnostic tests. The therapeutic keys provide a quick reference for symptomatic or specific therapy.

The most commonly encountered dermatologic entities will receive the most detailed attention. This book is not meant to be an exhaustive review of veterinary dermatology and clinical allergy; therefore, it should be supplemented when necessary with other more detailed references which are listed at the end of each chapter.

It is anticipated that the Appendices including the diagnostic and therapeutic keys, color plates of morphologic lesions, representative lesions of specific diseases, and client education series will provide the pertinent information in a simplified, systematic and readily accessible manner so that it can serve as a quick reference for the clinician. The chapters, which amplify the information incorporated in the diagnostic and therapeutic keys, will serve as an introductory clinical dermatology and allergy text for the student of veterinary dermatology.

I am most grateful to the staff of The Animal Medical Center who have played a part in making this book possible. The critiques of the diagnostic and therapeutic keys by many of the interns and residents have been most helpful. My dermatology residents, Drs. Gregg Kedan and Paul Caciolo, have been most supportive of this project, and deserve a special thanks.

Doctors Richard Anderson and Lloyd Reedy have carefully reviewed and critiqued the text. Their thoughtful suggestions were most timely and appreciated.

Several clinicians have allowed me to use their illustrations. Credit lines under these prints indicate the contributions; their cooperation was most helpful.

The many hours spent by Ms. A. Christine MacMurray in editing the manuscript were vital in the preparation of this book. Her unselfish devotion to this task is gratefully acknowledged.

A special thanks is due Mr. I. Sidney Bard for typing the manuscript.

The close cooperation of the staff at Lea & Febiger including Mr. Christian C.F. Spahr, Jr., Mr. Tom Colaiezzi, Ms. Dorothy DiRienzi, and Ms. Janet Nuciforo have allowed this project to move to completion in an orderly and timely way.

I am especially grateful for the encouragement and understanding of my wife, Sue, during the preparation of this book. Without her unselfish support, this project would not have been possible.

New York   GENE H. NESBITT

Contents

1
Structure and Function of the Skin

The clinician must have a basic knowledge of the skin's structure and function in order to understand the pathologic mechanisms associated with diseases of the skin. This background is essential before the clinical skills of observation, interpretation, and correlation of history, clinical findings, and diagnostic tests can be used best to arrive at a diagnosis and to formulate a therapeutic plan.

The structure of canine and feline skin has been well studied. However, many of the physiologic mechanisms discussed in this chapter are based on studies conducted in other animals and in man. It is thought that these mechanisms are similar to those of the dog and cat in most instances.

Skin is usually considered in terms of two principal layers—the epidermis and the dermis—not only in association with their development and functional morphologic factors, but also in terms of disorders and disease processes. These two layers are intimately related functionally and remain mutually interdependent throughout life. The epidermis is a composite of cells of different types, function, and developmental origin. The dermis is a dense, fibroelastic, connective tissue stroma that encloses the extensive vascular and neural networks as well as the specialized glands and appendages derived from the epidermis. Beneath the dermis is a subcutaneous layer or panniculus

of variable thickness. The skin is normally thickest over the dorsal anterior trunk, becoming progressively thinner posteriorly and ventrally. The integration of structure and function of canine and feline skin is summarized in Table 1–1.

EPIDERMIS

The epidermis is an organized, stratified epithelium with appendages, including hair follicles and apocrine and sebaceous glands, all of which project deep into the dermis (Figs. 1–1 and 1–2). The major cellular epidermal component is the keratinocyte, which is of ectodermal origin. Other cellular components include melanocytes, derived from the neural crest, and Langerhans' cells, of mesenchymal origin.

The primary function of the epidermis is protection from the external environment. The epidermis forms the barrier layer of the skin which prevents the entrance of toxic substances and microorganisms and the loss of water and electrolytes. The epidermal keratinocyte produces keratin, a highly resistant, insoluble, fibrous protein that is largely responsible for the mechanical protective function of the epidermis.

Most of the canine and feline epidermis is divided histologically into four layers (Figs. 1–3 and 1–4): the germinal basal cell layer; the stratum spinosum, which is composed of several strata of

TABLE 1–1. INTEGRATION OF STRUCTURE AND FUNCTION OF CANINE AND FELINE SKIN

Anatomic Structure	Principal Functions	Biologic Process	Description
Epidermis			
Stratum corneum	Protection, permeability to entrance of toxic substances and microorganisms and to loss of water and electrolytes	Desquamation	Dead, flattened keratinocytes in lamellar pattern
Stratum lucidum	Unknown	Unknown	Fully keratinized compact, thin layer of non-nucleated dead cells; present only in foot pads
Stratum granulosum	Permeability barrier to prevent loss of water and electrolytes	Keratinization	Flattened nucleated cells containing keratohyaline granules
Stratum spinosum	Synthesis of keratin precursors	Keratinogenesis and keratinization	Several layers of polyhedral nucleated cells; no blood vessels or nerves; not mitotically active
Germinal or basal cell layer	Precursor cells for keratinocytes	Mitosis	Single row of columnar cells
Melanocytes	Synthesis of melanin resulting in pigmentation and protection from sunlight	Melanogenesis and transfer of melanosomes	Neural crest derivation; dendritic cells that lie on the basal lamina packed between basal cells
Langerhans' cells	Involved in cell-mediated immune reactions	Antigen recognition and processing	Dendritic cells in upper stratum spinosum usually identified by electron microscopy
Dermis			
Fibrous portion Collagen Reticulin Elastin	Passively protects body from external injury; main support structure of skin	Synthesis and maturation of fibers	Matrix of loose connective tissue compound of fibrous proteins embedded in a ground substance
Ground substance	Water binding; barrier to bacterial penetration; provides reservoir and diffusion medium for regulating the distribution of water and salts	Undefined	Amorphous matrix of connective tissue derived from blood elements and metabolic products of parenchymal and connective tissue cells
Cells			
Fibroblasts	Precursors for collagen, elastin, and ground substance; wound healing	Collagenogenesis	Mesenchymal origin; most numerous cells in connective tissue; flat elongated cell with cytoplasmic processes at each end and elongated oval nucleus
Macrophages	Phagocytosis	Immune defense mechanism	Transformed blood monocytes or lymphocytes; eccentrically located indented nucleus, often with concentration of chromatin at periphery and one or two nucleoli
Mast cells	Release of vasoactive amines (histamine and heparin)	Inflammation	Round ornucleus with prominent nucleolus; prominent cytoplasm with spherical basophilic and metachromatic granules
Subcutis	Heat insulation; mechanical protection	Fat synthesis and storage	Connective tissue with collagen and elastin, nerves, blood vessels, and lipocytes
Vasculature	Thermoregulation; reducing heat loss by vasoconstriction; delivers nutrients and oxygen to the skin	Inflammation and wound healing	Simple and mixed cutaneous arteries and vascular plexus
Lymphatics	Drainage system; transports capillary transudates	Inflammation and circulation	Arise from capillary networks in superficial dermis

TABLE 1–1. *Continued*

Anatomic Structure	Principal Functions	Biologic Process	Description
Nerves			
Somatic sensory	Sensory perception; mediation of touch, pain, temperature, and itch	Afferent impulse transmission	Lie in subcuticular area and continue by a nerve plexus that extends through dermis to epidermis innervating epidermis, glands, muscles, and hair follicles
Autonomic	Secretomotor; control of blood vessels, glands, and pilosecretion	Efferent impulse transmission	Motor nerves to blood vessels, arrector pili muscles and myoepithelial cells around apocrine glands
Appendages			
Hair follicle	Precursor for hair	Formation of hair	Invagination of epidermis into the dermis; usually compound
Sebaceous glands	Lubrication	Secretion of lipids	Simple alveolar holocrine glands
Apocrine sweat glands	No known function in normal conditions; minor heat regulation in abnormal conditions	Secretion of proteins	Coiled secretory tubule extending deep into dermis and subcutis; may be globoid shaped in cats
Eccrine sweat glands	Possible lubrication	Gland secretions	Found only in footpads; small, tightly coiled, and tubular, located deep in the skin; secretory duct to the surface

polyhedral cells lying above the germinal layer; the stratum granulosum, a layer of flattened nucleated cells containing distinctive keratohyaline granules, which marks the transition to the overlying keratinized lamellae of the fourth layer, the stratum corneum. The stratum granulosum is not prominent in many microscopic sections of feline skin. A fifth layer, the stratum lucidum or clear layer, is present only in the footpads between the granular and corneal layers (see Fig. 1–19).

Although the exact structural components of the epidermal barrier have not been agreed upon, it is generally accepted that the stratum corneum constitutes the major protective barrier. Recent evidence suggests that the stratum granulosum or granulosum-corneum junction is also an important element of the epidermal barrier. Evidence shows that together with the transformation of viable nucleated cells into cornified cells, there is also complete sealing of the intercellular environment, which provides absolute control of the pas-

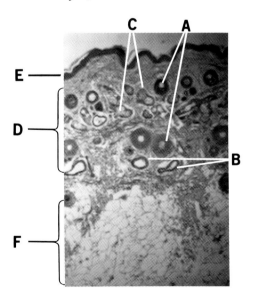

Fig. 1–1. Canine skin: Microscopic section of normal canine skin. Note epidermis *(E)*, multiple appendages (hair follicle *(A)*, apocrine glands *(B)*, and sebaceous glands *(C)*) in the dermis *(D)*, and subcutis *(F)* (low power).

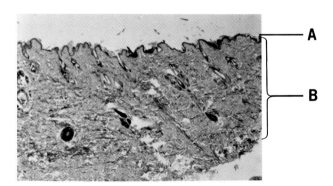

Fig. 1–2. Feline skin: Microscopic section of normal feline skin. Note the thin epidermis *(A)*, hair follicles, and adnexal structures throughout the upper two thirds of the dermis *(B)* (scan power).

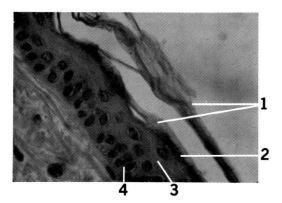

Fig. 1–3. Epidermal layers (canine): Microscopic section of normal canine skin. Note the four layers: (1) stratum corneum; (2) stratum granulosum; (3) stratum spinosum; and (4) basal cell layer (high power).

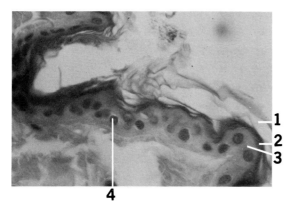

Fig. 1–4. Epidermal layers (feline): Microscopic section of normal feline skin. Note the four layers: (1) stratum corneum; (2) stratum granulosum; (3) stratum spinosum; and (4) basal cell layer (high power).

sage of aqueous solvents from both within and without the epidermis.

A chemical interface between the basal cell layer and the dermis is referred to as the basal lamina. The specific function of the basal lamina embryologically or postnatally is not known, although it is considered an important substrate for the basal cells, and acts as a barrier to the exchange of cells and large molecules.

Melanocytes are pigment-producing cells of neural crest origin found in the basal cell layer (Fig. 1–5). The only known function of melanocytes is the synthesis of pigment granules or melanosomes, which are subsequently transferred to the surrounding keratinocytes. The melanin released from the granules acts as a screen against solar, ultraviolet radiation.

Langerhans' cells are dendritic cells seen in the upper layers of the stratum spinosum. Their origin is obscure but probably mesenchymal. Their func-

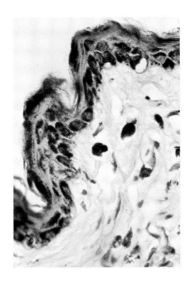

Fig. 1–5. Hyperpigmentation: Microscopic section of skin with increased melanogenesis in basal cell layer and melanin-laden macrophages in dermis.

tion in man is thought to be immunologic, and they are involved with the uptake and processing of antigenic material. It has been suggested that Langerhans' cells are special macrophages that function as the initial receptors for the cutaneous response to external antigens. These cells can be identified with certainty only by electron microscopy.

DERMIS

The dermis is located between the epidermis and the subcutaneous panniculus (Fig. 1–6). It consists of a matrix of loose connective tissue composed of the fibrous proteins—collagen, elastin, and reticulin—embedded in an amorphous ground substance. The matrix is traversed by blood vessels, nerves, and lymphatics, and is penetrated by the epidermal appendages including the apocrine glands and pilosebaceous units (see Fig. 1–2).

Arrector pili muscles are the major muscles in the dermis (Fig. 1–7). Variable numbers of smooth muscle fibers are present.

Collagenous fibers are the largest and most numerous type of fiber in the dermis, constituting approximately 90% of all fibers. The appearance of the fibers varies according to their depth in the dermis as well as the function of the dermis. The reticular fibers, or precollagen, are finely branched; these fibers are present throughout the ground substance at birth and gradually decrease in number within four weeks postnatally. They become concentrated around blood vessels, hair follicles,

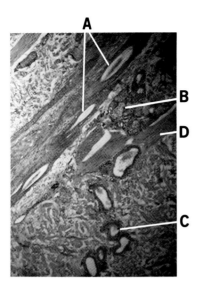

Fig. 1–6. Dermis (canine): Microscopic section of the dermis of normal canine skin. Note hair follicle unit (compound hair follicle (A), sebaceous glands (B), apocrine glands (C), arrector pili muscle (D)) surrounded by connective tissue matrix (low power).

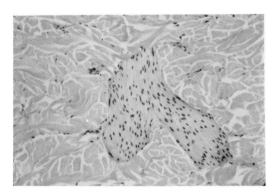

Fig. 1–7. Arrector pili muscle: Microscopic section of normal canine skin. Note large smooth muscle bundle in dermis (low power).

glands, and arrector pili muscles, and beneath the basal cell layer of the epidermis. With age, the reticular fibers closely approximate collagen fibers.

Elastic fibers, composed of single fine branches, are more abundant in the deeper part of the dermis. An inverse relationship exists between the abundance of terminal hairs in an area and the quantity of elastic fibers. Elastic fibers stretch easily with little loss of energy and resume their original shape when the stress is relieved. Fine elastic fibers in the upper dermis most likely function to anchor the epidermis to the dermis. The fiber content of the dermis plays a role in determining the presence and direction of tension lines in the skin.

The ground substance of the dermis is the structureless portion of connective tissue that lies out-

side the cells, fibers, blood vessels, and nerves. All other dermal components are embedded in this amorphous matrix. The ground substance appears to be a system of multiple components: substances derived from the blood, such as water, inorganic ions, blood sugars, blood proteins, and urea; metabolic products of parenchymal cells; and metabolic products of connective tissue cells. Thus the ground substance is considered the immediate environment of the cells and fibers of the dermis and an extension of the vascular system.

The cellular components of the dermis include fibroblasts, macrophages (Fig. 1–8), and mast cells (Fig. 1–9). Fibroblasts, the most numerous cells in connective tissue, are responsible for the formation of collagenous and elastin fibers and the amorphous ground substance. These cells develop from tissue mesenchymal cells.

Macrophages or histiocytes appear early in embryonic development. The phagocytic activity of these cells increases progressively throughout fetal and neonatal life. Controversy still exists about the origin and fate of tissue macrophages.

Mast cells vary in number among species as well as in different regions of the same animal. They are often arranged around the walls of small blood vessels. These cells probably have a hematogenous origin or arise from perivascular connective tissue cells. Mast cells degranulate under physical conditions such as cold, heat, and ultraviolet light, and in the presence of chemicals or various bacterial or animal toxins. Heparin and histamine contained within the granules are released. Mast cells are believed to participate in the regulation of lipid metabolism due to the effect of heparin accelerating lipid transportation or clearance. His-

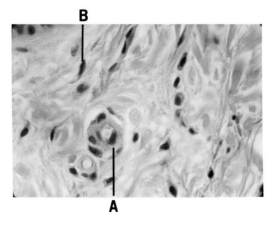

Fig. 1–8. Dermis (canine): Microscopic section of normal canine skin. Note blood vessels (A) and fibroblasts (B) with elongated nuclei (high power).

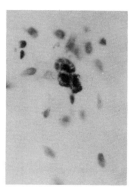

Fig. 1–9. Dermal mast cells: Microscopic section from a cat with allergic dermatitis. Note the three mast cells with granules in the cytoplasm. (Toluidine blue stain, high power.)

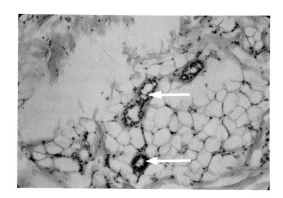

Fig. 1–10. Subcutis (canine): Microscopic section from normal canine footpad. Note the meshwork of the loose collagenous trabeculae and lipocytes. Eccrine sweat glands (arrows) are observed (low power).

tamine increases capillary permeability, causes smooth muscle fibers to contract, stimulates the phagocytic activity of blood and connective tissue cells, and promotes the secretion of various glands. It is thus responsible for the onset of inflammation, hyperemia, and the early increase in capillary permeability during the inflammatory process.

Several changes occur in the dermis with aging. In the fetal dermis, collagen fibers are fine and fibrillar, whereas in mature individuals they form coarse bundles. Collagen is synthesized continually, although its metabolic activities, including both synthesis and degradation, sharply decrease with age. Elastic fibers increase in number and diameter during aging. Dermal ground substance undergoes little histologic change.

The biologic functions of the dermis are many and complex. A primary function is to protect the body from external injury, The dermis is uniquely constructed to resist tearing, shearing, and localized pressure, but is also flexible enough to allow joint movement and local stretch. Both the amount and architecture of collagen determine the tensile strength of the dermis. It plays an important role as a substratum for the epidermis. The hyaluronic acid of the ground substance acts as a barrier to bacterial penetration. Hyaluronic acid also binds water and maintains dermal turgor in the tissues; thus, the dermis may function as a water storage organ. The dermis plays a minor role in cation exchange; it has a homeostatic function in maintaining proper levels of blood cations and in supplying mineral metabolism in general. Finally, the dermis is involved in thermal regulation by providing the supporting bed for the vasculature.

SUBCUTIS

The subcutis is composed of connective tissue, nerves, blood vessels, and lipocytes (Fig. 1–10).

The connective tissue consists of loose collagenous trabeculae that contain many elastic fibers that cross each other to form a meshwork; the spaces of the meshwork are further subdivided by smaller bundles. The adipose tissue can serve as a cushion or shock absorber, a filler, a sheath for easily injured parts such as nerves and vessels, and an insulator to protect the body from excessive heat loss. The degree to which the skin can be folded or displaced depends upon the development of the subcutis and the extensibility, length, and thickness of the fiber bundles.

VASCULAR SYSTEM

The kinds of cutaneous vascular beds are determined by the areas of skin they perfuse, the thickness of the various dermal and hypodermal layers, the types and numbers of appendages present, and the specific relation of the skin to the bones and muscle fascia under it. The primary function of the cutaneous vascular system is to deliver nutrients to the skin. The sources of the arteries and their large primary branches in the subcutaneous fascia are generally constant in all animals. The divisions and subdivisions of these arteries all run parallel to the skin surface, with no constancy in the arrangement of the smaller vessels and no pattern common to all dogs and cats.

There are two types of primary cutaneous vasculature: simple and mixed cutaneous arteries. The simple cutaneous arteries reach the skin by running between muscle masses and giving off small branches to the muscle tissue. The mixed cutaneous arteries pass through muscle beds, with large branches supplying the muscle before terminating in the skin.

There are three vascular plexus: the subcutaneous or deep; the cutaneous (middle or intermediate); and the superficial (subepidermal or subpapillary). These plexus lie parallel to the surface of the skin. The extensive microscopic plexus of the skin vessels appear to ensure a continuous and complete blood supply to the skin, even when there is temporary blockage of the main vessels coming from the deeper layers.

LYMPHATICS

Lymphatics of the skin arise from capillary networks that lie in the superficial area of the dermis and surround the follicles and glands. Their main function is to transport the capillary transudate.

NERVES

Nerves of the skin serve as sensory receptors and also control the sweat glands and arrector pili muscles (Fig. 1–11). The nerves lie in the subcutaneous area and are continuous with a nerve plexus that extends through the dermis to the epidermis, with branches from these plexus innervating the epidermis, glands, muscles, and hair follicles. Sensory nerve fibers have three types of terminal receptors: the dermal nerve network, the hair follicle network, and specialized end organs. The density of dermal nerve networks in the skin varies inversely with the hair coverage of the area. The dermal nerve network functions in pain perception and temperature variation.

The principal organ for touch perception is made up of sensory nerve fibers that form a double network around the primary hair. Every hair has a nerve ending associated with it. The nerve penetrates the follicle below the sebaceous gland duct, divides, and then lies parallel to the long axis of the hair. The mechanism of touch perception is more refined in the sinus or tactile hairs, where

engorgement of the vascular sinus surrounding the base of the hair follicle enhances sensory acuity.

In addition to the dermal and follicular networks, the hairless skin also contains many encapsulated nerve endings that make up the specialized receptors. These special end organs are found primarily at the mucocutaneous junctions and in the footpads. The skin also is supplied with adrenergic sympathetic motor nerves to blood vessels, arrector pili muscles, and myoepithelial cells around the apocrine sweat glands.

PILIARY APPARATUS

The pilosebaceous unit consists of the hair follicle, which is an epidermal appendage that penetrates the dermis, and the sebaceous glands that originate from the sides of the follicle (Fig. 1–12). Hairs consist of compactly cemented keratinized cells produced by the hair follicles.

Hair Follicle. The basic unit of hair production is the hair follicle (Fig. 1–13), which is made

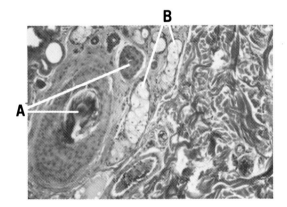

Fig. 1–12.   Pilosebaceous unit: Microscopic section of normal canine skin. Note the pilosebaceous unit consisting of a compound hair follicle (A) and sebaceous glands (B) (low power).

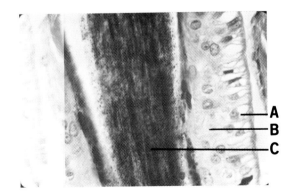

Fig. 1–13.   Hair follicle and hair: Microscopic longitudinal section of a normal canine hair follicle and hair shaft. Note the epithelial portion (outer root sheath (A) and inner root sheath (B)) and cortex of the hair (C) (high power).

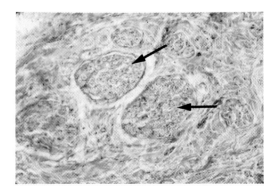

Fig. 1–11.   Nerves: Microscopic section of normal canine skin. Note multiple nerve bundles in the dermis (arrows) (high power).

up of a peripheral connective tissue portion and an inner epithelial part or root sheath. The connective tissue portion is derived from the dermis; the epithelial portion has an epidermal origin. The epithelial portion is divided into the outer root sheath, which is a continuation of the basal cell layer of the epidermis, and the inner root sheath, which grows upward with the hair from the hair bulb (Fig. 1–14).

At birth the hair follicles are simple or primary, with one hair per follicle. As the animal ages, accessory hairs develop in accessory or secondary follicles, which arise as buds from the original single follicle, forming a compound follicle (Fig. 1–15). There is a single follicular orifice with one primary cover or guard hair and a number of secondary hairs. The follicle and hair bulb of the guard hair in the compound follicle are larger and penetrate deeper into the subcutaneous tissue than those of the secondary hairs. Each secondary hair is also accompanied by sebaceous glands and an arrector pili muscle.

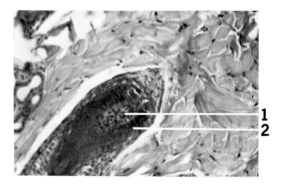

Fig. 1–14. Hair bulb: Microscopic section of normal canine skin. Note hair bulb with dermal papilla (1) and hair matrix (2) (low power).

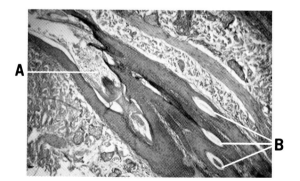

Fig. 1–15. Compound hair follicle: Microscopic section of normal canine skin. Note multiple hair follicles with the larger primary follicle (A) and several accessory follicles (B) (low power).

Hair. Hairs are epidermal structures (Fig. 1–13). The free portion is called the hair shaft and the proximal portion is called the root. The root is usually set obliquely to the skin. The root is attached to the underlying dermal papilla. The shaft is composed of medulla, cortex, and cuticle. The cortex is composed of tightly packed keratin cells that form the major portion of the hair. Hair color is determined by pigment in these cells.

Several classifications that exist for hair types in dogs are summarized in Table 1–2. Two types of hair coats are described for cats: Persian or long hair, and domestic or short hair. The short hair is the dominant gene.

Hair has several functions, including the first line of external defense against physical, chemical, and ultraviolet or actinic trauma. It also performs sensory functions and plays a significant role in the thermoregulatory mechanism.

Hair Cycle. The hair grows cyclically, with alternating periods of growth and quiescence. During the growth phase, follicles are in the anagen stage; during the subsequent resting phase, they contain club hairs and are in the telogen stage (Fig. 1–16). The catagen stage is the transition period when the follicles are reorganizing into an inactive state.

Several factors affect the hair growth cycle. The photoperiod plays a significant role. As the daylight hours increase, the rate of shedding increases and the hair coat becomes coarser and less dense. As the photoperiod decreases, the coat is again shed and there is a stimulation of hair growth that produces a dense hair coat accompanied by decreased sebum production. Poor health or generalized disease shortens the period of anagen and results in a larger percentage of body hairs being in telogen at one time. Anagen is stimulated by thyroxine, adrenocorticotropic hormone (ACTH), and testosterone, while estrogens have an inhibitory effect on anagen.

GLANDS

Sebaceous Glands. Sebaceous glands are simple, alveolar holocrine glands associated with the pilosebaceous apparatus (see Fig. 1–12). There are a few body regions where these glands are not associated with the hair follicle, including the external ear canal, anus, prepuce, vulva, and the tarsal glands of the eyelids. These glands tend to be larger and more numerous along the dorsal part of the neck, back, and tail.

Sebaceous glands are evaginated from the hair follicle and are connected to the upper part of the

TABLE 1–2.   CLASSIFICATION OF HAIR TYPES

Reference	Classification
Lovell and Getty, 1964	Protective hair 　Straight hair 　Bristle hair 　Wavy bristle hair
	Components of undercoat 　Bristle wavy 　Large wavy 　Fine wavy
Schwartzman and Orkin, 1962	Tactile hairs 　Feelers 　Whiskers 　Vibrissae
	Guard hairs from primary follicles 　Spines 　Bristles
	Fine soft underhairs from accessory or second- 　ary follicles 　Wool 　Fur 　Lanugo
Muller and Kirk, 1976	Normal (German Shepherd, Welsh Corgi)
	Long 　Fine (Cocker Spaniel, Pomeranian) 　Wooly or coarse (Poodle, Kerry Blue Terrier) Short 　Coarse (Rottweiler) 　Fine (Boxer, Dachshund)

follicle by a short duct. These glands have a peripheral basal cell layer with the central part of the gland consisting of large, foamy, lipid-filled cells (Fig. 1–17).

Apocrine Glands.   Apocrine glands are large, loosely coiled sweat glands that are distributed over the entire skin as an appendage of the hair follicles (Fig. 1–18). Greater numbers are found on the face and between the toes. Specialized apocrine glands are also present in the external ear canal (ceruminous glands), in the eyelids in association with the cilia (glands of Moll), and in the mammary glands. One apocrine gland is associated with each follicle complex in the form of a coiled secretory tubule that extends deep into the dermis and subcutaneous tissue. The apocrine secretory duct empties into the follicle above the opening of the sebaceous gland duct.

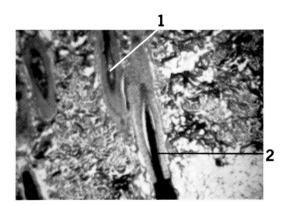

Fig. 1–16.   Hair follicles: Microscopic section of hair follicles in normal canine skin. Note the telogen follicle with the epithelial strand at the base (1) and the anagen follicle with the new hair shaft (2) (low power).

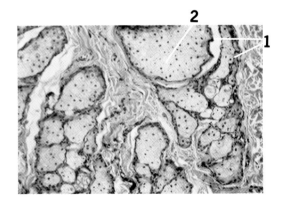

Fig. 1–17.   Sebaceous glands: Microscopic section of sebaceous glands from normal canine skin. Note the peripheral basal layer (1) and the foamy lipid-filled cells in the central part of the gland (2) (low power).

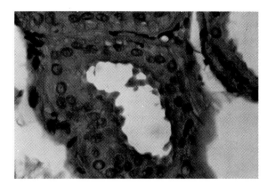

Fig. 1–18. Apocrine sweat glands: Microscopic cross section of apocrine sweat gland in normal canine skin. Note the secretory cuboidal epithelial cells (high power)

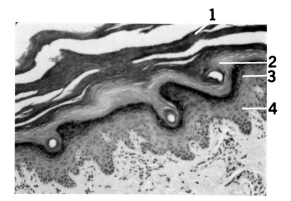

Fig. 1–19. Footpad (feline): Microscopic section of normal feline footpad. Note the thick stratum corneum (1), stratum lucidum (2), prominent granular layer (3), and the thick stratum spinosum (4) (low power).

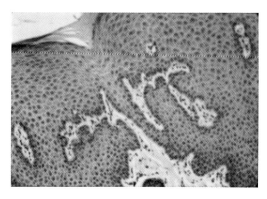

Fig. 1–20. Planum nasale (canine): Microscopic section of normal canine planum nasale. Note the thick stratum spinosum and absence of stratum lucidum and stratum granulosum (low power).

The apocrine sweat glands do not appear to function under normal conditions; however, they do respond to the application of local heat and to circulating catecholamines. The apocrine sweat glands of the dog do not actively participate in the central thermoregulatory mechanism; they mainly serve to protect the skin from an excess temperature rise. The apocrine secretion is a proteinaceous, white, odorless, milky fluid that is slowly and continuously formed.

Eccrine (Merocrine) Sweat Glands. These glands are found only in the footpads of the dog and cat, located deep in the dermis at its junction with the hypodermis (see Fig. 1–10). The excretory duct follows a tortuous path through the dermis and epidermis to a pore on the surface of the pad. The secretion of the eccrine sweat gland is watery. These glands have no thermoregulatory function.

Tail Glands. The tail gland area of a dog is located on the dorsal surface of the tail about 2 in. (5 cm) from the base of the tail. The hair coat over the glands is composed of coarse hairs emerging from single follicles. Numerous, large sebaceous and apocrine glands composing the tail glands extend deep into the dermis and subcutaneous tissue.

Circumanal and Perianal Glands. These glands are complexes found near the anal orifice. The circumanal glands are superficial sebaceous glands whose secretory ducts empty into hair follicles and onto the mucocutaneous anal surface. Perianal or deep circumanal glands make up the deeper, nonsebaceous part of the complex. The perianal glands do not have any secretory activity.

FOOT PADS

The footpads are characterized by a thick stratum corneum and a prominent stratum lucidum or clear layer (Fig. 1–19). There are numerous eccrine (merocrine) sweat glands in the lower dermis and hypodermis (see Fig. 1–10).

NASAL SKIN

Nasal skin (planum nasale) is characterized by only three layers in the epidermis: stratum corneum, stratum spinosum, and basal cell layer (Fig. 1–20). There is an absence of hair and glandular structures in the dermis. Pigment granules are usually prominent in the lower epidermis.

BIOLOGIC OR PHYSIOLOGIC PROCESSES OF SKIN

Five biologic or physiologic processes have great impact on clinical veterinary dermatology. The veterinary clinician must be familiar with the mechanisms involved and the factors influencing these processes to appreciate the historical, clinical, and diagnostic findings of many cutaneous diseases or syndromes.

Keratinization. Three distinct phases occur in the life cycle of keratinocytes: mitosis in the basal cell layer; differentiation in the stratum spinosum and stratum granulosum; and exfoliation of the corneal layer.

Since the surface layers are continuously being shed, the constant thickness of the epidermis depends upon a consistent rate of mitotic reproduction in the basal layer. The regulation of basal cell proliferation involves both intrinsic and extrinsic factors, which are summarized in Table 1–3.

Intrinsic factors are not well delineated at this time. In human and in pig skin, a tissue substance called an epidermal chalone has demonstrated antimitotic activity on basal cells; epinephrine is required to produce this effect. Prostaglandins can stimulate epidermal cell proliferation.

Extrinsic factors that influence basal cell proliferation include the dermis, which provides a substratum of suitable texture and produces factors that promote basal cell proliferation. An epidermal growth factor (EGF) and vitamin A have been shown to stimulate mitosis, although hydrocortisone inhibits epidermal mitotic activity. Trauma such as radiation, scraping, or incision on the surface of the epidermis results in a sudden burst of mitotic activity in the basal cell layer. There must be a complex interplay of these many intrinsic and extrinsic regulatory factors to ensure that the epidermis maintains the proper proportion of proliferating and differentiating cells sufficient to maintain a constant thickness in relation to the rate of surface desquamation. Several factors that affect the desquamation process are summarized in Table 1–4.

Pigmentation. The process of pigment development and the regulation of pigmentation in the hair and skin is not fully understood. The melanocytes are the basic structural units of the melanin pigmentary system. They lie on the basal lamina tightly packed between basal cells. Dendrites from the melanocytes project into the epidermis. The melanocytes synthesize melanosomes or pigment granules. In a manner not completely understood in man or animals, the melanosomes are transferred to keratinocytes. Some evidence in man shows that keratinocytes actively phagocytize the dendrites containing melanin.

Melanin pigmentation depends on the interaction between melanocytes and keratinocytes, the rate of pigment production (melanogenesis), the transfer to keratinocytes, and the final disposition of melanosomes within the keratinocytes. A functional epidermal-melanin unit consists of a melanocyte and a constant population of satellite keratinocytes. An example of the interaction of the components of this unit is the pigmentation of hair, in which melanocytes synthesize and transfer pigment to the keratinocytes of the hair shaft only during the anagen stage of the hair cycle.

Genetic and hormonal factors are thought to be the major regulators of melanocyte activity. Melanocyte-stimulating hormone (MSH) from the intermediate lobe of the pituitary gland causes increased pigmentation in man by influencing a greater dispersion of melanosomes and an increase in the number of melanosomes in the keratino-

TABLE 1–3. FACTORS INFLUENCING OR REGULATING KERATINIZATION

Factor	Effect	Target
Intrinsic		
Epidermal chalone and epinephrine	Antimitotic	Basal cells
Prostaglandins	Proliferation	Epidermal cells
Extrinsic		
Dermis	Substrate for proliferation	Basal cells
Epidermal growth factor	Proliferation	Basal cells
Vitamin A		
Normal	Proliferation	Basal cells
Excessive	Inhibition of keratinization	Epidermis
Deficient	Stimulation	Epidermis
Corticosteroids	Inhibition of keratinization	Epidermis
Copper deficiency	Weak hair	Hair
Estrogens	Stimulation of keratinization	Epidermis
Zinc deficiency	Lack of maturation of keratinocytes	Epidermis

TABLE 1–4. FACTORS AFFECTING DESQUAMATION

Factor	Effect
Accelerated epithelial proliferation	Hyperkeratosis (obvious scaling)
Failure to disintegrate	Marked hyperkeratosis (heavy scaling)
Persistent minor trauma	Inhibition (no scaling)
Low humidity	Drying of stratum corneum (mild scaling)

cytes. Increases in estrogen, progesterone, and MSH are associated with hyperpigmentation during pregnancy and with hyperestrogenism or ovarian imbalance I syndromes. The mode of action is unknown. ACTH also increases pigmentation.

The role of melatonin from the pineal gland in pigmentation is unclear. Conditions of darkness stimulate melatonin production. It may be an antagonist to MSH.

Hyperpigmentation is a clinical entity associated with an increase in melanin pigment in the basal layer of the epidermis and in the upper dermis. The intensity of hyperpigmentation depends on the amount of melanosomes produced and the number of melanosomes transferred to the keratinocytes. Two general categories of hyperpigmentation are defined: melanosis develops without preceding inflammatory skin disease; melanoderma is associated with or follows inflammatory disorders or lesions. Lentigo is a clinical finding characterized by focal hyperpigmented macules.

Clinical hypopigmentation, vitiligo, is also observed. Albinism is associated with a genetic trait causing a lack of tyrosinase to synthesize melanin. Hypopigmentation is associated with discoid lupus erythematosus, nasal solar dermatitis, burns, trauma, and ionizing irradiation presumably due to depression or destruction of the melanocytes.

Sebum Production. Sebum is an oily secretion composed of the products of the degenerated and disrupted cells of the sebaceous gland. Sebum tends to keep the skin and hair soft and pliable by forming an emulsion (lipid film) on the skin and hair surface to retain moisture. Approximately 90% of the lipid film results from sebum production, and 10% is derived from cytoplasmic contents of the epidermal cells and the apocrine sweat glands. The flow of sebaceous glands is thought to be continuous and the quantity of sebum released in a given time per unit area is proportional to the total glandular volume.

Both the size and the rate of maturation of sebaceous glands are regulated by hormones. Human studies have shown that androgens are the primary trophic hormone, estrogens have a suppressive ef-

fect, and progesterone and glucocorticoids have little direct effect on sebaceous gland secretion. In women, sebum production is thought to be stimulated by ovarian and adrenal androgens. The apparent decrease of sebum production in women following prednisone administration is possibly the result of suppression of ovarian androgens. Large doses of exogenous progesterone have a stimulatory effect on the sebaceous glands.

Pruritus. Pruritus is defined as an irritating, nonadapting cutaneous sensation that evokes the impulse to scratch. A wide variety of stimuli and noxious agents are believed to liberate peripheral chemomediators. The major mediators of pruritus in the dog and cat are thought to be proteolytic enzymes. Proteases are released by both fungi and bacteria, by mast cell degranulation following an antigen-antibody reaction, and by leukocytes in inflammatory infiltrates. Extracellular proteases such as plasmin are released as a result of capillary dilatation. Cathepsin from epidermal cells has proteolytic activity. This may account for the persistence of the itch sensation after epidermal damage induced by scratching. The role of kinins and prostaglandin E_1 has not been well defined. Pruritus may be initiated or potentiated by boredom and neuroses. Factors such as foreign bodies, insect bites, parasitisms, allergic reactions, infections, inflammation, or vasodilatation may facilitate access to proteases and thus potentiate pruritus.

The mediators of pruritus act on a finely arborizing, complex network of myelinated and nonmyelinated nerve endings, believed to be the fundamental cutaneous sensory receptor organ. In man, itch perception is localized in the area of the dermoepidermal junction and is independent of the presence of the epidermis. These sensory or "itch points" are specific areas that vary in number from animal to animal and from site to site. After skin damage, they may change in number and respond to a lower threshold of stimulation.

Two types of pruritus described are: physiologic itch, which is a spontaneous, well-localized itch believed to be conducted by myelinated, rapid-

TABLE 1–5. ETIOLOGIC FACTORS AND MECHANISMS OF REVERSIBLE
OR POTENTIALLY REVERSIBLE ALOPECIA

Etiologic Factors	Mechanisms
Endocrine disorders Hypothyroidism Hyperadrenocorticism Growth hormone deficiency Ovarian imbalance Estrogen excess in male dogs	Direct suppressive effect on hair follicle in a resting (telogen) state
Bacterial infection	Superficial folliculitis with neutrophilic exudate and hyperkeratosis of the infundibular portion of hair canal alters intrafollicular environment resulting in shedding of hair from the infected follicle
Dermatophytes	Fungal hyphae invade and proliferate within the hair shaft, weakening its structure and causing subsequent fracture of hair shaft
Parasitic infestation Nematode (Pelodera strongyloides)	Hyperkeratosis of hair canal and displacement of hair; facilitation by self-trauma resulting from irritation and inflammation associated with the presence of larvae
Fleas (hypersensitivity)	Self-trauma and immunologic mechanisms
Sarcoptic mange	Self-trauma associated with mites burrowing through the epidermis
Demodicosis	Stimulation of hyperkeratosis within the hair canal by proliferating mites with subsequent displacement and dislodgement of hair shafts, inflammation, and immunologic responses
Chemical and drug- induced alopecia Antimitotic drugs	Inhibit hair synthesis in anagen follicles; hair shaft becomes constricted and breaks off
Thallium	Converts follicles from anagen to telogen with subsequent shedding, inflammation, and parakeratotic hyperkeratosis
Nonscarring cutaneous disease Seborrheic syndrome	Faulty keratinization with increased epidermal turnover time and parakeratotic hyperkeratosis, edema, and perivascular infiltration
Acanthosis nigricans	Faulty keratinization due to increased epidermal turnover time, direct or indirect suppression of hair follicles by hormone influences
Alopecia areata	Antitissue antibodies directed against hair follicles resulting in follicular atrophy and hair shedding
Telogen effluvium	Variety of stress factors (fever, fright, parturition, shock, and other traumatic episodes)

conducting delta A fibers; and pathologic itch, which is an unpleasant, poorly localized itch conducted by unmyelinated, slow-conducting C fibers. The itch perception travels from the subepidermal nerve plexus by way of the dorsal root and the anterolateral spinothalamic tract to the thalamus and then through the internal capsule to the sensory cortex.

The predisposition to pruritus by neuroses and boredom in man has been attributed to the modification of the perception of itching at the higher cortical levels of the nervous system. Mental distraction may depress consciousness of itching, although boredom may greatly intensify pruritus.

Alopecia. Alopecia is defined as the loss or lack of hair in any amount up to complete baldness. The cause of alopecia may be divided into external and internal factors. Internal factors are further divided into primary (genetic) and secondary (consequence of other internal disease). Conroy (1979) has categorized the external factors as nutritional, biologic agents (parasites, microorganisms), physical and chemical factors, stress, inappropriate therapy, and trauma. The external factors, acting alone or in combination, can alter the external or internal environment to produce or enhance susceptibility.

Alopecias may be classified on the basis of permanence of the hair loss: irreversible or permanent effect and reversible or potentially reversible, a temporary effect.

The pathomechanism operative in alopecias is related to etiologic factors and may involve faulty development, suppression of the hair follicle, destruction and displacement, acute loss of telogen hairs, irritation and self-trauma, leukocytic activ-

TABLE 1–6. ETIOLOGIC FACTORS AND MECHANISMS OF IRREVERSIBLE ALOPECIA

Etiologic Factors	Mechanisms

Genetic alopecia
 Hypotrichosis
 Epitheliogenesis
  imperfecta
 Hereditary black hair
  follicular dysplasia
 Congenital ectodermal defect
 Color mutant alopecia
	Genetically controlled faulty growth and development (dysplasia), or complete absence (defect) of some, many, or all hair follicles

Necrotizing processes Physical or chemical injury	Destruction of dermal tissue including hair follicles with subsequent lack of piloglandular appendages and replacement of normal dermal tissue with scar tissue
Deep bacterial and fungal infection	Excessive inflammatory response, which destroys hair follicles by necrosis; intrafollicular bacteria or fungi attract leukocytes that are liberating proteolytic enzymes which destroy the follicular epithelium with subsequent scarring
Nasal solar dermatitis Lupus erythematosus	Repeated necrotizing inflammatory response and scar tissue formation
Cutaneous neoplasms and granulomas	Replacement of the follicular and glandular appendages by proliferating neoplastic cells or granulation tissue

ity, invasion and weakening of the hair shaft, necrosis and fibrosis of tissue, and immune-mediated responses. Tables 1–5 and 1–6 summarize the etiologic factors and mechanisms associated with reversible and irreversible alopecias.

SELECTED READINGS

Anderson, R.K.: Canine acanthosis nigricans. Compend. Cont. Ed. Pract. Vet. 1:466,1979

Breathnach, A.S., and Wolff, K.: Structure and development of skin. In Dermatology in General Medicine. 2nd Ed. Edited by T.B. Fitzpatrick, et al. New York, McGraw–Hill, 1979.

Conroy, J.D.: The etiology and pathogenesis of alopecia. Compend. Cont. Ed. Pract. Vet. 1:806, 1979.

Halliwell, R.E.W.: Pathogenesis and treatment of pruritus. J. Am. Vet. Med. Assoc. 164:793, 1974.

Lorincz, A.L.: Neurophysiologic reaction of the skin: pathophysiology of pruritus. In Dermatology in General Medicine. 2nd Ed. Edited by T.B. Fitzpatrick, et al. New York, McGraw-Hill, 1979.

Lovell, J.E., and Getty, R.: The integument. In Anatomy of the Dog. Edited by M.E. Miller, G.C. Christensen, and H.E. Evans. Philadelphia, W.B. Saunders, 1964.

———: The hair follicle, epidermis, dermis and skin glands of the dog. Am. J. Vet. Res. 18:1873, 1957.

Montagna, W., and Parakkal, P.F.: The Structure and Function of Skin. 3rd Ed. New York, Academic Press, 1974.

Mueller, G.H., and Kirk, R.W.: Small Animal Dermatology. 2nd Ed. Philadelphia, W.B. Saunders, 1976.

Schwartzman, R.M., and Orkin, M.: A Comparative Study of Skin Diseases of Dog and Man. Springfield, Ill., Charles C Thomas, 1962.

Strickland, J.H., and Calhoun, M.L.: The integumentary system of the cat. Am. J. Vet. Res., 24:1018, 1963.

Swaim, S.F.: Surgery of Traumatized Skin: Management and Reconstruction in the Dog and Cat. Philadelphia, W.B. Saunders, 1980.

2

Fundamentals of Dermatologic Diagnosis

The skin has a relatively limited number of pathologic responses to injury, manifested by various lesions consisting of one type or aggregates of several types. These lesions may be solitary or multiple, superficial or deep, and may have a distribution pattern that is localized, regionalized, or generalized. Some lesions may be of primary concern to the pet owner even though they do not alter the normal physiologic functions of the skin.

The component of the skin that is primarily affected, e.g., the epidermis, dermis, or hair follicle, should first be identified. This requires that the clinician be familiar with the anatomy and function of the skin. He must also be able to recognize types of skin lesions based on the morphologic structure and the arrangement and distribution of lesions as they relate to specific or general disease patterns. A working knowledge of these basic facts makes it easier to arrive at a definitive diagnosis and a specific therapeutic plan.

DESCRIPTION OF GENERAL DERMATOLOGIC DIAGNOSTIC KEY

The Dermatologic Diagnostic Key (Appendix 1:1) places all canine and feline skin diseases into one of nine etiologic classifications (see Appendices 1:2 to 1:14).

Dermatologic diagnostic keys can be the most important aid in achieving maximum efficiency when working with any skin disease. The diagnostic keys assist the clinician by focusing on pertinent history, clinical signs, and screening diagnostic tests that will help to establish a list of differential diagnoses in a minimal amount of time. The diagnostic keys can also serve as a basis for an organized, indepth discussion with the pet owner about the various aspects of the differential diagnoses. Steps for a systematic approach to a dermatologic diagnosis are outlined in Table 2–1.

HISTORY

The initial dermatologic history includes age, sex, and breed, the owner's complaint (how the problem is perceived), date of onset of signs, original location of lesions, and course of disease. Previous treatment administered and the clinical response elicited (drug history) often have diagnostic value. The intensity and frequency of pruritus, observation of external parasites, and history of possible contagion to other animals or man should also be noted.

The three historical points most useful in making the initial list of differential diagnoses are absence of pruritus, presence of external parasites, and drug history. The interpretation of these key historical points is given in Table 2–2. Pruritus must be considered in conjunction with other his-

TABLE 2–1. STEPS FOR A SYSTEMATIC APPROACH TO DERMATOLOGIC DIAGNOSIS

1. Obtain an adequate history.
2. Complete a thorough physical examination.
3. Correlate the historical and clinical findings.
4. List all possible general etiologic classifications (differential diagnoses) based on dermatologic diagnostic key.
5. Complete screening diagnostic tests to rule in or rule out the etiologic classifications listed in step 4.
6. Make a new differential diagnoses list based on step 5.
7. List possible specific etiologic classifications based on the individual etiologic diagnostic keys (history and clinical findings).
8. Complete the definitive diagnostic tests to rule in or rule out specific etiologic classifications or diagnoses.

TABLE 2–2. INTERPRETATION OF KEY HISTORICAL POINTS

History	Differential Diagnoses	
	Include	Exclude
Pruritus	Allergic Parasitic Bacterial Fungal Bullous Neoplastic Seborrheic Endocrine	None
External parasites	Parasitic	None
100% Response to cortico-steroids	Allergic Bullous (if high-dose) Neoplastic Seborrheic Nodular panniculitis	Endocrine Fungal Bacterial (primary) Parasitic Neoplastic
100% Response to antibiotics	Bacterial (primary)	Parasitic Fungal Endocrine Neoplastic Bullous
100% Response to parasiticides	Parasitic Allergic Seborrheic (secondary) Bacterial (secondary)	Endocrine Bacterial (primary) Fungal Bullous Neoplastic

torical and clinical findings in order to be of initial diagnostic value. Although endocrine diseases are generally nonpruritic, mild pruritus may be related to other primary diseases (e.g., allergy) or secondary to complications of a primary disease (e.g., pyoderma). There is a wide variation in frequency and intensity of pruritus in most etiologic classifications.

Although a history of external parasites indicates parasitic disease, failure of the pet owner to observe them does not rule out parasitic disease.

History of a previous response to corticosteroids may have been a result of dosage and/or type of drug used. All animals in a given etiologic clas-

sification do not respond equally to the same drug. A complete failure of clinical response to corticosteroids suggests endocrine, fungal, neoplastic and bullous skin diseases. A good response to a high dose (2 to 4 mg/kg/day) suggests autoimmune bullous disease. A good clinical response to antibacterial therapy does not indicate whether the infection is primary or secondary. History of partial response to antibiotics or parasiticides indicates the possibility of concurrent disease.

PHYSICAL EXAMINATION

A complete physical examination should be performed that includes all organ systems. Systemic signs are commonly seen with some endocrine, bullous, neoplastic, and fungal diseases, whereas with allergic and bacterial diseases, systemic signs are not characteristic.

When examining the skin include all areas of the body. Primary and secondary morphologic lesions, as well as miscellaneous skin lesions, should be identified and recorded. The various types of lesions are defined in Tables 2–3 (primary), 2–4 (secondary), and 2–5 (miscellaneous). Primary lesions are visualized in Plate 1. Secondary and miscellaneous lesions are shown in Plate 2. The distribution pattern and extent of alopecia and erythema should be noted and carefully correlated with other historical and clinical findings. The interpretation of key clinical findings is given in Table 2–6.

SCREENING DIAGNOSTIC TESTS

Screening diagnostic tests are those tests that are easily completed as part of a routine office procedure, or for which samples are obtained on an outpatient basis and sent to a reference laboratory. These tests may also be definitive, yielding confirmation of a specific diagnosis. The screening diagnostic tests include skin scraping, Wood's lamp (ultraviolet lamp), potassium hydroxide (KOH)) preparation, fungal and bacterial culture, direct smear, hematologic and biochemical testing, hormonal assay, cutaneous biopsy, and therapeutic trial. Interpretation of positive findings of screening diagnostic tests are given in Table 2–7.

Skin Scrapings. This simple procedure is indicated in all dermatologic diagnostic workups (Fig. 2–1). The basic technique requires the use of a No. 10 scalpel blade or a blunted tartar scraper, mineral oil, glass slide, and microscope (Fig. 2–1A). Place a drop of mineral oil on the lesion. Hold the scalpel blade or tartar scraper with the thumb and first finger close to the point for max-

TABLE 2–3. PRIMARY GROSS MORPHOLOGIC SKIN LESIONS

Lesion	Definition	Causative Mechanism
Macule	Circumscribed area of change in normal skin color of ≤ 1 cm without elevation or depression of the surface	Hypopigmentation, hyperpigmentation, or permanent vascular abnormalities of the skin
Patch	Circumscribed area of change in normal skin color of > 1 cm without elevation or depression of the surface	Same as above
Papule	Solid, elevated lesion < 1.0 cm diameter with most of the lesion above the plane of the surrounding skin	Metabolic deposits, localized hyperplasia of cellular components of the epidermis or dermis, or localized cellular infiltrates in the dermis
Nodule	Palpable, solid, round, or ellipsoidal lesion deeper than a papule in the dermis or subcutis	Neoplasia, inflammation, or metabolic deposits
Plaque	Elevation above the skin surface that occupies a relatively large surface area in comparison with its height above the skin	Confluence of papules
Tumor	Neoplastic mass of any structure at any depth	Neoplastic growth
Pustule	Circumscribed elevation of the skin that contains purulent exudate	Inflammation
Wheal	Rounded or flat-topped elevation in the skin of any size	Dermal edema
Vesicle	Circumscribed, elevated lesion ≤ 0.5 cm that contains fluid	Separation of epidermal cells or of cells at the dermoepidermal junction and infiltration with fluid
Bulla	Circumscribed, elevated lesion > 0.5 cm that contains fluid	Enlargement of a vesicle or confluence of vesicles

TABLE 2–4. SECONDARY GROSS MORPHOLOGIC SKIN LESIONS

Lesion	Definition	Causative Mechanisms
Sclerosis	Almost transparent epidermis; circumscribed or diffuse hardening of the skin	Dermal or subcutaneous edema, cellular infiltration, or collagen proliferation
Excoriation	Superficial excavations of epidermis that may be linear or punctate	Trauma, such as scratching, biting, or rubbing (friction)
Scale	Accumulation of loose fragments of the stratum corneum	Abnormal keratinization
Crust	Dried exudate on the surface of a lesion	Results when serum, blood, or purulent exudate dries on the skin surface
Scar	Area of fibrous tissue that has replaced normal layers of skin	Healing process following an ulceration
Ulcer	Destruction of the epidermis and upper dermis	Trauma, tissue infarction, or parasites
Fissures	Linear cleavages in the skin	Excessive drying of the skin or trauma
Hyperpigmentation	Excessive coloration of the skin	Increased melanin deposition
Lichenification	Thickening and hardening of the skin characterized by an exaggeration of the superficial skin markings	Chronic irritation
Hyperkeratosis	Increase in thickness of the stratum corneum	Abnormal keratinization

TABLE 2–5. MISCELLANEOUS GROSS SKIN LESIONS

Lesion	Definition	Causative Mechanisms
Erosion	Loss of the epidermis to a depth of the basal layer; moist, slightly depressed lesion	Ruptured vesicle or mild trauma
Furuncle	Deep necrotizing form of folliculitis with pus accumulation	Deep bacterial infection
Carbuncle	Coalescing of several furuncles	Deep bacterial infection
Abscess	Localized accumulation of purulent material so deep in the dermis or subcutis that the pus is not visible on the surface of the skin	Deep bacterial infection
Sinus	Tract leading from a suppurative cavity to the surface, or between cystic or abscess cavities	Chronic deep infection
Cyst	Sac that contains liquid or semisolid material	Plugging of an orifice

TABLE 2–6. INTERPRETATION OF KEY CLINICAL FINDINGS

	Suggested Etiologic Classification of Dermatologic Disease
Primary Lesions	
Most Commonly Observed	
Macule	Nonspecific
Papule	Nonspecific
Plaque	Nonspecific
Pustule	Bacterial
Most Helpful in Making Diagnosis	
Nodule	Neoplasm or cyst
Tumor	Neoplasm
Wheal	Allergic
Vesicle	Bullous and allergic
Pustule	Bacterial
Secondary Lesions	
Scale	All lesions nonspecific
Crust	
Excoriation	
Lichenification	
Hyperpigmentation	
Hyperkeratosis	
Other Clinical Signs	
Erythema	Usually associated with acute or active inflammation, nonspecific unless correlated with other signs
Alopecia	Nonspecific unless correlated with other signs

imum control. Rest the hand on the animal's body so that sudden movement will force the hand and instrument away from the body and avoid trauma (Fig. 2–1B). Direct the scraping instrument away from the eye or mouth.

The depth of the scraping varies depending on the history and clinical appearance of the lesion and the suspected parasite. If scaling (dandruff) is present with minimal alopecia and pruritus, scrape some scale onto the slide along with some hair (suspect Cheyletiella) (Fig. 2–1C). If the coat is long, clipping the area prior to scraping is indicated. If there is partial to total alopecia on a small focal area or a diffuse area with minimal pruritus, pinch the specific area to be scraped with the thumb and first finger (Fig. 2–1D). Then scrape a small area of the pinched skin until it bleeds and carry a small amount of blood-tinged material to the slide (suspect Demodex). If there is crusting with pruritus, a large area (1 to 3 cm) should be scraped, removing all crust (Fig. 2–1E, F) (suspect Sarcoptes). Examine the slides under scanning ($\times$ 4) or low power ($\times$ 10) objectives for the presence of external parasites. The crust may need to be broken up and/or digested with KOH prior to the examination.

The absence of parasites on skin scrapings does not rule out all parasitic disease. Multiple scrapings should be performed before a negative diagnosis can be made.

Wood's Lamp (Ultraviolet Light, Black Light). The diagnostic value of the Wood's lamp is limited to a screening and definitive test for Microsporum canis. The lamp must be used in a totally darkened room (Fig. 2–2). The characteristic fluorescent color is a bright apple green. Individual broken hairs are examined; both the extrafollicular and intrafollicular portions of the hair shaft will fluoresce. Scales and many topical medications have a diffuse, dull white or blue color under the Wood's lamp. Negative fluorescence does not rule out M. canis, since only about 50% of these infections routinely fluoresce.

Potassium hydroxide-Dimethyl sulfoxide preparation (KOH-DMSO). This procedure is occasionally used to identify fungal arthrospores and/or hyphae. Much experience is necessary to accurately interpret a KOH preparation. Necessary materials include the KOH-DMSO mixture, a glass slide, coverslip, fine forceps, lactophenol cotton blue or new methylene blue stain, and a microscope.

TABLE 2–7. INTERPRETATION OF ROUTINE SCREENING DIAGNOSTIC TESTS

Screening Diagnostic Test (Positive)	Differential Diagnoses	
	Include	Suggestive
Skin scrapings	Parasitic	
Wood's lamp	Fungal (Microsporum canis)	
Potassium hydroxide (KOH) preparation	Fungal	
Fungal culture	Fungal	
Direct smear	Neoplasia Bacterial	Neoplasia Bacterial Bullous
Bacterial culture	Bacterial	
Blood screens (CBC, biochemical profile)	Neoplasia	Endocrine Neoplasia
Hormonal assays Thyroid Cortisol Sex hormones	 Endocrine (hypothyroidism) Endocrine (hyperadrenocor- ticism)	 Endocrine (gonadal dermatoses)
Cutaneous biopsy	Parasitic Bacterial Fungal Bullous Neoplasia	Allergic Seborrheic Endocrine Nodular panniculitis Bullous Neoplasia

	Clinical Response					
	Complete		Partial		None	
	Include	Exclude	Include	Exclude	Include	Exclude
Therapeutic trials Corticosteroid	Allergic Parasitic Bullous Neoplasia Nodular panniculitis	Endocrine Fungal Bacterial (primary)	Allergic Seborrheic Bacterial Parasitic Bullous Neoplasia Acral lick gran- uloma		Endocrine Fungal Bacterial Bullous Parasitic Seborrheic Neoplasia	Allergic
Antibiotic	Bacterial (pri- mary)	Endocrine Fungal Neoplasia Bullous Seborrheic (primary) Parasitic	Bacterial Allergic Seborrheic Acral lick granuloma Fungal Bullous Parasitic	Endocrine	Fungal Endocrine Bullous Neoplasia Parasitic Nodular panniculitis Allergic	
Parasiticide	Parasitic Seborrheic (secondary) Allergic Bacterial (secondary)	Endocrine Fungal Bullous Neoplasia	Allergic Parasitic Bacterial Seborrheic	Neoplasia Bullous Endocrine Fungal	Endocrine Bullous Neoplasia Fungal Parasitic Bacterial Allergic Seborrheic	

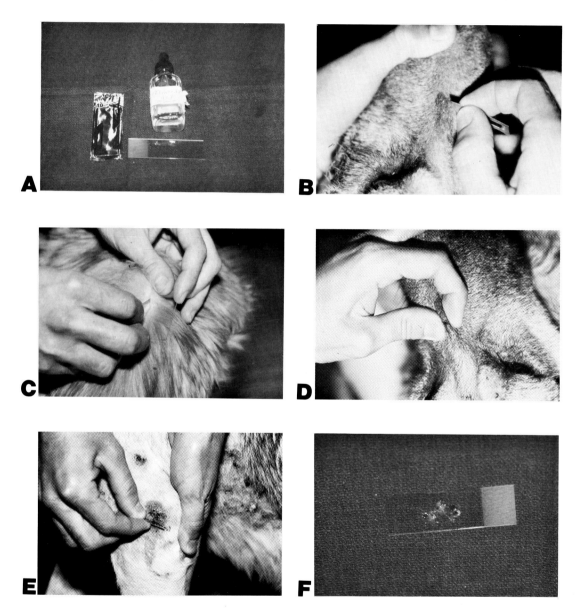

Fig. 2–1. Skin scraping technique: *A*, Use the following materials for skin scrapings: mineral oil, clean glass slide, No. 10 scalpel blade, or blunted tartar scraper. *B*, Hold scalpel blade between thumb and first finger close to point and rest hand on the animal's body. Direct blade away from the body. *C*, Cheyletiella: Place drop of oil on skin, scrape superficially to transfer dandruff to a glass slide. *D*, Demodex: Place drop of oil on skin and pinch a focal area of skin prior to scraping to depth of blood. *E*, Sarcoptes: Place drop of oil on skin and remove all crust over large area. *F*, Sarcoptes: Place all crust and debris onto glass slide for microscopic examination.

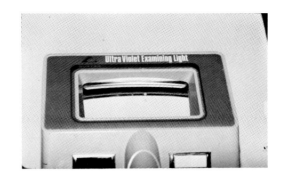

Fig. 2–2. Wood's lamp (ultraviolet lamp) with magnifying glass to use as a screening diagnostic test for Microsporum canis.

Take hair and scale from the periphery of the lesion and place on a glass slide. Place a drop of KOH-DMSO and a drop of stain on the specimen with a coverslip. After 30 to 60 seconds, examine the broken or distorted hairs on the preparation under low power for arthrospores. Hyphae are occasionally seen in the scale and cleared debris. A negative KOH-DMSO preparation does not rule out fungal disease.

Fungus Culture. There are two types of media routinely used for fungus cultures: dermatophyte test medium (DTM) and Sabouraud's medium.

A sample for fungus culture is obtained by selecting individual, representative hairs or scale. Broken hair shafts or fluorescent hairs or scale from nails are also satisfactory specimens. Large amounts of hair should be avoided. There should be minimal preparation of the skin prior to sampling since the fungal spores and hyphae are in the keratin layers of the epidermis and hair. A light disinfection with alcohol may be used to remove surface contamination. For best results the hair or scales should be lightly embedded in the culture medium by cutting the specimen into the medium with a sterile scalpel blade.

DTM is Sabouraud's medium with cycloheximide and chloramphenicol to inhibit selected fungal and bacterial growth and phenol red to act as a pH indicator. The pathogenic fungi utilize protein initially, giving off alkaline metabolic products which turn the medium red. Nonpathogenic fungi usually use carbohydrates first and then use protein after the carbohydrates are used up; thus, there is a larger amount of growth before the medium turns red. The DTM is a useful medium if used correctly. A culture positive for dermatophyte growth must show colony growth and color change from yellow to red simultaneously (Plate 6:*H*). This may occur from 1 to 21 days, although it usually occurs within the first 7 days. Therefore, the cultures must be observed daily. The 3 common dermatophytes of dogs and cats all have white colonies. Contaminant fungi show colony growth, which is usually dark in color prior to a medium color change. All old DTM culture media change from yellow to red (Plate 6:*I*).

Sabouraud's medium without color indicator may also be used. Each pathogenic and contaminant fungus has characteristic surface colony growth. The reverse side (bottom of plate) also shows characteristic color changes. Gross colony appearance and growth characteristics are often sufficient to make a specific genus and species identification on both Sabouraud's medium and DTM if the technician has had sufficient experience. The pathogens can be easily differentiated from contaminant growth by microscopic examination. See Chapter 7 for specific details of fungi identification.

An acetate tape technique is a simple method for obtaining a satisfactory mount for microscopic examination. Place a few drops of lactophenol cotton blue or new methylene blue stain on a clean glass slide. Attach a strip of clear acetate to the end of a tongue depressor with the sticky surface to the outside. Touch the tape lightly to the surface of the colony, remove the tape from the tongue depressor, place sticky side down on the glass slide over the drop of stain, and smooth out (Fig. 2–3*A, B, C, D*). The slide is examined under low power for the presence of macroconidia or microconidia (Fig. 2–3*E*).

Bacterial Culture and In Vitro Antibiotic Sensitivity Testing. Pyoderma is a frequently encountered dermatologic problem associated with many different diseases and syndromes. Whether the pyoderma is superficial or deep and primary or secondary, identification of the causative organism and determination of sensitivity of the bacteria to specific antibiotics may be important to the successful diagnosis and/or treatment of the condition. Specific indications for bacterial cultures are discussed in Chapter 6.

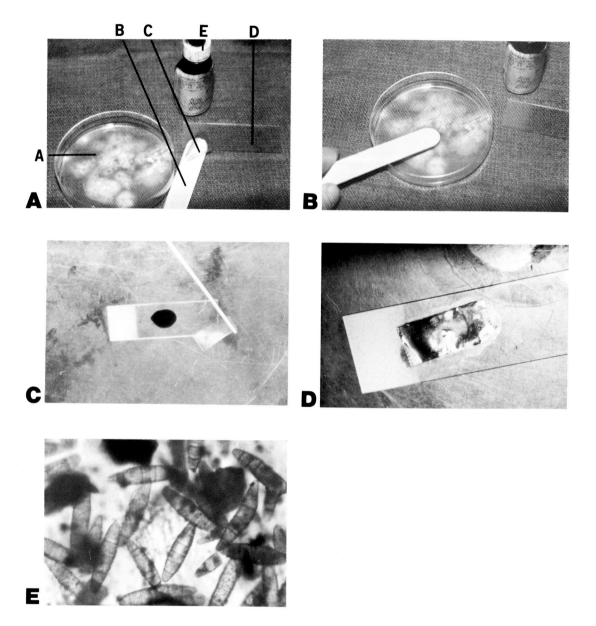

Fig. 2–3. Acetate tape technique for fungus identification: *A*, Use the following materials for acetate tape technique: fungus culture (*A*), tongue depressor (*B*), acetate tape (*C*), glass slide (*D*), lactophenol cotton blue (*E*), or new methylene blue. *B*, Gently touch tape, which is attached to end of tongue depressor with the sticky tape surface to outside, to the surface of the culture. *C*, Place tape with sticky surface down onto glass slide over drop of stain. *D*, Smooth tape on glass slide and examine under microscope. *E*, Macroconidia of Microsporum gypseum (low power).

TABLE 2–8. BACTERIAL SAMPLING TECHNIQUES

Type of Lesion	Technique

Superficial pustule	1. Clip hair around lesion, if necessary, avoiding trauma to surface of pustule.
	2. Gently wipe surface of pustule with alcohol and let dry.
	3a. Open pustule with No. 10 or No. 11 sterile scalpel.
	  b. Force exudate to surface by carefully squeezing opened pustule.
	  c. Touch sterile swab to the exudate avoiding contact with surrounding skin or hair.
	
	or
	
	4a. Aspirate exudate from pustule using a fine needle and syringe.
	  b. Place exudate from syringe and needle onto sterile swab.
	5. Streak directly onto agar plate or place in transport media.

Crusty lesion	1. Clip hair around lesion, if necessary, leaving crust intact. 2. Gently wipe surface of crust and surrounding area with alcohol and let dry. 3. Remove crust with forceps using as aseptic a technique as possible. 4. Rub sterile swab over the moist surface directly beneath the crust avoiding contact with surrounding area. 5. Streak directly onto agar plate or place in transport media.
Deep pyoderma with tract but no pustule	1. Clip hair from site of lesion. 2. Wipe surface of lesion with alcohol and let dry. 3. Apply pressure to deeper layers of skin forcing the exudate onto the surface. 4. Touch sterile swab to exudate avoiding contact with surrounding skin or hair. 5. Streak directly onto plate or place in transport media.

Deep pyoderma with unruptured pustule	1. Clip hair from area, if necessary, avoiding trauma to pustule.
	2. Gently wipe surface with alcohol and let dry.
	3a. Open pustule with No. 10 or No. 11 sterile scalpel.
	  b. Insert swab into cavity and rub vigorously.
	
	or
	
	4a. Aspirate exudate from pustule using a fine needle and syringe.
	  b. Place exudate from syringe and needle onto sterile swab.
	5. Streak directly onto agar plate or place in transport media.

Deep pyoderma with ulcerated skin	1. Clean area of lesion with soap and water. 2. Swab area with alcohol. 3. Infiltrate lesion subcutaneously with local anesthetic. 4. Use 6-mm biopsy punch to obtain plug of skin at the site to be cultured. 5. Carefully split the plug longitudinally, cutting from the bottom to the surface with No. 10 or No. 11 sterile scalpel. 6. Place sterile swab into the midsection of the split biopsy and rub vigorously avoiding contact with the surface. 7. Streak directly onto agar plate or place in transport media.

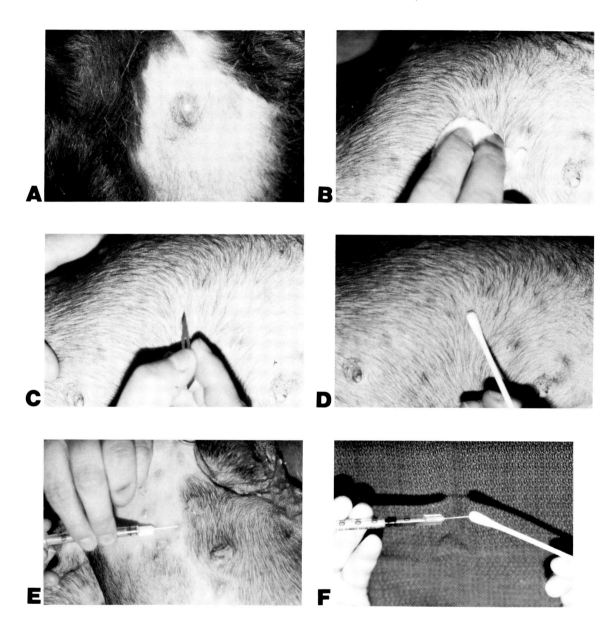

Fig. 2–4. Bacterial sampling technique—superficial or deep unruptured pustule: *A,* Superficial pustule. *B,* Gently wipe surface of pustule with alcohol and air-dry. *C,* Open pustule carefully with sterile scalpel blade, *D,* and carefully touch sterile swab to exudate forced onto surface and avoid contact with surrounding skin or hair. If the pustule is large, insert swab into cavity and rub vigorously. Another method is to aspirate the pustule with a fine needle, *E,* and place aspirated material on sterile swab and streak onto agar, *F.*

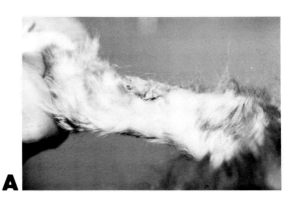

Fig. 2–5. Bacterial sampling technique—crusty lesion: *A*, Bacterial lesion with thick crust on surface. *B*, Gently wipe surface of crust and surrounding area with alcohol and air-dry. *C*, Carefully lift crust from surface with forceps and rub sterile swab over moist surface beneath crust; avoid contact with surrounding skin and hair.

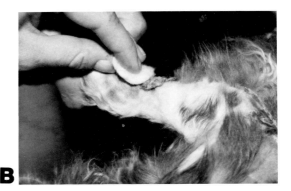

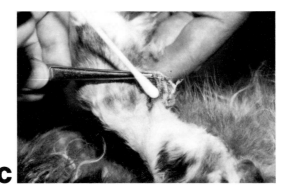

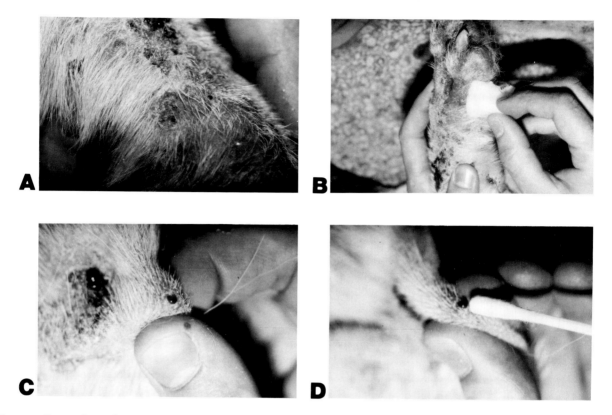

Fig. 2–6. Bacterial sampling technique—deep pyoderma with tract: *A*, Deep pyoderma with sinus (tracts). *B*, Carefully wipe surface with alcohol and air-dry. *C*, Apply pressure to deeper layers of skin forcing exudate onto cleaned surface. *D*, Carefully touch sterile swab to surface of exudate; avoid contact with surrounding skin or hair.

The proper technique of obtaining a specimen for bacterial culture is important. An intact superficial pustule is sampled differently than a crusty lesion or deep pyoderma. The clinician and technician should be familiar with the various techniques that are used to obtain a representative sample from different types of bacterial lesions. These techniques are outlined in Table 2–8 and visualized in Figures 2–4 through 2–7. Commercially available transport media have made possible the preservation of bacterial specimens for sending to a reference laboratory.

Culturing of bacteria has been simplified by commercially available culture plates that contain several selective media. These multimedia culture plates include Mueller-Hinton agar, an all purpose medium used for antibiotic sensitivity testing; MacConkey agar, which supports gram-negative bacteria and inhibits gram-positive bacteria; brain-heart infusion agar, which supports all common aerobic pathogens; mannitol salt agar, which inhibits most bacteria except Staphylococcus spp; and streptosel agar used for the isolation of streptococci. Tellurite glycine agar has been recommended for the initial isolation of Staphylococcus

aureus, coagulase positive. This agar inhibits most bacteria except this species of Staphylococcus. It also contains a coagulase indicator that facilitates isolation of pathogenic colonies.

Pathogenic bacteria can be tentatively identified by their characteristic behavior on these selective media (Fig. 2–8). In addition, gram stains and microscopic examinations can be used to help identify bacteria growth. Refer to the manuals that accompany commerically prepared multimedia culture plates for guidelines on identification.

Antibiotic sensitivity discs and dispensers are also readily available. Most of the multimedia plates are adapted for use with these discs. Refer to the laboratory manuals accompanying the plates and discs for specific techniques and interpretations. In vitro antibiotic sensitivity testing should only be done on single isolates, not on mixed bacterial growth. This diagnostic test is often reserved for S. aureus isolates. Remember that sensitivity to antibiotics in vitro does not assure they will be effective in vivo.

Blood Screens. Hematologic testing including a differential white blood cell count and serum biochemical testing are helpful for some differ-

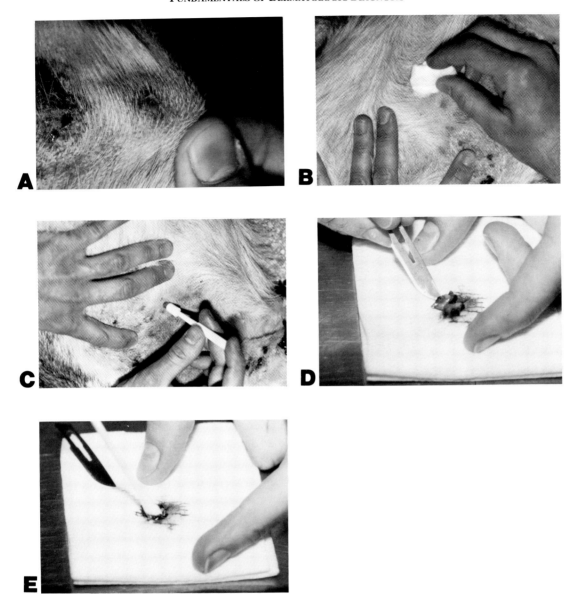

Fig. 2–7. Bacterial culture technique—deep pyoderma with ulcerated surface: *A*, Deep pyoderma. *B*, Clean surface well with soap and water and alcohol; then air-dry. *C*, Use biopsy punch to remove full-thickness plug of skin. *D*, Place plug of skin on a sterile surface, with the epidermal surface down; split plug longitudinally with sterile scalpel blade. *E*, Place sterile swab in center of split tissue and rub vigorously; avoid contact with the edges.

Fig. 2–8. Multimedia bacterial agar plate (Bactassay, Pitman-Moore).

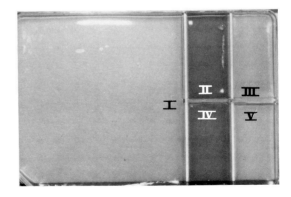

TABLE 2–9. CUTANEOUS BIOPSY TECHNIQUES

Biopsy Technique	Procedure	Indications
Punch	1. Equipment and supplies: 4-mm or 6-mm disposable biopsy punch, needle holder, skin suture, smooth thumb forceps, fine sharp-sharp scissors, 2 × 2 gauze sponges, formalin. 2. Carefully clip (not close) lesion only if needed, avoiding removal of scale or crust on surface. 3. Do not wash or disinfect the biopsy site since the diagnostic value of specimen may be on the surface. 4. Inject 0.5 ml of local anesthetic subcutaneously. 5. Place biopsy punch on exact site to be biopsied and drill into tissue with rotary motion in one direction applying moderate pressure. There will be less resistance when punch reaches subcutis. 6. Withdraw punch. The plug should follow punch to surface if cut to an adequate depth. 7. Carefully lift plug with fine smooth forceps or a fine needle and cut off base of plug including some fat with scissors or scalpel. 8. Close wound with one or two skin sutures. 9. Place specimen in 10% buffered formalin and submit to laboratory.	All types of solid skin lesions if total excision is not indicated All small lesions, up to 5 mm, which can be totally excised
Needle aspiration	1. Equipment and supplies: Syringe (6 ml to 12 ml), hypodermic needle (25 to 20 gauge), clean glass slides, stain, microscope. 2. Carefully clip hair from lesion, avoiding trauma to surface. 3. Prepare biopsy site with surgical scrub. 4. Insert sterile needle attached to syringe into the lesion while creating a firm vacuum with syringe. (Needle and syringe sizes depend on size of lesion and density of tissue or content). When material is aspirated into the syringe, withdraw the needle after allowing the pressure to equalize. 5. If initial aspiration is nonproductive, carefully move needle back and forth several times within the tissue while aspirating. 6. Place aspirate in the needle and syringe on the clean glass slides; spread it to make a thin film. 7. Select appropriate stain. 8. Examine with microscope.	To characterize cell type or contents of a mass (tumor, nodule) or cavity (cyst, vesicle, pustule) without surgical invasion
Excisional	1. Equipment and supplies: sterile surgical pack (drape, scalpel, hemostats, needle holder, suture needles, smooth thumb forceps, scissors, gauze sponges, suture), formalin. 2. Carefully clip hair from lesion and surrounding area avoiding trauma to skin. 3. Clean surgical site with soap and water, rinse, apply 70% alcohol avoiding vigorous scrubbing. 4. Inject local anesthetic subcutaneously, using ring block or general anesthetic. 5. Make an elliptical excision of the full depth of skin to the subcutis using a No. 10 or No. 15 scalpel blade. 6. Close the wound in a routine manner. 7. Submit specimen in 10% buffered formalin.	Total removal of small nodules, cysts, vesicles, and tumors
Incisional	1, 2, 3, and 4 same as excisional biopsy technique. 5. Select a biopsy site on basis of a representative tissue, access to biopsy site, and minimal postsurgical complications. 6. Be prepared to control excessive hemorrhage on large or active lesions. 7. Make a full-thickness incision to subcutis in form of a wedge or ellipse, removing a section at least 5-mm wide. 8. Close the wound in a manner to prevent postsurgical complications. 9. Submit specimen in 10% buffered formalin.	To obtain a specimen for histopathologic examination from a large mass which cannot be totally excised due to size, location, or for cosmetic reasons

TABLE 2–9. *Continued*

Direct impression smear	1. Equipment and supplies: microscope, glass slides, coverslips, stain, sterile cotton-tipped applicator sticks, and scalpel blade (optional).	To characterize cell type or debris on the surface of any lesion
	2. Carefully clean the area of debris and blot away excessive blood, serum, or contaminating exudate.	
	3. Obtain sample by: pressing a clean slide firmly against lesion to transfer cells to slide, or gently scraping the lesion with scalpel blade and transfer material to glass slide, or collecting material on a sterile cotton-tipped applicator and then rolling it onto slide.	
	4. Select appropriate stain.	
	5. Examine with microscope.	

ential diagnoses. There are no general etiologic classifications in which these blood tests are definitive. In the majority of conditions in both dogs and cats with primary skin disease, the blood cell indices and biochemical profiles are within the normal range if they are not influenced by therapy, such as the administration of glucocorticoids. More abnormalities are associated with endocrine diseases than most other disease classifications. Borderline anemia and hypercholesterolemia are sometimes associated with canine hypothyroidism. Hyperadrenocorticism is characterized by lymphopenia, eosinopenia, neutrophilia, and elevated alkaline phosphatase. A T-lymphocyte immunodeficiency is suspected if the absolute lymphocyte count is <1000 cells/mm^3.

Most thyroid and cortisol assays are readily available from reference laboratories. The thyroid assays (T$_3$ and T$_4$), with or without thyroid-stimulating hormone (TSH) stimulation (see Table 8–1), are routinely run as the first screening diagnostic test to determine the presence of endocrine dis-

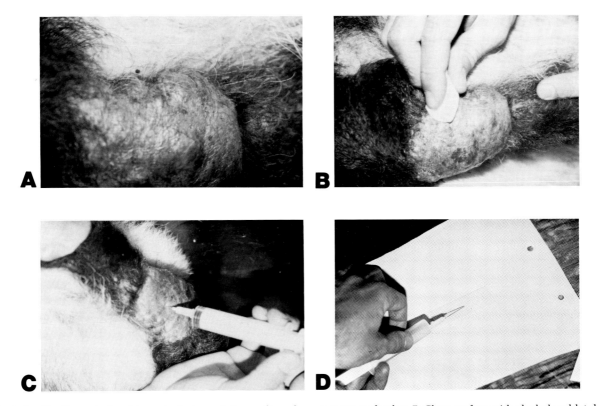

Fig. 2–9. Needle aspiration biopsy technique: *A*, Large, firm alopecic mass on foreleg. *B*, Clean surface with alcohol and let dry. *C*, Insert needle into mass and apply negative pressure in syringe, which will pull fluid and cells from mass into syringe. *D*, Place and spread mass aspirate onto clean glass slides.

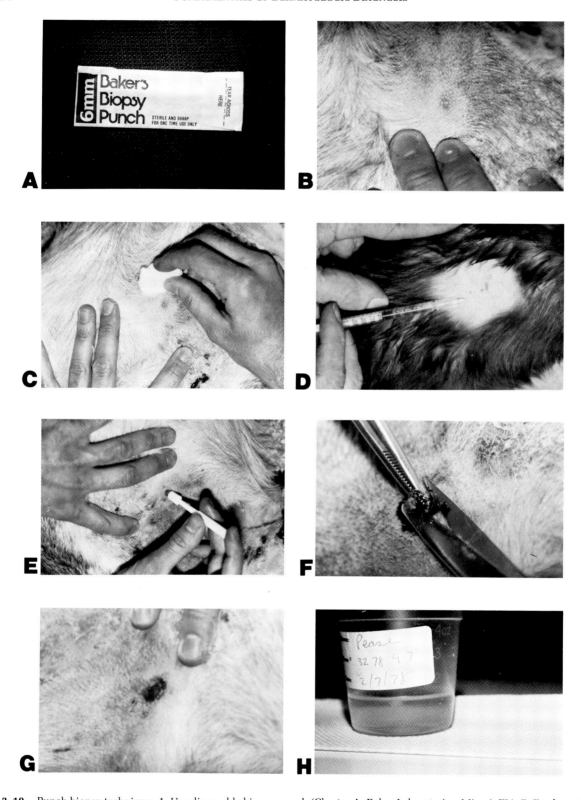

Fig. 2–10.   Punch biopsy technique: *A,* Use disposable biopsy punch (Chester A. Baker Laboratories, Miami, FL). *B,* Erythematous papule biopsy site. *C,* If needed, carefully remove gross debris from periphery of lesion with alcohol; avoid wiping the surface of the biopsy site. *D,* Inject local anesthetic subcutaneously beneath the biopsy site. *E,* Place biopsy punch perpendicular to the skin directly over the lesion. *F,* After cutting through the full thickness of the skin with the punch, carefully lift plug with forceps and cut through the subcutaneous tissue. *G,* Biopsy site following removal of plug of skin prior to placing suture. *H,* Place biopsy specimen in container with buffered formalin.

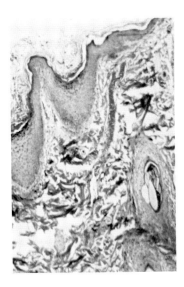

Fig. 2–11. Microscopic section of lesion in which anesthetic was injected intradermally. Note the upper dermal edema characterized by a separation and a disruption of the normal architecture of the collagenous fibers.

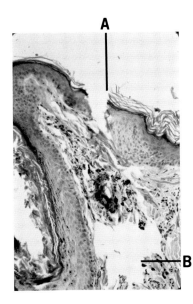

Fig. 2–13. Microscopic section of biopsy tissue that was stretched excessively when removed from the skin. Note the fissure through the epidermis (A) and the large open space in the dermis (B) due to artifactual separation of collagen fibers.

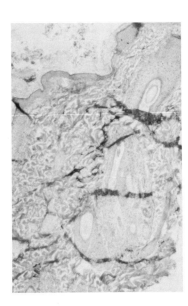

Fig. 2–12. Microscopic section of biopsy tissue that was crushed by forceps. Note the multifocal areas of folding dermal tissue.

TABLE 2–10.   GLOSSARY OF DERMATOPATHOLOGIC TERMS

Term	Definition	Correlation with Gross Morphologic Structure
Acantholysis	Loss of coherence between epidermal cells due to degeneration of intercellular cement substance and intercellular bridges	Vesicles, bullae
Acanthosis	Increase in thickness of the stratum spinosum	Lichenification, plaque
Bulla-vesicle	Cavity formed either within or beneath the epidermis and filled with fluid	Vesicles, bulla
Crust	Coagulated tissue fluid and blood plasma intermingled with degenerated inflammatory cells and epithelial cells	Crust
Dyskeratosis	Faulty keratinization of individual epidermal cells.	
Atrophy		
Epidermal	Thin epidermis with a decrease in the number of epidermal cells	Thin skin
Dermal	Decrease in the upper dermal connective tissue	Thin skin
Erosion	Superficial loss of epithelium; dermis is intact	Erosion
Granulation tissue	Newly formed, edematous collagenous tissue arising in wounds, healing ulcers, or inflammatory processes	Scar, sclerosis
Granuloma	Chronic proliferative lesion containing chronic inflammatory cells and epitheloid and/or giant cells	Nodule
Hyperkeratosis	Excessive thickness of the stratum corneum	Scale
Intercellular edema (spongiosis)	Edema between squamous cells causing an increase in the width of the space separating them	Edema
Liquefaction degeneration of basal cells	Type of degeneration causing vacuolation of basal cells	Vesicles, erosion, ulceration
Microabscess	Small accumulations of cells in the epidermis	Pustule, papule
Parakeratosis	Incomplete keratinization, showing retention of nuclei in the horny layer and absence of a granular layer	Scale
Ulcer	Area in which the epidermis and also part of the dermis are absent	Ulcer
Hyperpigmentation	Increase in melanin pigment in the epidermis, dermis, or both	Hyperpigmentation

ease. If the history and clinical signs are suggestive of hyperadrenocorticism, an ACTH-stimulation test or low-dose dexamethasone suppression test (see Table 8–3) should be performed as a screening and definitive diagnostic test. Sex hormone concentrations for testosterone, estradiol, and progesterone are performed by a limited number of reference laboratories. The clinical significance of many of the sex hormone blood concentrations is questionable in most animals at this time; thus, their usefulness as a screening or definitive diagnostic test is often limited.

Cutaneous Biopsies. *Indications.* Biopsies are indicated in any skin condition characterized by nodules, tumors, vesicles, bullae, or any lesions that are unresponsive to symptomatic therapy, or in those lesions in which specific etiologic factors have not been identified. Biopsies can help deny or confirm the presence of some parasites and fungi.

Cutaneous biopsies are diagnostically valuable if they provide a definitive diagnosis and deny or suggest a clinical diagnosis. The latter two indications require the clinician to correlate the history, clinical findings, and other laboratory data with histologic findings.

Contraindications. There are a few absolute contraindications for cutaneous biopsies, e.g., in animals that have uncontrollable hemorrhage. Sepsis should be considered in debilitated animals or in those receiving immunosuppressive drugs, although this is rarely a problem.

Choice of Biopsy Site. A small specimen taken from a carefully chosen site may yield more information about the dermatosis than a large piece of skin removed from a poorly chosen site. If the site chosen has clinically diagnostic features, the histologic features are more likely to be diagnostic.

General guidelines to follow for selection of the biopsy site include: (1) in generalized dermatoses, select a lesion that is typical, not subjected to trauma, not encrusted, and not modified by treat-

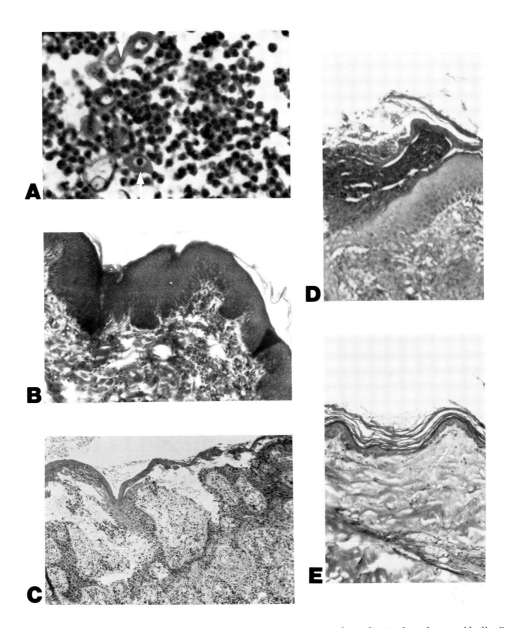

Fig. 2–14. Dermatopathologic lesions: *A*, Acantholysis: Note keratinocytes (arrow) lying free in the subcorneal bulla. *B*, Acanthosis: Increased thickness of stratum spinosum; associated with plaques and lichenification grossly. *C*, Bulla-vesicle: Large suprabasilar accumulation of fluid resulting in separation of superficial epidermis. *D*, Crust: Accumulation of densely staining debris, necrotic cells, and serum on the surface. *E*, Epidermal atrophy: Thin epidermis with a decrease in thickness of the stratum spinosum. Mild hyperkeratosis is observed.

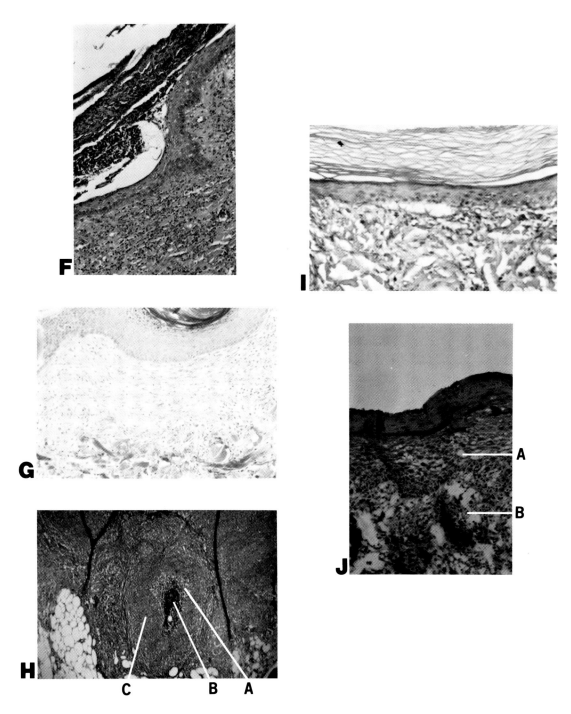

Fig. 2–14 *(Continued).* *F,* Erosion: Superficial loss of epithelium. Note large crust on the surface. Associated with excoriation grossly. *G,* Granulation tissue: New, edematous collagen with fibroblastic proliferation in the upper dermis; associated with scar grossly. *H,* Granuloma: Dense accumulation of mononuclear cells *(A)* surrounding a central core of necrosis with a mixed cellular infiltrate *(B)*. Fibroblastic proliferation encapsulates the lesion *(C)*; associated with nodules grossly. *I,* Hyperkeratosis: Increased thickness of lamellar stratum corneum. Note atrophy of epidermis and disruption of basal layer (liquefaction necrosis) and vesicle formation at dermoepidermal junction. Hyperkeratosis is associated with scale grossly. *J,* Intercellular edema (spongiosis): Diffuse edema in stratum spinosum with separation of keratinocytes *(A)*. Note marked dermal edema *(B)*. Associated with edema grossly.

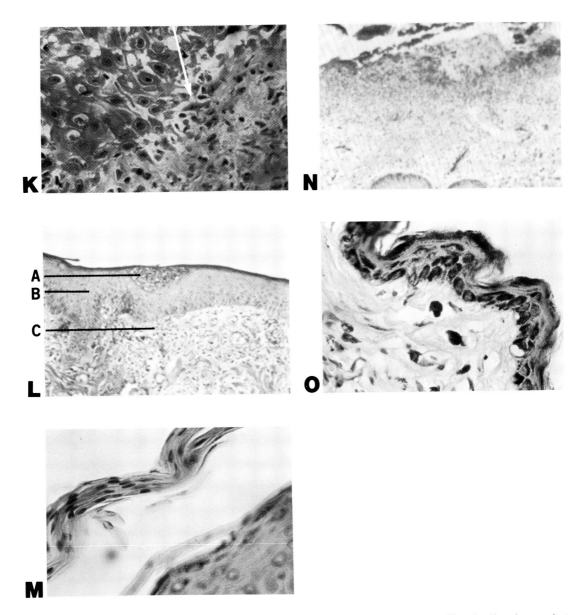

Fig. 2–14 *(Continued).* *K,* Liquefaction degeneration of basal cell layer. Note loss of continuity of basal cell with vacuolation and disintegration of basal cells (arrow). *L,* Microabscess: Small accumulation of neutrophils in the superficial dermis *(A).* Note moderate acanthosis *(B)* and dermal edema *(C).* Associated with pustule or papule grossly. *M,* Parakeratosis: Retention of nuclei in the stratum corneum. Associated with scale grossly. *N,* Ulcer: Absence of epidermis and superficial dermis. Note accumulation of serum and dense inflammatory infiltrate on the ulcerated surface and dermal edema. *O,* Hyperpigmentation: Increased melanogenesis in basal layer of epidermis and pigment-laden macrophages in the dermis.

ment; (2) select a fully developed lesion, but if there are stages in the evolution of a lesion, multiple biopsies of the different stages should be obtained; (3) avoid scarred lesions; (4) remove small vesicles or bullae intact; and (5) when possible, obtain two biopsies: one pathologic specimen and one of normal tissue from similar locations.

Biopsy Techniques. There are five common methods of obtaining cutaneous biopsies including excisional, incisional, direct impression smear, needle aspiration, and cutaneous punch.

An excisional biopsy is a complete surgical excision of the lesion, which has the advantage of diagnosis and treatment in one procedure. A large sample can be obtained for a histologic examination. This technique is used routinely for removing small nodules, cysts, vesicles, and tumors.

An incisional biopsy is the partial excision of a lesion. This technique is used when the lesion is too large to totally excise easily. It is also indicated in those lesions that do not lend themselves to surgical removal. Both excisional and incisional biopsies may require general sedation or anesthesia if the lesion is large or in a difficult location.

Needle aspiration biopsy is the technique of removing cells or their contents from a lesion by negative pressure in a syringe. This is a simple, nonsurgical method of characterizing many cysts, nodules, tumors, and pustules. The staining and examining of cells or their contents yield a diagnosis or suggest one, often directing the clinician to another diagnostic procedure.

The impression smear is most helpful when there is potentially diagnostic material (cells or their content) on the surface of a lesion. It can also be used in conjunction with excision of larger masses by making a direct smear from a cut surface.

The punch biopsy technique is the most commonly used cutaneous biopsy procedure. In most instances, 4- to 6-mm biopsy specimens are obtained following the administration of a local anesthetic agent. A short-acting general anesthetic agent may be used. There are minimal trauma, hemorrhage, and postbiopsy problems. Disposable biopsy punches have made this procedure available to most practitioners.

Each type of biopsy procedure is outlined in Table 2–9. The step-by-step procedure for needle aspiration biopsy is visualized in Figure 2–9, and the punch biopsy technique is shown in Figure 2–10.

Handling the Biopsy Specimen. Care must always be exercised when handling a biopsy spec-

imen. The microscopic architecture of the tissue can be disrupted by injecting the anesthetic intradermally (Fig. 2–11), by crushing the tissue (Fig. 2–12), or by stretchng the tissue (Fig. 2–13). The tissue should be placed in individual containers and carefully labeled. Cutaneous biopsies submitted to the pathologist should be accompanied by the following information: age, sex, and breed; history; description of gross lesion(s); duration of lesion; clinical diagnostic test data; treatment; and clinical diagnosis or impressions (a list of differential diagnoses).

Interpretation of Histopathologic Findings. Familiarity with the common dermatopathologic terms can be invaluable when interpreting the histopathology report and the subsequent correlation with the history, clinical findings, and laboratory data as outlined in Table 2–10. Histopathologic findings associated with gross morphologic lesions are visualized in Figure 2–14.

All histopathology reports should include information concerning the depth of the lesion and the specific structures involved, what microscopic pathologic process was found including description, distribution, and if possible, the interpretation of the pathogenesis of the process. It is the clinician's responsibility to read the pathology report and to correlate the pathologic findings with the history, clinical findings, and therapeutic responses. Only then will the biopsy have the most diagnostic value.

Therapeutic Trials. Therapeutic trial is often the most valuable screening diagnostic test used in the rule in or rule out of differential diagnoses based on history and clinical signs (see Table 2–7). Glucocorticosteroids are widely used to differentiate between etiologic classifications of pruritus (see Table 3–3). Only the short-acting corticosteroids should be used. Clinical response must be carefully evaluated, taking into consideration the dosage used, the duration of therapy, and any concurrent diagnostic or therapeutic procedures.

Antibiotic therapeutic trials must also be carefully evaluated. The antibiotic of choice (see Table 3–6) for the test must be selected on the basis of the history of specific antibiotic therapy, the respective clinical response, the dosage and duration of antibiotics used, the clinical signs, and the concurrent diagnostic and therapeutic procedures.

Therapeutic trials with parasiticides (see Table 3–2) are indicated if a specific parasitic disease (e.g., sarcoptic mange, fleas) is suspected on the basis of history and/or clinical signs, and has not been identified with other screening diagnostic tests.

The clinician must have the systematic approach clearly defined before initiating any therapeutic trial. Concurrent use of corticosteroids and antibiotics does not allow differentiation of allergic disease from primary bacterial disease. Similarly, concurrent administration of corticosteroids and parasiticides does not differentiate primary parasitic and allergic disease; however, these drugs may be helpful diagnostic tests if used singularly. In some animals, the systematic approach will include the initial use of concurrent therapeutic trials with a discontinuation of one prior to the other.

The general Dermatologic Diagnostic Key (Appendix 1:1) should be used as a guide for initial history, physical examination, and selection of diagnostic tests, as well as for making a differential diagnoses list based on general etiologic classifications of skin disease. If the steps and procedures discussed in this chapter are understood and implemented, a definitive diagnosis will often be determined. Therapeutic trials frequently become the treatment of choice as well as a diagnostic test. If the specific etiologic factor has not been defined

and the problem is not resolved, a more definitive diagnostic workup using the specific diagnostic disease keys (see Appendices 1:2 to 1:14) is indicated as discussed in Chapters 4 to 12.

SELECTED READINGS

Allen, S.K., and McKeever, P.J.: Skin biopsy techniques. Vet. Clin. North Am. 4:269, 1974.

Austin, V.H.: Skin biopsies: when, where and why. Compend. Cont. Ed. Pract. Vet. 2:531, 1980.

Barton, C.L.: Biopsy and cytology in veterinary practice. Compend. Cont. Ed. Anim. Health Tech. 1:259, 1980.

Fitzpatrick, T.B.: Fundamentals of dermatologic diagnosis. In Dermatology in General Medicine. 2nd Ed., Edited by T.B. Fitzpatrick, et al. New York, McGraw-Hill, 1979.

Foote, E.B.: Practical bacteriology for the technician. Compend. Cont. Ed. Anim. Health Tech. 1:249, 1980.

House, J.A.: Bactassay bacterial test media: a method for direct sensitivity and tentative identification of common pathogenic bacteria. Washington Crossing, N.J., Pitman-Moore, Inc., 1972.

Ihrke, P.: Skin scraping techniques for ectoparasites in small animal practice. Compen. Cont. Ed. Anim. Health Tech. 2:5, 1981.

Lever, W.F., and Schaumberg-Lever, G.: Histopathology of the Skin. 5th Ed. Philadelphia, J.B. Lippincott, 1975.

Nesbitt, G.H.: A practical approach to dermatological problems. In Proceedings of Region I of the American Animal Hospital Association. Hartford, Conn., 1979, p. 156.

Rojko, J.L., Hoover, E.A., and Martin, S.L.: Histologic interpretation of cutaneous biopsies from dogs with dermatologic disorders. Vet. Pathol. 15:579, 1978.

Withrow, S.J., and Lowes, N.: Biopsy techiques for use in small animal oncology. J. Am. Anim. Hosp. Assoc. 17:889, 1981.

3

Dermatopharmacology

The veterinarian can choose from a large number of topical and systemic drugs when treating canine and feline dermatologic disease. Each class of drugs has its own indications for use in treating particular problems. To determine the appropriate therapy, the clinician must first recognize and characterize the lesions and try to categorize their cause. For example, is the lesion moist or dry, scaly or exudative, and deep or superficial? The veterinarian must also know the characteristics of the specific drugs so that the desired therapeutic effect on the lesion may be matched with the drug most likely to produce that effect.

Most skin conditions require routine monitoring by the veterinarian or pet owner to assess the success or failure of the treatment regimen. Many therapeutic failures are caused by poor or inadequate communication between the pet owner and the veterinarian. Another common cause of ineffective therapy is failure to pursue a systematic approach to definitive diagnosis, which results in administering medications that are not the best choice. Inadequate or excessive doses as well as discontinuance of medications prior to total resolution of the problem may also result in treatment failure.

Dermatologic drugs can be divided into two groups: topical and systemic. The purpose of this chapter is to review these drugs with respect to classification, general modes of action, and indications for use. The specific drugs, indications,

and dosages are given in the Therapeutic Keys in Appendix 2.

TOPICAL DERMATOLOGIC DRUGS

Forms. Topical dermatologic agents are available in many forms. Table 3–1 gives the mode of action, indications, and disadvantages of each of the seven most common forms.

Classes. Topical dermatologic agents are classified according to their mode of action based on active components. There are usually many specific formulations in each class. The common drugs and agents and their modes of action included in the nine classes of topical dermatologic agents are given in Table 3–2. Specific indications are also listed for some drugs.

SYSTEMIC DERMATOLOGIC DRUGS

The two most frequently used classes of systemic dermatologic drugs are glucocorticosteroids and antibiotics. Other classes include hormones, antihistamines, antifungal, antiparasitic, immunotherapeutic, and chemotherapeutic drugs.

Glucocorticosteriods. The most used and often abused class of systemic dermatologic drugs are glucocorticosteroids. When treating dermatologic disease, familiarity with the actions, indications, side effects, and treatment protocols for the various types of corticosteroids is necessary.

A practical classification for corticosteroids is based on the length of adrenal suppression. Table

TABLE 3–1. COMMON FORMS OF TOPICAL DERMATOLOGIC AGENTS

Form	Action/Characteristics	Indication	Disadvantages
Wet dressings	Cleans, maintains drainage, soothes; keratolytic, anti-inflammatory, antimicrobial, analgesic, antipruritic	Acute moist dermatoses with edema, erythema, pustules, vesicles, exudate, ulcers, and pain Subacute dermatoses with erythema, minor exudation, and ulceration	Requires frequent or prolonged application; penetrates poorly; often drying to skin
Gels, creams, ointments	Protects, soothes, softens, penetrates; antipruritic; vehicle for specific agents	Chronic nonpainful dermatoses with dry scale, lichenification, acanthosis	Occlusive, greasy, messy
Powders	Cools, soothes, protects, reduces friction; absorbent; vehicle for residual agents	Intertriginous lesions	Nonpenetrating; tends to form a dry, occlusive covering that must be removed before each new application; cannot use on open lesions
Lotions	Cools, soothes, dries, protects, allows some drainage, astringent; anti-inflammatory, antipruritic	Acute moist dermatoses	Poor penetration; somewhat occlusive; may be drying and irritating; leaves deposit; not indicated on chronic lesions
Rinses (dips)	Vehicle for residual agent	Parasitic dermatoses; seborrheic dermatoses (emollient bath oils)	Parasitic rinse: odiferous, may be irritating; Emollient rinse: oil film on hair if too concentrated

3–3 gives the length of adrenal suppression for each type of glucocorticosteroid, the commonly used drugs included within each type, and the relative anti-inflammatory effect of these drugs. Table 3–4 is a guideline for dosage of short-acting corticosteroids. Table 3–5 lists the relative frequency of occurrence and the pathogenesis of side effects of long-term daily and alternate-day corticosteroid therapy. The advantages of achieving control of signs with alternate-day therapy are readily recognized. The actions, indications, and dosages of specific systemic corticosteroids are given in the Therapeutic Keys (Appendices 2:3 to 2:5).

Antibiotics. The antibiotic of choice in treating dermatologic problems is often different from those commonly selected for systemic disease. Table 3–6 lists the common types of antibiotics, specific drugs, actions, efficacy, and dosages.

The selection of the antibiotic of choice is based on drug history, clinical signs, and in vitro bacterial culture and antibiotic sensitivity testing. In general, ampicillin, penicillin, and the tetracyclines are not routinely recommended for treating either primary or secondary pyoderma because of their relatively lower clinical efficacy (Table 3–6). Bacterial resistance to these antibiotics is commonly observed. Bactericidal antibiotics should be used to treat deep pyoderma and chronic or recurrent superficial pyoderma.

Therapeutic dosages of an efficacious drug should continue to be administered for a minimum of 7 to 10 days following a complete clinical response. If there is a minimal clinical response in 5 to 7 days, the treatment protocol should be re-evaluated. A more detailed discussion of the use of antibiotics is found in Chapter 6. The Bacterial Disease Therapeutic Key (Appendix 2:9) lists specific antibiotics, indications, and suggested dosages.

Antihistamines. Antihistamines have been only minimally effective in masking pruritic signs. To achieve a true antihistaminic effect, the drug should be administered prior to an expected histaminic reaction (e.g., hyposensitization injection) or immediately following histamine release (e.g., insect sting). In most pruritic conditions, antihistamines must be given at a dosage that produces a sedative effect in order to achieve some control of the pruritus. Table 3–7 lists examples of antihistaminic drugs, their major actions, and suggested dosages.

Hormones. Hormonal therapy is used primarily as a replacement for a specific or relative deficiency. Thyroid hormone is the most widely used hormonal drug in the dog. There are several thyroid preparations available, and the veterinarian should be familiar with the different types of drugs and their indications. These are given in Table 3–8. More detailed information on indications for various thyroid medication is found in Chapter 8 and in the Endocrine Disease Therapeutic Key (Appendix 2:11).

TABLE 3–2. CLASSES OF TOPICAL DERMATOLOGIC AGENTS

Class	Drugs or Agents	Action/Characteristics	Specific Indications
Antipruritic	Menthol 0.12–1%; camphor 0.12–5%; hot or cold water	Substitutes itch sensation with heat or cold	Pruritus/temporary relief
	Ointments, creams, petrolatum	Protects skin from external influences	Focal pruritic lesions
	Local anesthetics (dibucaine 0.5%)	Anesthetizes peripheral sensory nerves	Focal pruritic lesions
	Glucocorticosteroids: hydrocortisone 1–2.5%; prednisolone 0.5%; methylprednisolone 0.25%; desoximetasone 0.25%; triamcinolone acetonide 0.1%; betamethasone 0.1%; fluocinonide 0.05%	Anti-inflammatory	Focal pruritic, erythematous, or excoriated lesions
Keratolytic	Salicylic acid 5–40%; coal tar 1–10%; resorcinol 2–30%; sulfur 2–10%; benzoyl peroxide hydrous 5%	Helps remove stratum corneum or reduces thickness by hydration, softening, and peeling	Seborrheic lesions; bacterial dermatitis
Keratoplastic	Salicylic acid 1–2%; coal tar 1–5%; sulfur 2–10%	Helps normalize keratinization by unknown mechanism	Seborrheic lesions; bacterial dermatitis
Antiseborrheic	Sulfur 2–5%; coal tar 1–5%; benzoyl peroxide hydrous 2.5–5%	Reduces scaling, greasiness, inflammation, and pruritus by keratolytic or keratoplastic actions	Seborrheic lesions; bacterial dermatitis
Antiparasitic	Sulfur 1.0–5%	Kills adults, larvae, or ova by direct contact or ingestion	Mites, lice, chiggers
	Pyrethrins 0.05–0.4%	Acts as contact poison resulting in the release of acetylcholine	Lice, flies, mosquitos, fleas
	Rotenone 2–10%	Glutamic acid inhibitor	Mites, fleas, lice, chiggers
	Lindane 4–9%	Destabilizes neuronal membranes	Fleas, lice, mosquitos
	Organophosphate Malathion 0.5% Delnav 5%	Cholinesterase inhibitor	Flies, lice, mosquitos, mites, fleas, ticks
	Carbamates 5–8%	Acts as contact poison by cholinesterase inhibition	Mosquitoes, lice, flies, fleas, ticks
Antimicrobial	Povidone-iodine	Bactericidal, fungicidal, and sporicidal; liberates hypochlorous acid	Bacterial dermatitis; dermatophytosis
	Cuprimyxin 0.5%; chlorhexidine	Bactericidal and fungicidal	Bacterial dermatitis; dermatophytosis
	Sulfur 1–10%	Bacteriostatic and antifungal	Bacterial dermatitis; dermatophytosis
	Benzoyl peroxide hydrous 2.5–5%	Antibacterial and antiseborrheic	Bacterial dermatitis; dermatophytosis; acne
	Neomycin sulfate, bacitracin, polymyxin B, nitrofurazone, thiostrepton	Antibacterial	Bacterial dermatitis
Antifungal	Miconazole nitrate 2%; clotrimazole 1%; haloprogin 1%; thiabendazole	Fungicidal; acts on cytoplasmic membrane of fungus	Dermatophytosis; yeast infections
	Tolnaftate 1%	Fungistatic	Microsporum gypseum only
	Nystatin	Anticandidal; causes cells to lose potassium ions	Candidal infections
Emollient oil rinses	Bath oil	Softens stratum corneum, protects, soothes; vehicle for other drugs; artificial sebum	Seborrhea sicca; dry skin
Astringent	Aluminum acetate; tannic acid 5%	Precipitates protein; decreases cell permeability	Moist, weeping lesions

TABLE 3–3. SYSTEMIC DERMATOLOGIC DRUGS: CORTICOSTEROIDS

Type	Length of adrenal suppression	Drug	Relative anti-inflammatory effect*
Short-acting	<36 h	Hydrocortisone	1
		prednisone	4
		prednisolone	4
		methylprednisolone	5
		triamcinolone	5
Long-acting	≥60 h	Dexamethasone	10–20
		betamethasone	10–20
		flumethasone	20 or more
Residual	2–4 wk	Triamcinolone acetonide methylprednisolone acetate betamethasone dipropionate	

*When compared to hydrocortisone on a mg to mg basis.

TABLE 3–4. SHORT-ACTING CORTICOSTEROID DOSAGE GUIDELINES FOR ORAL ROUTE

Corticosteroid treatment	Size of Dog					
	Small (< 9 kg)		Medium (9 to 23 kg)		Large (> 23 kg)	
	Initial	Maintenance	Initial	Maintenance	Initial	Maintenance
Pruritus						
Minimal	5 mg q2d	taper*	5 mg q24h	5 mg q2d and taper*	10 mg q24h	10 mg q2d and taper*
Moderate	5 mg q12h or q24h	5–10 mg q2d and taper*	10 mg q12h or q24h	10 mg q2d and taper*	10–20 mg q12h or q24h	20 mg q24h and taper*
Marked	10 mg q12h or q24h	10–15 mg q2d and taper*	10–20 mg q12h or q24h	20–30 mg q2d and taper*	25 mg q12h or q24h	25–50 mg q2d and taper*

*Try to decrease dosage 50% each week, either in frequency or quantity.

TABLE 3–5. SIDE EFFECTS OF CHRONIC DAILY AND ALTERNATE DAY SHORT-ACTING CORTICOSTEROID THERAPY

Clinical Sign	Frequency of Treatment		Pathogenesis
	Daily	Alternate Day	
	Relative Frequency of Occurrence*		
Polyuria/polydipsia	+ + + +	±	Unknown
Alopecia	+ +	−	Atrophy of hair follicles, sebaceous glands, and epidermis
Thin skin	+	−	Atrophy of epidermis, collagen, and fibroelastic tissue
Hepatomegaly	+ +	−	Glycogen accumulation within hepatocytes
Distended abdomen	+	−	Muscle weakness, hepatomegaly, and intraperitoneal fat deposition
Calcinosis cutis	+	−	Altered dermal protein matrix with dystrophic binding of calcium
Hyperpigmentation	+ +	−	Unknown
Infection	+	−	Anti-inflammatory and immunosuppressive effects
Anestrus/testicular atrophy	+	−	Probable inhibition of gonadoptropin release

*If on continuous long-term therapy (months to years) using prednisone, prednisolone, or methylprednisolone.

Most androgens and estrogens are used in therapeutic trials because of a lack of specific assays and standards for interpretation of blood levels. Preliminary studies have not shown a consistent correlation of serum hormone concentrations and clinical signs. Modes of action and indications are listed in the Endocrine Diagnostic Therapeutic Key (Appendix 2:11). A progestational drug (megestrol acetate, Ovaban, Schering) has been used extensively in the treatment of several feline syndromes of unknown etiologic origin. Remember, this drug is not approved for cats in the United States and has been shown to have side effects.

Antifungal Drugs. Systemic antifungal drugs

TABLE 3–6. SYSTEMIC DERMATOLOGIC DRUGS: ANTIBIOTICS

| Type | Drug | Action | % Relative Efficacy in Pyoderma* | | Dosage/Route |
			Gram (+)	Gram (−)	
Penicillin	Cloxacillin sodium	Bactericidal	87	9	22 mg/kg bid-tid PO
	Nafcillin	Bactericidal	92	0	22 mg/kg bid-tid PO
	Oxacillin sodium	Bactericidal	92	0	22 mg/kg bid-tid PO
	Ampicillin	Bactericidal	38	61	22 mg/kg bid PO
	Penicillin G, potassium	Bactericidal	19	9	20,000 U/kg PO qid
Cephalosporin	Cephalexin	Bactericidal	95	27	20–30 mg/kg bid PO or 20 mg/kg tid PO
	Cephadrine	Bactericidal	NA†	NA†	20–30 mg/kg bid PO or 20 mg/kg tid PO
Aminoglycoside	Gentamicin sulfate	Bactericidal	96	90	4.4 mg/kg bid (day 1); then SID SC
	Kanamycin sulfate	Bactericidal	93	48	6–8 mg/kg bid SC
Tetracycline	Tetracycline	Bacteriostatic	46	13	15–20 mg/kg tid PO
Macrolide	Erythromycin	Bacteriostatic	84	9	10–15 mg/kg tid PO
	Troleandomycin	Bacteriostatic	86	0	20 mg/kg tid PO
Miscellaneous	Chloramphenicol	Bacteriostatic	93	52	20–50 mg/kg tid PO
	Lincomycin hydrochloride	Bacteriostatic	78	15	20 mg/kg bid PO
Sulfonamide and sulfonamide potentiator	Trimethoprim and sulfadiazine	Bactericidal	52‡	36‡	30 mg/kg sid or divided bid PO

Data were extrapolated from Ihrke, P.J., Halliwell, R.E.W., and Deubler, M.J.: Canine pyoderma. In Current Veterinary Therapy VI: Small Animal Practice. Edited by R.W. Kirk. Philadelphia, W.B. Saunders, 1977, p. 518 and Nesbitt, G.H., and Schmitz, J.A.: Chronic bacterial dermatitis and otitis: A review of 195 cases. J. Am. Anim. Hosp. Assoc. 13:446, 1979.

*Relative efficacy was based on in vitro antibiotic sensitivity tests.

†NA means no data are available.

‡These percentages may be abnormally low due to an inhibition of antibiotic activity by thiamine which is present in blood agar. Mueller-Hinton agar plates should be used for in vitro antibiotic sensitivity testing with trimethoprim and sulfadiazine.

TABLE 3–7. SYSTEMIC DERMATOLOGIC DRUGS: ANTIHISTAMINES

Subclass	Generic Name	Trade Name	Action/Characteristic	Dosage/Route
Phenothiazine	Promethazine hydrochloride	Phenergan HCl (Wyeth)	Markedly antipruritic	0.2–1 mg/kg tid-qid PO
	Trimeprazine tartrate	Temaril (SmithKline)	Markedly sedative	1–2 mg/kg bid PO
Ethanolamine	Diphenhydramine HCl	Benadryl HCl (Parke-Davis)	Antipruritic, anticholinergic	1–2 mg/kg bid-tid PO
Alkylamine	Chlorpheniramine maleate	Chlor-Trimeton (Schering)	Antipruritic, weakly sedative	0.5–2 mg/kg bid-tid PO

are limited in their indications (Table 3–9). Griseofulvin is the only approved systemic antifungal agent used in treating dermatophytes. Nystatin is only indicated for candidal infections; sodium iodide is used in treating sporotrichosis, and amphotericin B is used for deep mycotic infections. Ketoconazole is a new antifungal agent effective in dermatophytosis and deep mycotic infections in man. It is still an experimental drug in small animal medicine. Specific drugs, indications, and dosages are given in Table 3–9 and in the Fungal Disease Therapeutic Key (Appendix 2:10).

Antiparasitic Drugs. Systemic antiparasiticides are the most limited of all of the classes of systemic dermatologic drugs (Table 3–9). Proban cythioate is the only antiparasitic drug presently on the market that is approved and efficacious. Indications include fleas and ticks.

Immunotherapeutic Drugs. The efficacy of the immunotherapeutic drugs is controversial. They have been most widely used as adjunct therapy in treating cancer and chronic staphylococcal infections. The most commonly used immunotherapeutic agents include staphylococcus and mixed bacterins, levamisole, and Bacillus Calmette-Guerin (BCG). The indications and therapeutic protocols are given in Table 3–9. Refer to the Bacterial (Appendix 2:9) and Neoplastic Disease (Appendix 2:14) Therapeutic Keys for more specific indications, dosages, and side effects.

TABLE 3–8.   SYSTEMIC DERMATOLOGIC DRUGS: HORMONES

Type	Drug or Hormone	Hormone Replaced	Dosage/Route
Thyroid	Sodium levothyroxine	Thyroxine (T_4)	0.02 mg/kg sid-bid PO
	L-triiodothyronine	Triiodothyronine (T_3)	4–5 µg/kg tid PO
	Combination drugs	T_3 and T_4	Dosage calculated on basis of T_4 content (0.02 mg/kg bid) PO
Androgen	Methyltestosterone	Testosterone	0.5 mg/kg sid (dogs) PO
	Repositol form testosterone	Testosterone	12.5 mg q6wk (cats) IM
Estrogen	Diethylstilbestrol	Estrogens	0.1 mg/5 kg sid or q2d PO (dogs)
	Repositol form stilbestrol	Estrogens	0.625 mg q6wk IM (cats)
Progesterone	Megestrol acetate	Unknown action (probably anti-inflammatory)	5 mg sid × 7 days tapering to q7d or longer PO (cats only)
	Repositol form progesterone	Progesterone	2.2–20 mg/kg q6wk IM
	Medroxyprogesterone acetate	Progesterone	100–350 mg/kg q6wk IM

TABLE 3–9.   SYSTEMIC DERMATOLOGIC DRUGS: ANTIFUNGAL, ANTIPARASITIC, IMMUNO-THERAPEUTIC, AND CHEMOTHERAPEUTIC

Class	Drugs and Agents	Action/Characteristics	Dosage/Route	Side Effects
Antifungal	Griseofulvin	Fungistatic for dermatophytes	50–100 mg/kg divided bid PO	Teratogenic anomalies; bone marrow depression (cats), anorexia (cats)
	Nystatin	Anticandidal	100,000 U q6h PO	
	Sodium iodide, 20%	Antisporotrichosis	1.0 mg/5 kg q8h to q12h PO	Lacrimation, dandruff
	Amphotericin B	Sporocidal (deep mycoses)	0.15–1 mg/kg in 5% dextrose q2d IV	Vomiting, nephrotoxicity
	Ketoconazole	Fungicidal; acts on cytoplasmic membrane	11.0 mg/kg q8hr to q12hr PO	Insufficient drug experience
Antiparasitic	Proban cythioate	Cholinesterase inhibitor	3.3 mg/kg q3d or q4d PO	Excessive lacrimation, vomiting, muscle twitching, weakness
Immunotherapeutic	Bacillus Calmette-Guerin (BCG) bacterin	Nonspecific lymphocyte stimulation	Variable at local site of lesion ID	Fever, malaise, induration
	Corynebacterium parvum bacterin	Nonspecific lymphocyte stimulation	1–2 mg/kg q1wk or q2wk SC	
	Levamisole HCl	Nonspecific lymphocyte stimulation	5 mg/kg q2d or q3d PO	Vomiting, anorexia
	Staphylococcal bacterins	Nonspecific lymphocyte stimulation	Variable protocols (see Bacterial Disease Therapeutic Key, Appendix 2:9)	
Chemotherapeutic	Cyclophosphamide	Alkylating agent	50 mg/m² sid 4 days of each week PO, IV	Vomiting, leukopenia, hemorrhagic cystitis
	Chlorambucil	Alkylating agent	2 mg/m² sid PO	Minimal to none
	Vincristine sulfate	Alkaloid; antimitotic	0.5 mg/m² q1wk or q2wk IV	Anemia, leukopenia, stomatitis
	Methotrexate	Antimetabolite; folic acid antagonist	2.5 mg/m² sid IV, IM, PO	Anemia, gastrointestinal disturbances
	Azathioprine	Antimetabolite	1.0–1.5 mg/kg sid (dogs) q2d (cats)	Leukopenia

Chemotherapeutic Drugs. These drugs are widely used in treating systemic neoplasia, but have limited benefit in treating most primary cutaneous neoplasms. They are also used routinely with corticosteroids in treating immune-mediated bullous diseases. The most commonly used chemotherapeutic drugs, their indications, and average dosages are given in Table 3–9 and in the Neoplastic Disease Therapeutic Key (Appendix 2:14).

SELECTED READINGS

Dillon, A.R., Spano, J.S., and Powers, R.D.: Prednisolone induced hematologic, biochemical and histologic changes in the dog. J. Am. Anim. Hosp. Assoc. 16:831, 1980.

Eyre, P.: Pharmacology of antipruritic drugs. In Current Veterinary Therapy VII: Small Animal Practice. Edited by R.W. Kirk. Philadelphia, W.B. Saunders, 1980.

Halliwell, R.E.: Antibiotic therapy in canine skin disease. Biweekly Small Animal Vet. Med. Update Series. Princeton, N.J., Veterinary Publications, 12:1, 1978.

———: Steroid therapy in skin disease. In Current Veterinary Therapy VI: Small Animal Practice. Edited by R.W. Kirk. Philadelphia, W.B. Saunders, 1977.

Ihrke, P.J.: Topical therapy—uses, principles and vehicles: Dermatologic therapy (Part I). Compend. Cont. Ed. Pract. Vet. 2:28, 1980.

———: Topical therapy-specific topical pharmacologic agents: Dermatologic therapy (Part II). Compend. Cont. Ed. Pract. Vet. 2:156, 1980.

———: Antibiotic therapy in canine skin disease: Dermatologic therapy (Part III). Compend. Cont. Ed. Pract. Vet. 2:177, 1980.

Ihrke, P.J., Halliwell, R.E.W., and Deubler, M.J.: Canine pyoderma. In Current Veterinary Therapy VI: Small Animal Practice. Edited by R.W. Kirk. Philadelphia, W.B. Saunders, 1977.

Madewell, R.B., and Theilen, G.H.: Chemotherapy. In Veterinary Cancer Medicine. Edited by G.H. Theilen and B.R. Madewell. Philadelphia, Lea & Febiger, 1979.

Meijer, J.C.: Canine hyperadrenocorticism. In Current Veterinary Therapy VII: Small Animal Practice. Edited by R.W. Kirk. Philadelphia, W.B. Saunders, 1980.

Nesbitt, G.H., and Schmitz, J.A.: Chronic bacterial dermatitis and otitis: A review of 195 cases: J. Am. Anim. Hosp. Assoc. 13:442, 1977.

Peterson, M.E.: Canine cushings syndrome. In Proceedings of Annual Meeting of Region I of the American Animal Hospital Association, Hartford, Conn., 1979, p. 328.

Scott, D.W.: Therapeutics. J. Am. Anim. Hosp. Assoc. 16:434, 1980.

———: Systemic glucocorticoid therapy. In Current Veterinary Therapy VII: Small Animal Practice. Edited by R.W. Kirk. Philadelphia, W.B. Saunders, 1980.

———: Topical cutaneous medicine. Proceedings of 46th Annual Meeting of the American Animal Hospital Association, 1979.

Theilen, G.H. and Madewell, B.R.: Immunotherapy. In Veterinary Cancer Medicine. Edited by G.H. Theilen and B.R. Madewell. Philadelphia, Lea & Febiger, 1979.

4

Allergic Diseases

Canine allergic diseases have been well documented, whereas feline allergic disorders have been less commonly recognized. The Allergic Diagnostic Key (Appendix 1:2) lists the most pertinent historical and clinical findings and diagnostic tests that help to differentiate the common etiologic factors of canine and feline allergic diseases.

CANINE ATOPIC DERMATITIS

Canine atopic dermatitis is an inherited predisposition to allergic disease that is mediated by immunoglobulin E (IgE). Synonyms include allergic inhalant dermatitis (AID), canine atopy, atopic disease, and atopic inhalant dermatitis.

Etiologic Factors. The causes of canine atopic dermatitis may be divided into 3 groups: *inhalant* allergens, such as weed, tree and grass pollens, molds, house dust, animal danders, sheep wool, feathers, kapok, cottonseed, and tobacco; *intrinsic* allergens, such as estrogen and progesterone; and *miscellaneous* causes, such as ingestants (food), injectants (insect saliva), and endoparasites (hookworm, roundworm, whipworm). The exact pathophysiologic mechanisms involving the last mentioned group are unknown. It is common to have multiple causes of clinical signs, e.g., flea saliva and inhalant allergens.

Pathogenesis. The pathogenesis of canine atopic disease involves a Type I hypersensitivity reaction to an antigen. This is an immediate re-

action in which there is an excess of IgE in the dermis, and this skin-sensitizing antibody becomes fixed to tissue mast cells. The coupling of the specific antigen and antibody results in the degranulation of the mast cells and the subsequent release of low molecular weight vasoactive amines including histamine, slow-release substance of anaphylaxis (SRS-A), and many macromolecular mediators, such as lysosomal and polymorphonuclear leukocyte enzymes. Smooth muscle contraction, capillary dilatation, increased capillary permeability, and pruritus follow. The respiratory system is considered to be the most common route of entry of the allergen. Inherited susceptibility, rather than the degree of exposure to the antigen, is thought to be the determining factor in developing hypersensitivity.

History. The history of a dog with canine atopic dermatitis is characteristic. The average age of onset is 1 to 3 years; however, there is a range of 6 months to greater than 6 years.

The list of breeds reported to be predisposed to atopic dermatitis has lengthened or changed over the last several years, due partially to differences in breed popularity and to specific genetic lines within the various breeds. The breeds with a higher incidence than expected for the general population include Wirehaired Fox Terrier, West Highland White Terrier, Dalmatian, Cairn Terrier, Golden Labrador Retriever, and Irish Setter.

Face rubbing, foot licking, and axillary pruritus

are the most common allergic signs reported. Many dogs, especially when young, have a seasonal pattern with severe signs in warm weather. These seasonal patterns vary depending on geographic location, growing season of pollen-producing plants, and environmental factors such as humidity, wind, temperature, and degree of exposure to the allergen(s). Some dogs have fall and winter seasonal patterns, which often correlate with low humidity and forced air heating systems. As the dog ages, it is common to see an increase in severity and duration of allergic signs. Some atopic dogs have a year-round (nonseasonal) history of allergic disease from the onset of clinical signs, especially in climates with minimal seasonal changes.

A decrease in pruritus is usually reported when corticosteroids are administered daily or on alternate days at a dosage of 0.5 to 1 mg/kg. Also, a change in environment may result in temporary improvement or worsening of signs depending on exposure to the allergen(s). Because of the amnestic response, an atopic dog may have an allergic reaction with infrequent exposure to the allergen.

Clinical Manifestations. Dogs with atopic dermatitis have variable clinical manifestations. The lesions may be acute or chronic, localized or generalized, and are commonly found periorbitally and on the feet, ear pinnas, flank, perineum, ventral abdomen, and axillae. Most lesions are secondary to pruritus and are usually characterized by various secondary morphologic changes. Alopecia is variable. Signs of acute inflammatory reaction include erythema and edema of the skin (Plate 3:A,B) and ears (Plate 3:C). Chronic inflammation is characterized by acanthosis, hyperpigmentation (Plate 3:D), and occasionally lichenification. Common concurrent problems associated with atopic dermatitis include dry skin, seborrheic and bacterial dermatitis, and salivary staining of the hair (Plate 3:E).

Definitive Diagnostic Test (Intradermal Skin Testing). Intradermal (ID) skin testing is the only practical method of identifying inhalant allergens. A positive ID reaction only indicates that the dog or cat has IgE antibodies to the allergen injected. It does not necessarily mean that the dermatologic problem is caused by atopic disease. A history of exposure to the allergens must be confirmed.

The client must fully understand the procedures of skin testing and hyposensitization before testing is initiated. A dissatisfied or misinformed client is the first step toward short- and long-term problems in managing an atopic dog or cat.

It is important to consider the time of year when performing ID testing. An animal's intensity of reaction to the specific ID test may be directly correlated to the degree of exposure to the allergen(s). Generally, the best time to test for seasonal allergens is within 1 to 2 months after exposure, or postseasonally. Weaker or negative ID skin test reactions may be expected if several months have elapsed following exposure to a seasonal allergen.

At the time of testing, the dog or cat must not be under the influence of immunosuppressive drugs. It is often difficult to determine the waiting time necessary after the last medication has been administered because of variable factors including type of medication, route, dosage, and duration of treatment. A guideline for the waiting time following daily administration of oral short-acting glucocorticoids is a minimum of 3 weeks or until a marked increase in pruritus is observed. The longer the duration of treatment, the more prolonged the waiting time needs to be. Following injectable corticosteroids, the waiting time is unpredictable. A reasonable guideline is to wait at least 3 weeks following the expected duration of the effect of the drug or until the animal shows a marked increase in pruritus. Wait at least 1 day following tranquilization and 3 days following antihistamine administration. The duration of action of megestrol acetate may be prolonged since cortisol response following ACTH administration has remained suppressed for up to 4 months after discontinuing chronic megestrol acetate therapy.

ID skin testing has proved to be an effective diagnostic test in experienced hands. However, there are reports of less than satisfactory results by clinicians or technicians who have not mastered the techniques because of infrequent testing or lack of familiarity with the many potential problems related to selection and handling of antigens. Lack of uniformity of injections or difficulty with grading and interpreting test results can also render the procedure ineffective. It is recommended that one technician or veterinarian in a group practice be designated to do all of the ID skin testing. If there is insufficient volume in the practice for the individual to develop the necessary skills, the dog should be referred for the diagnostic procedure.

Technique. Place the dog or cat in lateral recumbency without the use of any chemical restraint. Gently clip the lower lateral thoracic wall with a No. 40 blade avoiding excessive heat or trauma to the skin. Mark the injection sites with a felt pen, leaving ³/₄ to 1 in. between sites and avoid areas that are irritated or otherwise look abnormal. Use a 1.0 ml tuberculin syringe and a 26-gauge, $^3/_8$-in. needle with the bevel dorsal to make the ID injections. The recommended volume of each allergen injected varies from 0.02 to 0.05 ml or a minimum bleb. The smaller volume is generally used by the clinician or technician experienced with the procedure. The injection of an equal volume of allergen in each site is more important than the volume itself. Unequal volume at the different sites makes interpetation difficult. It is equally important to place each injection at the same shallow depth in the dermis.

Grading of ID Reactions. Grading may be subjective or objective. Subjective grading is based on the criteria listed in Table 4–1. A reaction of 2 or more is considered positive. Objective grading is based on actual measurements of the negative control and individual reactions. The most widely accepted criterion is that a positive reaction measures at least 3-mm larger in diameter than the negative control. Another suggested method of objective grading is to average the diameter of the positive and negative control wheals and consider a positive reaction to be greater than or equal to the average. Read the tests 15 to 20 minutes after injection with the dog or cat held in lateral recumbency. Most tests are easier to read in a darkened room using indirect lighting (pen light). The grading of the reactions in cats is usually more difficult than for dogs since the wheal tends to be flatter

TABLE 4–1. CRITERIA FOR GRADING INTRADERMAL SKIN TEST REACTIONS

I. Subjective
  1. Compare size and color of wheal and steepness of wall.
  2. Compare positive and negative controls to allergen reaction.
  3. Grade individual reactions 0 through 4:
    a. Negative control = 0
    b. Positive control = 4
    c. 2 × size of negative control = 1
    d. 3 × size of negative control = 2
    e. 4 × size of negative control = 3
    f. Equal to size of positive control = 4
  4. Increased erythema and/or steep walls has positive influence on the grade.
  5. Known mild irritant reaction of allergen has negative influence on grade.
II. Objective
  1. Measure diameter of negative control.
  2. Measure diameter of individual reactions.
  3. Grading:
    a. Negative reaction = < 3 mm larger than negative control.
    b. Positive reaction = > 3 mm larger than negative control.
      or
    c. Average the diameter of negative and positive controls. Any wheal greater than the above average is a positive reaction.

and borders are less defined, which is probably a result of a thinner dermis and epidermis.

False negative ID skin test reactions may be caused by improper injection techniques such as subcutaneous injections, or injection of air instead of the allergen, influence of immunosuppressive agents, and the use of outdated, impotent, or improperly prepared test antigens. The dilution effect of mixed antigens for ID skin testing may result in false-negative reactions. A contaminated or irritant negative control (i.e., glycerin) may result in a larger wheal being used for comparison. If there is a greater reaction than expected associated with the negative control, the test should be repeated using fresh buffered saline solution. The negative control wheal should measure no more than 4 mm in diameter 15 minutes following the injection of 0.05 ml of sterile buffered saline solution.

False-positive ID skin test reactions may be a result of contamination of diluted extracts, irritant reactions to the allergen or diluent used, excessive concentration or volume of test allergens, or cross reactivity with related allergens.

Interpretation. Several factors are important to consider when interpreting ID skin test results. It is imperative that positive ID reactions correlate with a history of exposure. For example, a positive wool reaction must be discounted if there is a reliable history of no wool exposure. Generally, there is a poor correlation between the grade of the positive reaction and the degree of hypersensitivity. Factors that influence the severity or grade of the ID reaction include the time of testing relative to exposure, and the antigenicity of the testing extract.

Concentration of Allergens. Only aqueous antigens are used for ID skin testing. Antigen concentration is defined in protein nitrogen units (PNU). When measuring, 1 mg of protein nitrogen is equivalent to 100,000 PNU. The final concentration of antigen routinely used is 1000 to 1500 PNU/ml. Another common measurement is weight per volume (w/v). Most testing concentrations are a 1:10 w/v. A 1:10 w/v is defined as 1 gram of raw material extracted in 10 ml of extracting or diluting fluid.

Selection of Testing Allergens. Allergens are generally grouped on the basis of the taxonomic classification of plants and organisms. The 3 most common groupings include first, pollen types: the trees, weeds, and grasses; the second, molds; and the third, epidermals. A mixed, inhalant group includes several nonrelated antigens: silk, pyrethrins, orris root, and kapok. Each group contains variable percentages of the individual antigens (e.g., 5 to 40%). In addition, several single antigens are routinely used, such as house dust and tobacco.

The selection of allergens for testing is based on several factors including the source of the allergens, the geographic location, the history (seasonal, perennial), and the maximum number of allergens to be used.

Several manufacturers of human allergens also package and market allergens specifically for veterinary use. Other manufacturers sell human allergens to veterinarians upon request. ID testing kits for veterinary use are generally regionalized to reflect the geographic distribution of various pollens. Molds and other nonseasonal allergens are usually the same for all regions. These testing kits provide the veterinarian with a convenient source of allergens that are ready to use without diluting. There is a disadvantage, however, in the lack of flexibility to adapt the testing materials to the individual animal's exposure or local geographic areas. Also, the total number of allergens in the testing kit is limited. A specific plant may be prevalent in a limited geographic area, but may not be included in the kit. False-negative and false-positive ID reactions discussed previously may occur.

Prior to selecting the allergens to be used in any given area, the most common problems in the area for both man and animals should be identified. A human allergist should be consulted since the allergens that cause human inhalant allergies are the same as those that affect dogs. If there are veterinary colleagues in the area with ID skin testing experience, they should also be consulted. The most common regional allergens are listed in Table 4–2. The use of groups of antigens versus individual antigens for testing is controversial. There is limited to no cross-reactivity among some allergens within the same family. Johnson and Bermuda grass contain distinct antigens that do not cross-react with the other common grasses in the grass group. Most weeds are also antigenically distinct. It is thought that the various animal fibers (epidermals) do have some cross-reactivity. Molds are usually grouped. Since the concentration of the testing antigen is usually standardized at 1000 or 1500 PNU or 1:1000 w/v, dilution is a factor to consider with grouped antigens. A 10 tree mix with equal parts of 10 tree antigens at a concentration of 1500 PNU/ml of mixture will only contain 150 PNU/ml of each antigen. If one of the tree

pollens was the only allergen of clinical importance, a false-negative reaction could occur due to an inadequate concentration of that antigen.

The number of allergens that can be tested at any given time is not standardized. The majority of testing kits use 10 to 15 grouped and individual allergens. If the clinician uses an expanded testing battery, 20 to 30 allergens are usually included. There has been no increase in side effects or alterations in reactions when I have used 55 individual and grouped antigens for testing. Since standardization is lacking, I suggest using the guidelines in Table 4–3 when selecting allergens for ID skin testing.

Some antigens are irritating, possibly resulting in a false-positive reaction at the higher concentrations. The antigens that are normally more irritating include house dust, wool, feathers, and horse dander. If strong reactions are routinely obtained with one or more individual or groups of antigens, especially if most other reactions are negative or there is no history of exposure to these antigens, a weaker concentration of antigen should be used. A 250 to 500 PNU/ml concentration of house dust and a 500 PNU/ml of wool and feathers are often used.

All allergens tend to become less stable, biodegrading more rapidly as they are diluted; thus, testing concentrations must be replaced frequently. If a commercial test kit is used, observe the dating closely and discard all outdated materials. The allergens also lose antigenicity on exposure to heat; thus, they must be kept refrigerated except for short periods of time for testing.

Management. General considerations in managing the atopic dog include: avoid allergens whenever possible, use topical and/or systemic medications when needed, consider hyposensitization, and treat all concurrent problems.

The clinician and client should be aware of the "allergic threshold" concept. An allergic load may be tolerated by a dog without disease manifestations; however, a small increase in the load may push the dog over the threshold and initiate clinical signs. Combined stresses of immunologic, genetic, climatic, and physiologic origins may precipitate the allergic disease. The allergic threshold is not fixed and may be raised or lowered by various factors that may affect the dog, including the general condition of the skin, the nutritional state, infection, external parasites, and the environment.

Medical Management. All manifestations of disease in the atopic dog must be treated simultaneously (Allergic Disease Therapeutic Key,

TABLE 4–2. DISTRIBUTION OF MAJOR ALLERGENS BY REGION*

Nonseasonal allergens common to all regions of the United States
  Molds: Alternaria, Aspergillus, Fusarium, Helminthosporium, Cladosporium (Hormodendrum), Penicillium, Phoma, Rhizopus
  Epidermals: horse, cat and dog epithelium; chicken, duck, and goose feathers; human dander; sheep wool
  Miscellaneous: house dust, kapok, silk, orris root, pyrethrins, cottonseed

Seasonal pollens of highest incidence by region†

Region (states)	Grass pollens	Weed pollens	Tree pollens
Northwest (Oregon, Washington)	June, orchard, redtop, rye, timothy	Pigweed, plantain, thistle	Birch, box elder, walnut
California	Bermuda, Johnson, orchard, rye, redtop, timothy	Pigweed, plantain, sagebrush	Alder, birch, cottonseed, cypress, elm, walnut
Intermountain (Colorado, Idaho, Montana, Nevada, Utah, Wyoming)	June, orchard, redtop, timothy	Lamb's-quarters, pigweed, plantain, ragweed, sagebrush, thistle	Cottonwood
Southwest (Arizona, New Mexico, Texas)	Bermuda, Johnson, June, rye	Pigweed, plantain, ragweed, sagebrush, thistle	Cottonwood, juniper
North Central (Michigan, Minnesota, North Dakota, South Dakota, Wisconsin)	June, orchard, redtop, timothy	Pigweed, plantain, ragweed	Cottonwood, elm, hickory, maple, oak, walnut
Midwest (Illinois, Indiana, Iowa, Kansas, Missouri, Nebraska, Ohio)	June, orchard, redtop, timothy	Pigweed, plantain, ragweed, thistle	Ash, cottonwood, elm, hickory, oak, sycamore, walnut
South Central (Arkansas, Kentucky, Louisiana, Mississippi, Oklahoma, Tennessee, Texas)	Bermuda, Johnson, June, orchard, redtop, rye, timothy	Lamb's-quarters, marsh elder, pigweed, plantain, ragweed, thistle	Ash, elm, hickory, oak, pecan
Northeast (Connecticut, Delaware, New Hampshire, New York, New Jersey, Pennsylvania, Maine, Massachusetts, Rhode Island, Vermont)	June, meadow fescue, orchard, redtop, rye, sweet vernal, timothy	Lamb's-quarters, pigweed, plantain, ragweed	Ash, birch, cottonwood, elm, hickory, oak, walnut
Southeast (Alabama, Florida, Georgia, Maryland, North Carolina, South Carolina, Virginia, West Virginia)	Bermuda, Johnson, June, orchard, redtop, rye, timothy	Pigweed, plantain, ragweed	Ash, elm, oak, sycamore

*Adapted from Weiss, N.S., and Rubin, J.M.: Practical Points in Allergy, 2nd Ed. Medical Examination Publishing, Garden City, NY, 1980.
†There are differences in the specific plant populations among states in a given region and within individual states. This is not all-inclusive of important allergens in any given state.

Appendix 2:7). Antiseborrheic and antibacterial shampoos help remove excessive scales and reduce surface bacterial flora. Daily water soaks for 15 minutes followed by an oil rinse are indicated for treating dry skin. Antibiotics are indicated if there is bacterial dermatitis.

Corticosteroids are routinely used to relieve focal or generalized pruritus. Topical corticosteroid ointments or creams may help relieve pruritus or pain in a focal inflamed or excoriated area. These ointments and creams are not practical if lesions are generalized.

Short-acting oral corticosteroids are preferred to mask pruritic signs and relieve acute inflammation since they may be discontinued when pruritus stops. A loading dose of prednisone or prednisolone followed by a step-down dosage schedule,

preferably alternate day in the morning, is recommended (see Table 3–4). Intermediate, long-acting or residual injectable corticosteroids are not indicated for chronic nonseasonal pruritus. They may be used for short, seasonal pruritus when 1 or 2 injections are all that is required for the entire year, or if oral administration is not possible. Oral corticosteroids should not be used concurrently with the injections.

Antihistamines in large dosages (see Appendix 2:7) may be helpful in easing pruritus in some animals.

Biologic Management. Hyposensitization is the biologic method used to treat the atopic dog. The standard theory of the immunologic mechanism has been that hyposensitization stimulates IgG antibodies. These antibodies have a selective affinity

TABLE 4–3. GUIDELINES FOR SELECTING ANTIGENS TO USE FOR INTRADERMAL SKIN TESTING

I. Before starting skin testing identify all specific allergens that may cause allergic signs in dogs and man and their season of occurrence in your geographic area by consulting with human and veterinary allergists.

II. When testing small numbers of dogs (screening test):
1. Select a commercial skin testing kit that includes the most common allergens for your geographic area.
2. If there are one or more prominent allergens that are indigenous to the geographic area, or that have been suggested on the basis of history, and these are not included in the commercial kit, order them separately.
3. Use all allergens in the kit for both seasonal and nonseasonal pruritus.

III. When testing large numbers of dogs, it is economical to maintain a battery of stock antigens for ID skin testing and hyposensitization:
1. Divide antigens into two groups: seasonal (pollens) and nonseasonal (molds, dust, epidermals, mixed inhalants, miscellaneous). Refer to Table 4–2.
2. When possible, individual trees, grass, and weed pollens should be used. If pollen groups are being used, be sure that pollens indigenous to the geographic area are included. Epidermals (sheep wool, feathers, cat epithelium) should be individual rather than grouped. Molds are routinely used in small groups.
3. For a seasonal (spring, summer, or fall) or nonseasonal allergy, use both seasonal and nonseasonal allergens if testing during or within two months of the end of the pollen exposure.
4. For a winter allergy (in colder climates) use only nonseasonal antigens.
5. For a nonseasonal allergy tested at least two months after the end of pollen exposure, and prior to the next pollen exposure, use the nonseasonal group and then test with the seasonal antigens after the next pollen exposure has occurred up to 2 months following the termination of pollination. If poor or inconclusive reactions were obtained with the first test, repeat the nonseasonal group also.

for specific allergens, and thus block the IgE antibody-antigen reaction and prevent the release of chemical mediators from the target mast cells.

More recent investigations have shown that hyposensitization stimulates specialized T lymphocyte suppressor cells and helper cells. Suppressor cells prevent IgE production and helper cells turn on B lymphocytes that produce IgG.

Hyposensitization should be considered when the allergic signs last for 4 months or more each year, or when a dog exhibits side effects from medical treatment, regardless of the duration of allergic signs. Also, some dogs show no beneficial response to corticosteroids even when given at higher dosages.

The client must understand all aspects of hyposensitization, including the procedure, short- and long-term costs, and prognosis. Many dogs require booster injections for life. If a dog is sign-free for 1 year, it may be possible to discontinue injections with no recurrence of problems.

Several months may pass before maximal clinical response is observed. Occasionally, in the case of seasonal allergy, the best response is not observed until the second year of treatment. The prognosis varies depending on the individual animal, concurrent problems, and the experience of the clinician with testing and interpreting ID reactions. Approximately 50% of atopic dogs are well controlled with allergen boosters without corticosteroids, 25% improve markedly but still require low-dose corticosteroids intermittently or continually, and 25% do not improve appreciably. A better clinical response to hyposensitization is reported in dogs with primary pollen reactions compared to those with nonpollen reactions. The most common causes of hyposensitization failure include persistent flea infestation, secondary bacterial infection, newly acquired inhalant allergy, and concurrent allergies (e.g., food contact).

The two types of treatment antigens currently available are the aqueous and alum-precipitated types. The major considerations for selecting these antigens are given in Table 4–4. Aqueous antigens are used in most dogs for hyposensitization because of their availability and cost.

Initial treatment protocols for aqueous antigens vary among clinicians. A widely accepted treatment protocol is given in Table 4–5. Most treatment protocols for alum-precipitated antigens are similar to the schedule given in Table 4–6.

The selection of antigens to include in the treatment should be based on the correlation of positive ID reactions, history of exposure to the specific test-positive antigens, and inability to avoid exposure. If there is poor correlation between the positive ID test and the history of exposure, the allergen is not used for hyposensitization. Likewise, if the allergen can be eliminated from the environment, it should be excluded from treatment.

The total number of allergens or the total PNU load that an allergic dog can tolerate is variable and subject to discussion among veterinary allergists. Some clinicians use a maximum of 10 different allergens, individual or grouped, as the upper limit. Many clinicians include all allergens deemed clinically important regardless of the total number. Most treatment protocols use groups of antigens, especially pollens and molds, similar to those used for testing (see Table 4–2). If a limited number of dogs are being hyposensitized in a practice, it will be cost effective to order an individual

TABLE 4–4. COMPARISON OF AQUEOUS AND ALUM-PRECIPITATED TREATMENT ALLERGENS

Criteria	Aqueous	Alum-precipitated
Cost of vaccine per unit	Low	High
Assortment of antigens	Many	Limited
Average number of injections in initial series*	15–20	6–9
Frequency of injections for initial series	Every 3–7 days	Every 7–21 days
Frequency of booster injections	1–4 wks	1–3 mo
Side effects	Increased pruritus if over tolerance	Increased pruritus if over tolerance; nodule at injection site
Stability of vaccine	Loses potency in weak dilutions	Stable for dating

*The total number of injections may vary depending on the time of year hyposensitization was started and the clinical response.

treatment set from the manufacturers. However there is usually a minimum of 4 weeks or longer before specially ordered treatment sets are received. If there is sufficient volume, stocking the individual or grouped antigens is cost effective. The stock concentrated antigens are subsequently diluted for both testing and treatment.

TABLE 4–5. HYPOSENSITIZATION SCHEDULE FOR AQUEOUS ANTIGENS

Day	Vial No. 1 (ml)	Vial No. 2 (ml)	Vial No. 3 (ml)
1	0.1		
4	0.2		
7	0.4		
10	0.8		
13	1.0		
16		0.1	
19		0.2	
22		0.4	
25		0.8	
28		1.0	
31			0.1
34			0.2
37			0.4
40			0.8
43			1.0
50			1.0
57			1.0

Boosters as required (Use vial No. 3: 1.0 ml)

Vial No. 1: 10 ml of 10:1 dilution of vial No. 2 (100–200 PNU*/ml)
Vial No. 2: 10 ml of 10:1 dilution of vial No. 3 (1000–2000 PNU*/ml)
Vial No. 3: 10 ml of allergen mixture, i.e., 1 ml of 10,000 to 20,000 PNU solution of each single or grouped allergen up to a maximum of 10; if there is less than 10 ml of allergen, the difference is made up with sterile saline or sterile diluting solution.
Boosters are given whenever the dog begins to show more pruritic signs. If there is a seasonal allergy, the injections may be maintained year round with 1.0 ml doses of vial No. 3 administered every 4 to 8 weeks during the nonallergic season. If the injections are discontinued for several months, start with vial No. 2 (0.4 ml) when recommencing hyposensitization.

*PNU—protein nitrogen units

The protocol for allergen boosters for each atopic dog is based on response to the initial hyposensitization and the anticipated pattern of occurrence of clinical signs. The general guideline is to give an injection whenever there is an increase in pruritus. There is often an advantage to giving periodic boosters during the nonallergy season to dogs with a seasonal allergic pattern. If a long interval exists between injections, the booster may have to be reinitiated at a less than maximum dose to prevent exacerbation of pruritus. The major indication that an excessive amount of antigen was administered is a marked increase in pruritus within 24 hours after the injection. This response must be differentiated from a milder, transient increase in pruritus a few hours after the injection. A written treatment schedule (Fig. 4–1) and an instruction sheet should accompany every treatment program with the following instructions:

TABLE 4–6. HYPOSENSITIZATION SCHEDULE FOR ALUM-PRECIPITATED ALLERGENS

Week	Amount of Single Antigen or Group* Used (PNU)†
1	100
2	200
3	400
5	800
8	1,500
12	2,000
16	3,000
20	6,000
24	10,000

Boosters as needed‡

*Mixture of related antigens such as mixed molds
†Protein nitrogen unit
‡Given when pruritus starts to increase

Date: _____

ID number: _____   Referral veterinarian: _____

Client: _____   Address: _____

Animal name: _____   _____

Client phone: _____   Veterinarian phone: _____

Instructions for aqueous vaccine:

1. Vaccine must be refrigerated.
2. All vaccine is given subcutaneously (under the skin).
3. There will be vaccine left in vials No. 1 and 2. Do not discard until booster program is established.
4. Use 1-ml syringes and 25-gauge, $^1/_2$-in. needles for injections.

Injection schedule:

Vial No. 1				*Vial No. 2*				*Vial No. 3*		
Day	Date	Volume (ml)		Day	Date	Volume (ml)		Day	Date	Volume (ml)
1	_____	0.1		16	_____	0.1		31	_____	0.1
4	_____	0.2		19	_____	0.2		34	_____	0.2
7	_____	0.4		22	_____	0.4		37	_____	0.4
10	_____	0.8		25	_____	0.8		40	_____	0.8
13	_____	1.0		28	_____	1.0		43	_____	1.0
								50	_____	1.0
								57	_____	1.0

Vaccine booster schedule:

Booster injections should be given whenever scratching starts to increase, usually at 1- to 4-week intervals. Please record date and volume of injection on back of this sheet to help to determine the best booster program for your animal.

_____Use Vial No. 3. 1.0 ml/booster

_____Use Vial No. _____ : _____ ml/booster

The vaccine contains the following allergens:

Fig. 4–1. Aqueous Hyposensitization Schedule

INJECTION PROCEDURES

Give all injections subcutaneously.

Use 1.0-ml syringes and 25-gauge, $^1/_2$-in. needles.

Rotate injection sites each time.

HANDLING OF VACCINE

Keep all vaccine refrigerated.

Do not discard the vaccine left in vials No. 1 and 2 until a booster vaccine program has been established.

SIDE EFFECTS OF VACCINE

At times, the pruritus will increase within 24 hours after the injection. If this happens, decrease the dosage to the level given prior to the last injection, or to the dosage used 3 days before the dosage that caused the reaction.

If there is another increase in scratching at the reduced dosage, or if there was no significant decrease in the pruritic reaction, the dog should be re-evaluated to rule out concurrent problems.

The dosage or frequency of the injections may need to be changed.

If necessary, corticosteroids may be administered (short-acting, low-dose) to bring the acute pruritus under control.

BOOSTER VACCINE SCHEDULE

Give a booster injection when the animal's scratching first begins to increase. This may be in 1 week or 1 month. Use 1.0 ml of vial No. 3 unless otherwise directed.

Oral, short-acting corticosteroids may be given concurrently at the minimum dosage necessary to control the pruritus (see Appendix 2:7).

FELINE ALLERGIC DERMATITIS ASSOCIATED WITH AIRBORNE ALLERGENS

There is increasing evidence based on history and diagnostic tests that airborne allergens may be a cause of feline allergic dermatitis.

Etiologic Factors. Allergic reactions have been associated with grass and weed pollens, molds, house dust, animal danders, feathers, and kapok.

Pathogenesis. The proposed mechanism of the allergic reaction is based on positive ID testing. A Type I hypersensitivity reaction involving IgE similar to that seen in canine atopic dermatitis is thought to be involved. However, feline IgE has not been identified.

History. Pruritus and excoriation are the primary signs. In many cats there is a seasonal occurrence. The onset of pruritus may coincide with the turning on of indoor heat in the late fall. Other cats manifest a seasonal pruritus during the warmer months or during specific pollen seasons, such as ragweed season.

Clinical Signs. The clinical signs are variable depending on the intensity of pruritus. In most cats there is excoriation, erythema, and alopecia (Plate 3:F). Ulceration and crusting may also be present. The distribution of lesions is often localized or regionalized.

Diagnosis. Screening diagnostic tests help to rule out other differential diagnoses. Skin scrapings and fungal cultures are negative. Diet testing does not result in clinical improvement. Cutaneous biopsy findings are consistent with allergic dermatitis with dermal edema and increased numbers of mast cells and eosinophils. The diagnosis of allergic dermatitis due to airborne allergens is based on positive ID skin testing as described for canine allergic dermatitis.

Management. Managing a cat with allergic reactions to airborne allergens is similar to managing an atopic dog. Short-acting corticosteroids at daily or alternate-day dosages are commonly used to mask pruritic signs and relieve acute inflammation. Residual corticosteroids given subcutaneously have been used with minimal side effects every 4 to 6 weeks. Topical steroids may be used although they may predispose to increased licking of the lesions. Megestrol acetate has been used extensively to control pruritic signs even though it is not approved for use in cats. Refer to the Allergic Disease Therapeutic Key (Appendix 2:7) for specific drugs and dosages. Hyposensitization using the treatment protocol outlined in Table 4–5 has been used satisfactorily in cats.

ALLERGIC CONTACT DERMATITIS

Contact dermatitis is usually classified into two etiologic categories: irritant and allergic. It is often difficult to differentiate between the two entities clinically although different pathomechanisms are involved. Allergic contact dermatitis is immune-mediated, while irritant contact dermatitis is caused by nonimmunologic factors of a physical or chemical nature. The following discussion focuses on allergic contact dermatitis. Irritant contact dermatitis is discussed in Chapter 12, although differentiating characteristics of the two diseases are presented here.

Etiologic Factors. Many agents have been incriminated as causes of allergic contact dermatitis. These are listed in Table 4–7. Generally, wool, nylon, and other synthetic fibers are thought to cause an irritant rather than an allergic contact reaction. The dyes and finishes used in the manufacture of carpeting, blankets, and furniture may be the primary factors associated with allergic problems. The number of topical medications reported to cause allergic contact dermatitis is limited; in such cases it often is not clear whether the active drug or the vehicle is causing the problem. The reaction may be irritant or allergic, or a combination of both.

Incidence. The incidence of contact dermatitis in the dog and cat is not well documented, partially because it is difficult to differentiate between allergic and irritant etiologic factors. It has been reported that 1 to 5% of pruritic dogs have allergic contact dermatitis; the condition is rare in cats.

Pathogenesis. A delayed hypersensitivity (Type IV) reaction is the basis of allergic contact dermatitis. Contact allergens are usually substances of relatively low molecular weight. They are incomplete antigens or haptens, which attach to a structural epidermal protein forming a com-

TABLE 4–7. ETIOLOGIC FACTORS OF ALLERGIC CONTACT DERMATITIS IN DOGS AND CATS

1. Chemicals and ions
   Chrome
   Nickel
   Iodine
   Formaldehyde
   Dyes
   Finishes (floor, fibers)
   Oleoresins
   Sterols
   Antioxidants

2. Materials and products
   Wool
   Cotton
   Synthetic fibers
   Rubber
   Plastic
   Cleaning materials
   Polishes
   Leather
   Topical drugs (neomycin, parasiticides, bases)
   Flea collars
   Fertilizer
   Fish scale

plete antigen. A subpopulation of lymphocytes develops, which has been sensitized to the antigen. Subsequent cutaneous contact with the antigen results in the migration of sensitized lymphocytes to the contact site, where chemical mediators (lymphokines) are released, resulting in pruritus and inflammation.

Three clinical stages in the pathogenesis of allergic contact dermatitis have been identified. The *refractory phase* is characterized by no detectable evidence of skin change or immunologic activity. In the *incubation phase,* the contactant or antigen does not produce clinical evidence of a contact reaction; however, immunologic activity can be detected by in vitro methods. The third phase is that of *hypersensitivity* with clinical evidence of changes in the skin.

It is important to remember that all contact reactions that are allergic in nature require repeated exposure to the allergen. Thus, it is common for a substance to be a primary irritant on the first exposure and to cause an allergic response on subsequent exposure.

There are several factors that may predispose an animal to contact sensitivity. These include trauma or irritation to the skin, which results in a break of continuity of the protective epidermal surface; continued or repeated wetting of the skin, which softens the keratin layer; use of wetting agents; the dose-time relationship of exposure to the contactant, the vulnerability of the skin, environmental factors such as temperature, and humidity, and prior exposure. The nutritional status of the animal with mineral and vitamin deficiencies may alter the responsiveness of the skin. The epidermal protein in ichthyotic and defatted skin is more susceptible to conjugation with an incomplete antigen. Endocrine imbalances and metabolic disturbances may cause variations in the integrity of the skin. Once an allergic reaction has been established, the severity of signs associated with subsequent exposure to the contactant may be enhanced by irritants, abrasives, and skin alkalinity.

History. The single most important factor in the evaluation of an animal with contact dermatitis is the history. The age of onset varies since the development of an allergic response requires repeated exposure to the contactant. An immediate reaction on first exposure may be seen with an irritant contactant. The total length of the refractory and sensitizing periods is in excess of 2 years in 70% of the cases of allergic contact dermatitis, and is rarely less than 6 months. No specific breed

susceptibility to allergic contact dermatitis has been verified.

Most dogs and cats with allergic contact dermatitis have nonseasonal pruritus, although some seasonal patterns may be identified with solid contactants such as fibers. The distribution of lesions is regionalized and occurs on the ventral and lateral aspects of the body in most animals. When liquid contactants such as shampoos have been used, the distribution may be generalized. Frequently, pet owners observe increased pruritus associated with a particular area of the environment such as one room, one rug, or a dog run. Improvement of clinical signs and pruritis is often reported in association with a change in the environment such as that produced by traveling or boarding. Usually only one animal in a multiple animal household is affected. A history that reveals a sudden onset of pruritus and associated clinical signs correlated with recent exposure to potentially irritant chemicals is suggestive of an irritant rather than an allergic reaction.

Clinical Manifestations. A physical examination reveals variable signs that depend on many factors, such as severity of pruritus, location of lesions, and degree of secondary skin change. Acute, allergic contact dermatitis is usually characterized by erythema and a moist edematous lesion (Plate 3:G). The most common primary morphologic lesions are erythematous papules or macules, often lacking bilateral symmetry. Occasionally wheals are observed. Dogs with chronic allergic contact dermatitis usually have secondary morphologic lesions including excessive scaling, hyperpigmentation (Plate 3:H), and occasionally lichenification accompanied by varying degrees of alopecia. Excoriation and crusts are observed in self-traumatized lesions. Lesions localized to the ventral and lateral aspects of the trunk are suggestive of a reaction to floor cleaners, bedding, grass resins, or other ground or floor contactants. Generalized distribution of lesions is suggestive of a reaction to shampoo or insecticide. If allergic reactions occur with specific medications, the area of involvement tends to be localized or regionalized to the areas of contact with the medication. In long-haired dogs and cats, the lesions may be localized to the least protected areas of the body.

Concurrent skin disorders are common in dogs with allergic contact dermatitis. Distribution of lesions may be generalized in these dogs, and a secondary superficial pyoderma is frequently present.

Diagnosis. Diagnosis of allergic contact dermatitis is based on history, clinical signs, and screening and definitive diagnostic tests. The routine screening diagnostic tests and some definitive tests do not identify allergic contact dermatitis, but they do help to rule out other primary etiologic factors. These tests include skin scraping, fungal culture, bacterial culture, biopsy, intradermal skin testing, and diet testing. Results of hematologic and biochemical testing are generally normal. Cutaneous biopsy is not a specific test for either irritant or allergic contact dermatitis although some microscopic changes are consistent with a delayed hypersensitivity reaction.

Isolation followed by provocative exposure is the definitive diagnostic test for allergic contact dermatitis. The time that the dog or cat must be isolated from the suspected contactant is variable; some acute clinical signs resolve within 4 to 7 days, while 14 days of isolation is required for other animals. During this time there should be a marked reduction of pruritus and acute inflammation. Once the animal is clinically normal or stabilized in a less reactive state for 24 to 48 hours, maximum exposure to the suspected contactant should be given. Signs of an allergic reaction should return within 48 to 72 hours of re-exposure if continuous contact is maintained. It is not unusual to see obvious exacerbation of signs within 24 hours. If more than one contactant is suspected, isolate the dog or cat from all contactants initially; then provocatively expose the animal to each one individually until all suspected contactants have been ruled out as the cause of the skin problem. If there is a reaction to one contactant, isolate the animal again until the clinical signs resolve; then provocatively expose the animal to the next suspected contactant.

Hospitalizing or boarding the dog or cat is often a satisfactory alternative to isolation at home. If an animal shows improvement in a hospital environment, maximum provocative exposure to some allergens can be achieved by placing remnants of the material in the cage with the animal.

Patch testing is a definitive diagnostic test for allergic contact dermatitis, although it is seldom needed or used. An open patch test using chemical extracts of vehicles may be used. The major problem is obtaining the extracts of vehicles of suspected contactants in a concentration that will produce an allergic reaction and be nonirritating. The reader is referred to lists of suggested concentrations and vehicles (Walton, 1977). Select an area of normal skin on the trunk and mark clearly with a felt-tip pen. Part the animal's hair and soak the skin with the test solution. Examine the test site daily for 5 days for evidence of irritation and local inflammatory change. If the tested substance requires sunlight for activation, then the hair at the test site should be clipped.

The closed patch test is not generally accepted as a practical diagnostic test for the dog or cat. It is reserved for situations in which treated fibers such as rugs are suspected, but isolation is impossible and open patch testing for the various possible chemicals is not practical. The technique involves the following: carefully clip an area on the lateral thorax; place a 2-in. square of material on the clipped area with the fiber side adjacent to the skin, and a gauze sponge of the same size beside the suspected allergen as a control; and secure the suspected contactant and gauze firmly to the clipped area of skin with elastic tape around the thorax. Every 24 hours cut the chest tape at the top edge of the samples, pull back the wrap sufficiently to observe for irritation at the contact site, and then carefully replace the material exactly on the original contact site. Then place another layer of tape around the chest. After 72 hours remove the patches and make a comparison of the control and test sites.

Management. Treatment alternatives for allergic contact dermatitis are limited. The best method is to avoid exposure to the contactant material or chemical. If complete avoidance is not possible, every effort should be made to minimize exposure, such as using a cover over the carpet to reduce direct contact. In many cases the life style of the dog or cat must change in order to reduce to a minimum the contact time with the primary allergen. When it is not possible to avoid the offending material or chemical, a low alternate-day maintenance dose of corticosteroids is usually required (see Appendix 2:7).

All concurrent problems must be treated at the same time to achieve maximum control of clinical signs.

Prognosis. The prognosis for most allergic contact dermatitis problems is guarded since continuous avoidance is usually difficult and many of the contactants are commonly encountered in the animal's environment. Also, many pet owners are reluctant to change the life style of the dog or cat to maximize avoidance of the primary allergen. The requirement for corticosteroids usually increases with the chronicity of the problem.

FOOD ALLERGY

Food allergy or food hypersensitivity is a clinical entity that may affect several target organs and manifest in a variety of clinical signs.

Etiologic Factors. Most basic food components have the potential to cause an allergic reaction; these include proteins (especially proteins of greater than 10,000 MW), lipoproteins, glycoproteins, lipopolysaccharides, and carbohydrates. The antigenicity of an allergen is often altered by pre-ingestion cooking or processing or by digestion, which either enhances or destroys its allergenic character. Artificial flavors, dyes, and preservatives may act as direct allergens or as haptens. Some specific foods reported to cause food allergies in dogs and cats include milk, wheat, raw and cooked beef, dog biscuits, eggs, chicken, cat food, rabbit food, pork, fish, horsemeat, mutton, and cod liver oil.

Incidence. Reportedly, from 1 to 30% of dogs and cats with pruritus have allergies to food.

Pathogenesis. All types of hypersensitivity reactions have been incriminated as causative factors, with types I and III the most common. Type III reactions are probably involved in the acute intestinal reactions that occur several hours after the ingestion of an allergen. If the time of onset in relation to the ingestion of the allergen is immediate (occurring within minutes), soluble, whole food molecules are incriminated. If there is a delay of one to several hours after the ingestion of an allergen before clinical signs occur, insoluble molecules that require digestion are suspected. These degradation products are most likely to be the allergens. Hypersensitivity reactions to foods must be differentiated from food intolerance that results from enzymatic deficiencies, reduced gastric hydrochloric acid, reduced bile secretions, and mechanical factors.

History. There are no breed or sex predilections. Most food allergies are observed in adult dogs and cats. Over 70% of all animals with food allergies may have had constant exposure to the specific antigen(s) for at least 2 years. There may be recent history of a dietary change, but this is rare. Nonseasonal pruritus is usually the primary sign. If the animal is fed a varied diet with intermittent exposure to the allergen, a seasonal or intermittent pattern of clinical signs may be observed.

Stress may lower the allergic threshold, and other concurrent allergies may predispose to exacerbation of clinical signs caused by food allergies. Occasional gastrointestinal signs may be a concurrent problem, but this occurs more often in the dog than the cat. Rarely, respiratory signs of sneezing and rhinitis are reported.

The clinical signs are often responsive to the administration of corticosteroids in both the dog and cat and to megestrol acetate in the cat.

Clinical Signs. *Canine.* A dry, thin, or lusterless hair coat may be observed. Urticaria and wheals may be present, and angioedema occasionally occurs in puppies. The most common, primary morphologic changes include papules and erythematous macules (Plate 3:I). There may be many secondary morphologic changes including hyperpigmentation, hyperkeratosis, crusts, scale, and frequently focal or generalized excoriation. Erythema and alopecia are variable, depending on the degree of pruritus. In chronic food allergies, a secondary seborrhea or pyoderma may be noted. The distribution of lesions is variable and indistinguishable from contact or atopic dermatitis.

Gastrointestinal signs may vary from mild flatulence to acute, profuse watery or hemorrhagic diarrhea. There is usually minimal general depression associated with the gastrointestinal signs, which may help to differentiate food allergy from other systemic diseases. In chronic food allergies vomiting may be observed. The feces are often intermittently or chronically soft.

Respiratory signs include sudden onset of rhinitis and sneezing without concurrent evidence of conjunctivitis. These signs usually appear within a few minutes of ingestion of the food allergen and resolve within 1 to 2 hours without treatment.

Feline. Several different clinical signs have been associated with feline food allergies. These include pruritic, ulcerative, or erosive dermatitis of the head (Plate 3:J), neck, and axillae; pruritus without lesions; a miliary eczema-like eruption; and pruritic, urticaria-angioedema. Focal ulcerative or plaque lesions on the abdomen have also been observed (Plate 3:K). Excoriations, crusts, and variable alopecia and erythema are frequently seen.

Diagnosis. The diagnosis of food allergy is based on the history, clinical signs, and screening and definitive diagnostic tests. The routine diagnostic tests do not identify a food allergy, but they do rule out other primary etiologic factors. These include skin scraping, fungus and bacterial cultures, biopsy, isolation and provocative exposure, and ID skin testing. Results of hematologic and biochemical testing are generally within normal limits. Cutaneous biopsy is not specific for food allergy, but may be consistent with the diagnosis of allergic dermatitis. ID skin testing for food allergens is generally considered unreliable and not recommended in dogs and cats.

Diet Testing (Test Meal Investigation.) The basis of diet testing is to avoid ingestion of the allergen. Since many components of the normal diet may be the cause, it is generally recommended to limit the test diet to foods to which the dog or cat has not been previously exposed. In some instances this is not possible due to a number of reasons, such as lack of knowledge of basic components of the normal diet, expense of feeding an elimination diet, and unwillingness of the owner to subject the dog or cat to a restricted diet.

Diet testing may be started by withholding all food for 3 days and then administering a saline cathartic prior to starting a test meal. Most diet testing for dogs is initiated by feeding lamb or mutton and rice, proportioned $^1/_3$:$^2/_3$ for 14 to 21 days. Other foods that have been recommended as a substitute for lamb, if there has been no previous exposure, include cottage cheese, chicken, and hamburger. Most commercial diets, however, contain beef and poultry by-products as well as milk proteins.

Diet testing in cats is usually achieved by feeding cooked chicken or lamb with rice, proportioned $^1/_2$:$^1/_2$. The client may be given the option of purchasing lamb or mutton from the store and preparing the diet, or using a commercial prescription diet (D/D, Riviana Foods). There will be a marked improvement within 7 to 14 days characterized by decreased pruritus and inflammation if a food allergy is the primary problem.

Good client education and communication is an integral part of a successful diet testing program, since strict compliance to the nonallergenic diet is essential. All other foods, snacks, and treats must not be fed during the trial. Bottled spring water is recommended by some veterinary allergists to eliminate algae.

At the end of the test period, individual components of the normal diet may be provocatively tested (i.e., beef, chicken, vegetables). If there are multiple components to the normal diet, try to provoke an exacerbation of clinical signs by feeding only one new pure food component every 7 to 14 days. If there is no exacerbation of clinical signs, add one more component for an additional 1 to 2 weeks, repeating the process until each component of the normal diet, including table foods, supplements, and treats have been ruled in or ruled out as the cause of the clinical signs. Limit the meat portion to approximately one-third of the total food intake. If the dog or cat reacts to one of the components, with exacerbation of clinical signs, revert back to the previous diet that did not provoke a reaction. When the clinical signs subside, add a different component. If all of the basic ingredients of the normal diet have been added with no exacerbation of clinical signs, try the commercial diet again. If a reaction is provoked, preservatives or degradation products associated with processing are most likely involved. If one of the components of the diet, other than the commercial diet, is strongly suspected, the regular commercial diet may be added first. If there is no exacerbation of clinical signs after 1 week, add the other individual foods, snacks, or chewables, one at a time.

Management. The only satisfactory method of treating a food allergy is complete and permanent removal of all allergenic foods and substances causing the reaction. If this is not possible, glucocorticoids may be administered, preferably on an alternate-day basis, to control the pruritus and self-trauma. In cats, megestrol acetate has also been used (see Appendix 2:7). Concomitant allergies and other problems should also be treated.

Prognosis. The prognosis is generally good if the allergen(s) is identified and avoided. However, it must be remembered that the dog or cat may develop allergies to other food components at a later time.

FLEABITE ALLERGIC DERMATITIS

Fleabite allergic dermatitis is an immune-mediated reaction to the saliva of the flea. The condition is also known as flea allergy dermatitis (FAD) and fleabite hypersensitivity.

Etiologic Factor. The common dog and cat fleas, Ctenocephalides canis and C. felis, are the causative parasites.

Incidence. The incidence of fleabite allergic dermatitis is geographically related. It is a major, clinical dermatologic problem in areas with moderate temperatures and moderate to high humidity and is uncommon in altitudes greater than 5000 feet with low humidity. In many areas of the United States, fleabite allergic dermatitis is the most commonly recognized canine and feline allergic disease.

Pathogenesis. There are four basic reactions of a host to the flea: histaminic, enzymatic, hypersensitivity, and refractory. The first of these reactions is seen in all animals, but a sustained reaction occurs only in those that are immunologically competent and hypersensitive. Histamine or histamine-like compounds in the flea saliva are the initial mediators of this reaction. The enzymatic reaction is also mediated by the secretions of the parasite; the enzymes help to dissolve tissue and to provide the parasite with an avenue to its predilection site. When enzymes in the saliva are injected into the host tissues, they become antigenic as well as cytolytic. As a result of the absorption of the antigen at the site of infestation, animals may become sensitized, with the hypersensitivity becoming apparent on subsequent exposure. In some dogs, a state of immune tolerance is observed following a state of hypersensitivity, although this does not happen frequently.

Experimentally C. felis infestation in guinea pigs elicited a five-stage sequence of events in the skin of the host. Stage one is the induction of hypersensitivity with no observable skin reaction from days 1 to 4. Stage two is delayed hypersensitivity reaction from days 5 to 9. The third stage is immediate hypersensitivity followed by delayed reaction from days 10 to 60. Stage four is characterized only by the immediate hypersensitivity lasting from days 61 to 91. Stage five is a period of no skin reactivity after 90 days. Following the daily exposure of previously unexposed guinea pigs to fleabites, reactions were not observed until the fifth day, at which time the previously exposed but nonreactive bite sites reacted. This same phenomenon appears to occur in dogs, with the exception that few dogs reach stage five, or desensitization.

History. Pruritus is nearly always the primary clinical sign. There is no breed, sex, or haircoat-type predisposition. The majority of dogs with fleabite allergic dermatitis that live in an area endemic for fleas develop clinical signs between 1 and 4 years of age. In areas with seasonal flea infestations, the age of onset of hypersensitivity reactions is variable, as it is partially dependent on the indoor flea population. There is more variability in age of onset in cats with fleabite allergic dermatitis.

Flea infestations are usually observed by the owners, preceding or concurrent with an increase of pruritus. In some cases, the owner has not observed fleas nor have any been seen on the dog or cat on previous examination. Fleabite allergic dermatitis commonly occurs simultaneously with other allergic disease, especially atopic dermatitis in dogs. The clinical signs attributable to the fleabite may be severe, even though only a small number of fleas or only flea excrement are observed. Frequently only one dog or cat in a multiple animal household manifests signs of fleabite allergic dermatitis.

Clinical Findings. *Canine.* The lesions are most commonly distributed over the dorsal caudal back, tail, and perineum. They are found frequently on the flanks and the caudal ventral area

of the abdomen, and less commonly in the axillae and on the cranial trunk. A few dogs manifest a generalized distribution, most commonly associated with atopic dermatitis. Fleas and/or flea excrement are usually seen.

The primary morphologic lesions most frequently observed are erythematous papules on the ventral abdomen and occasionally in the axillae. Diffuse erythema of the dorsal cranial tail region (Plate 3:L) is commonly accompanied by secondary morphologic signs including scaling, excoriation, hyperpigmentation, hyperkeratosis, and occasionally lichenification (Plate 3:M). Alopecia is variable, from mild to marked, although the distribution may be localized or involve the entire posterior half of the trunk and perineum. Superficial folliculitis is associated with approximately 10% of fleabite allergic dogs.

Feline. The most common signs are those of miliary dermatitis with papules and crusts (Plate 3:N). Fleas and flea excrement are usually present. Other signs associated with the pruritus include excoriation, ulcers, and variable alopecia and erythema. The distribution is predominantly on the dorsal caudal trunk, dorsal neck, perineum, and ventral abdomen. Occasionally a generalized distribution is observed.

Diagnosis. History or observation of flea infestation correlated with a distribution of lesions regionalized to the dorsal caudal back, perineum, and caudal ventral abdomen and accompanied by intense pruritus, is suggestive of canine fleabite allergic dermatitis. Lesions on the dorsal neck and back are frequently observed in cats.

Screening diagnostic tests are mainly used to rule out other causes of the clinical signs. Skin scrapings are negative for mites. A flea egg or larvae may occasionally be seen in the scraping. Skin biopsy is not specific for fleabite allergic dermatitis, although it is consistent with allergic dermatitis; many tissue eosinophils are seen on microscopic examination of the biopsy specimen.

The reliability of ID skin testing as a definitive diagnostic test for fleabite allergic dermatitis in the dog is controversial; it is seldom used in the cat. Both glycerinated and nonglycerinated whole flea extracts (antigens) are commercially available for testing, although the glycerinated products are not recommended because of irritation and consistent false-positive reactions. The antigenic strength of flea antigens varies among manufacturers. Many flea antigens must be diluted to 1:1000 w/v or more to avoid false-positive reactions caused by irritation or excessive concentrations. The procedure is the same as for other antigens (see pp. 48–49); 0.02 to 0.05 ml of diluted flea antigen injected intradermally. The immediate reaction is read at 15 to 20 minutes postinjection, observing the characteristics of the wheal reaction compared to the positive histamine and negative buffered saline controls. The site should also be observed at 24 and 48 hours for a delayed hypersensitivity reaction characterized by a small area of erythema with minimal swelling at the site of the injection.

A high percentage of positive reactions to ID flea antigen has been observed in flea endemic areas, thus raising some question as to the value of the test for diagnostic purposes. If there is a consistent pattern of positive reactions in most dogs, the antigen should be further diluted. It is often advantageous to use at least 2 dilutions, 1:1000 w/v and 1:4000 w/v, on the same dog. The 2 dilutions are generally part of a larger battery of ID injections used to identify atopic dogs.

The most widely used diagnostic test for fleabite allergic dermatitis is a therapeutic trial with parasiticides. A complete flea control program must be initiated and maintained including fumigation of the animals's indoor environment, and continuous flea control on all animals in the household (Parasitic Disease Therapeutic Key, Appendix 2:8). A 100% clinical response to the flea control program is considered diagnostic for fleabite allergic dermatitis. If the response is less than complete, other concurrent problems must be considered.

Management. An effective control program for fleabite allergic dermatitis in the dog and cat must include three objectives: to break the flea life cycle in the environment, minimize infestations of all animals in the environment, and control the allergic reaction to the fleabite. Control of fleas in the environment may necessitate fumigation, thorough vacuuming of carpets, removal of debris and old bedding, disinfection of hard surfaces, and spraying of some kennels and yards (see Appendix 2:8). To minimize infestation, the prophylactic treatment of all animals on a continuous basis is required. The use of powder and spray 2 to 3 times per week is usually effective on small, short-haired dogs and most cats. Flea collars or medallions may be used on cats and small dogs; powder may need to be used concurrently. An insecticidal dip every 1 to 2 weeks is often a satisfactory method of continuous flea control for medium to large dogs and for long-haired dogs. A few insecticidal dips are approved for cats; these are usually effective although often more difficult to use than powders.

Systemic insecticides are not effective in the fleabite allergic animal since they do not prevent fleabites and deposition of the antigen in the tissue.

There may be problems with any of these methods of flea control. Powders and sprays are often difficult to work through hair to the skin; sprays and dips may evaporate rapidly in areas of high environmental temperatures, resulting in a shortened residual effect. There is potential for systemic side effects from the storage of insecticides in the body if absorbed through the skin following application of sprays and dips, although this is seldom a problem. Local dermatitis may be associated with flea collars and medallions; these are generally ineffective on larger dogs.

One of the major problems is the development of resistance to the common insecticides, especially the carbamates, among the endemic flea population. It is often necessary to change the insecticide periodically, regardless of which method of flea control is used.

The control of the allergic reaction to the fleabite is most commonly achieved by using oral or injectable corticosteroids. Oral corticosteroids may be given for 1 to 2 weeks while good flea control is initiated (see Appendix 2:8). If there is good flea control and no concurrent problems, corticosteroids are usually not required for a prolonged time. Therefore, the injectable residual steroids are usually not indicated.

The use of flea antigen for hyposensitization is controversial. Most studies have not shown a significant clinical improvement over flea control alone. However, some dogs and cats with fleabite allergic dermatitis do respond well to the antigen. Flea hyposensitization is indicated in an animal that manifests fleabite allergic dermatitis historically and clinically, other causes of clinical signs have been ruled out, and good flea control in the environment and on the animal(s) has not resulted in a good clinical response. Duration of effect of flea antigen is relatively short, often requiring booster injections every 1 to 3 months. Flea antigen may be given intradermally, subcutaneously, or both. Recommendations of the manufacturer for dosage and treatment schedules should be followed.

Prognosis. If a diligent control program is maintained, the prognosis is good for many animals. However, in flea endemic areas, 100% flea control is often impossible. In these dogs and cats the prognosis for good control of fleabite allergic dermatitis is fair to guarded.

DRUG ERUPTION

A drug eruption is any dermatologic manifestation that results from administering a drug orally, parenterally, topically, or as an inhalant.

Etiologic Factors. Only a limited number of pharmacologic agents have been reported to cause drug eruption in dogs and cats. Those reported for dogs include acepromazine, povidone-iodine, Betadine (Purdue-Frederick), selenium sulfide, propylene glycol, and a variety of insecticidal agents.

Drug eruption in cats has been reported following the administration of sulfisoxazole, ampicillin, hetacillin, penicillin, tetracycline, neomycin, miconazole nitrate, panleukopenia vaccine, otic preparations, and following the use of dichlorvos collars.

Incidence. The reported incidence of drug eruption in animals is low, although the problem is thought to be more common than recognized.

Pathogenesis. Drug eruption may not be immune-mediated, manifesting as an irritant contact reaction. All four types of hypersensitivity reactions may be associated with immune-mediated drug eruption. The low molecular weight drugs act as haptens, combining with plasma or epidermal proteins. There is often a lag period of 5 to 21 days before humoral antibodies are formed or tissue lymphocytes become sensitized. Cross-reactions between drugs may occur.

History. Careful questioning of owners will reveal that the animal is on some medication, either topical or systemic, or that medication has recently been discontinued. In immune-mediated drug eruption, a history of repeated exposure or prolonged therapy is obtained. Pruritus is variable from none to severe. There may be a history of poor response to symptomatic treatment if the animal is still on the medication.

Clinical Signs. Lesions in the dog are variable from mild scales, erythema, and alopecia to edema, excoriation, and ulceration. The distribution of a drug eruption is often on the head and dorsal spine if a systemic reaction has occurred. A local reaction occurs when there is an allergic reaction to a topical drug. The hair epilates easily. Reported clinical signs associated with drug eruption in the cat include miliary eczema, urticarial-angioedema, contact dermatitis, and variable degrees of alopecia.

Diagnosis. The diagnosis of a drug eruption is based on the history of exposure to a drug, clinical signs, and negative findings on screening diagnostic tests which would identify other primary causes. A drug eruption is suspected when there is marked improvement of clinical signs within 7 to 14 days after discontinuing the drug and when there is no recurrence of clinical signs. Occasionally, clinical signs persist for several weeks. Provocative exposure to the suspected drug is not recommended to verify the probable cause of clinical signs. In most instances, provocative testing is done inadvertently when a specific medication is repeated.

Management. Discontinuing the administration of a suspected drug is the primary treatment. Clinical signs are treated symptomatically. If there is pruritus, corticosteroids are given using a step-down dosage schedule (Allergic Disease Therapeutic Key, Appendix 2:7). Drugs of similar chemical structure to the suspected ones should be avoided, since cross-reactivity may occur.

Prognosis. Most skin lesions resulting from a drug eruption respond well to withdrawal of the drug and symptomatic treatment. However, there is high probability that the reaction will recur if the animal is re-exposed. This presents a problem for dogs and cats reacting to a medication indicated for a chronic condition.

SELECTED READINGS

August, J.R.: The reaction of canine skin to the intradermal injection of allergenic extracts. J. Am. Anim. Hosp. Assoc. 18:157, 1982.
———: The intradermal test as a diagnostic aid for canine atopic disease. J. Am. Anim. Hosp. Assoc. 18:164, 1982.
Austin, V.H.: Common skin problems in cats. Mod. Vet. Pract. 56:541, 1975.
———: The skin. In Feline Medicine and Surgery. 2nd Ed. Edited by E.J. Catcott. Santa Barbara, CA. American Veterinary Publications, 1975.
Baker, E.: Food allergy in the cat. Feline Pract. 5:18, 1975.
———: Food allergy. Vet. Clin. North Am. 4:79, 1974.
Baker, K.P.: Some aspects of feline dermatoses. Vet. Rec. 86:62, 1970.
Chamberlain, K.W. (ed.): Symposium on allergy in small animal practice. Vet. Clin. North Am. 4:1974.
Doering, G.G.: Feline dermatology. Vet. Clin. North Am. 6:463, 1976.
Gordon, B.J.: Essentials of Immunology. 2nd Ed. Philadelphia, F.A. Davis, 1974.
Halliwell, R.E.W.: Hyposensitization in the treatment of flea-bite hypersensitivity: Results of a double-blind study. J. Am. Anim. Hosp. Assoc. 17:249, 1981.
———: Flea bite dermatitis. Compend. Cont. Ed. Pract. Vet. 1:367, 1979.
———: Hyposensitization in the treatment of atopic disease. In Current Veterinary Therapy VI: Small Animal Practice. Edited by R.W. Kirk. Philadelphia, W.B. Saunders, 1977.
———: The immunology of allergic skin disease. J. Small Anim. Pract. 12:431, 1971.
Lorenz, M.D.: Allergic skin disease. In Current Veterinary Therapy V: Small Animal Practice. Edited by R.W. Kirk. Philadelphia, W.B. Saunders, 1974.
Nesbitt, G.H.: Contact dermatitis. In Current Views in Veterinary Allergy and Dermatology. Gainesville, FL, Division of Continuing Education, University of Florida, 1979.

———: Canine allergic inhalant dermatitis: A review of 230 cases. J. Am. Vet. Med. Assoc. *172*:55, 1978.

———: Contact dermatitis in the dog: A review of 35 cases. J. Am. Anim. Hosp. Assoc. *13*:155, 1977.

Nesbitt, G.H., and Schmitz, J.A.: Fleabite allergic dermatitis: A review and survey of 330 cases. J. Am. Vet. Med. Assoc. *173*:282, 1980.

Reedy, L.M.: Canine atopy. Compend. Cont. Ed. Pract. Vet. *1*:550, 1979.

———: Results of allergy testing and hyposensitization in selected feline skin diseases. J. Am. Anim. Hosp. Assoc., *18*:618, 1982.

Schultz, K.T.: Intradermal skin testing for canine atopy. Compend. Cont. Ed. Pract. Vet. *1*:160, 1980.

Scott, D.W.: Observations on canine atopy. J. Am. Anim. Hosp. Assoc. *17*:91, 1981.

———: Immunologic disorders. J. Am. Anim. Hosp. Assoc. *16*:377, 1980.

———: Immunologic skin disorders in the dog and cat. Vet., Clin. North Am. *8*:641, 1978.

———: Drug eruption in a cat due to a mitecide. Feline Pract. *7*:47, 1977.

———: Feline Dermatology. Proceedings of 43rd Annual Meeting of the American Animal Hospital Association, 1976.

Van Winkle, K.A.: An evaluation of flea antigens used in intradermal skin testing for flea allergy in the canine. J. Am. Anim. Hosp. Assoc. *17*:343, 1981.

Walton, G.S.: Allergic contact dermatitis in the dog and cat. Proceedings Kal Kan Symposium for the Treatment of Dog and Cat Diseases. Columbus, Ohio, 1980, p. 30.

———: Allergic contact dermatitis. *In* Current Veterinary Therapy VI: Small Animal Practice. Edited by R.W. Kirk. Philadelphia W.B. Saunders, 1977.

———: Skin responses in the dog and cat to ingested allergens. Observations on one hundred continual cases. Vet. Rec. *81*:709, 1966.

Weiss, N.S., and Rubin, J.M.: Practical Points in Allergy. Garden City, NY, Medical Examination Publishing, 1980.

5

Parasitic Diseases

The Parasitic Diagnostic Key (Appendix 1:3) lists the most pertinent historical and clinical findings and diagnostic tests used to help differentiate the common causes of canine and feline parasitic diseases.

FLEA DERMATITIS

Flea dermatitis is a reaction of the skin to the physical presence of the flea or to mechanical trauma of the fleabite, which is not immune mediated.

Etiologic Factors. The common dog and cat fleas, Ctenocephalides canis and C. felis, are the primary parasites. Other fleas reported to infest both dogs and cats include Pulex irritans (human flea) and Echidnophaga gallinacea (chicken stick-tight flea). Ceratophyllus spp. (bird and hedgehog flea) and Leptosylla segnis (rat flea) infest cats.

Incidence. Flea dermatitis is geographically dependent and is a major clinical dermatologic problem in areas with moderate temperatures, moderate to high humidity, and in areas where elevations are less than 5000 feet. In regions with a warm climate year-round, the flea problems are often nonseasonal, whereas in regions with seasonal temperature and humidity extremes, flea infestation generally occurs only during the warmer months. However, a nonseasonal incidence of flea dermatitis will be observed in any climate if there is indoor infestation.

Pathogenesis. The flea saliva that is deposited in the skin contains histamine or histamine-like compounds. These chemicals initiate an inflammatory reaction at the bite site, which is usually transient in duration. An enzyme reaction in the skin, which is mediated by the secretions of the flea, follows. These enzymes dissolve parts of tissues and provide the flea access to the predilection site. A concurrent fleabite allergic dermatitis results if the dog or cat develops a hypersensitivity reaction to the enzymes which act as antigens (see Chap. 4).

Flea Life Cycle. Knowledge of the flea life cycle is important for client education as well as for planning a protocol of treatment and control. The flea life cycle, including the egg, larva, pupa, and adult may be completed within 3 weeks, or it may persist for 2 years. The eggs are usually laid in dust, building cracks, or on damp ground. If they are laid on the host, they soon drop off. Approximately 3 to 18 eggs are laid at one time, with several hundred laid over a life span of 6 to 12 months. The incubation period varies greatly. With optimal conditions of 25°C and 80% relative humidity, the larvae may hatch in 2 to 4 days. The larvae ingest organic material (i.e., fecal pellets) as well as the egg of the tapeworm, Dipylidium caninum, and hide from light in places such as floor crevices and under carpets. They pass through 3 stages that can last from 9 to 200 days. A cocoon is spun during the third stage. The pupal stage can persist from 10 days to 1 year with low ambient temperature prolonging this stage. The adult flea must eventually feed on the host, but can usually survive 1 to 2 months separated from the host in the immediate environment. High humidity may prolong the survival time, while desiccation from low humidity may cause death of the adult in a few days.

History. There is no age, sex, or breed predilection for flea dermatitis. Pruritus and clinical signs vary from none to severe. The dog owner usually reports signs of biting over the dorsal caudal back and perineum with some alopecia and variable excoriation. Pruritus in the cat is most common over the lumbar and dorsal neck areas. Fleas or flea excrement are often observed by the owner. Bathing or flea control (powders, sprays) usually gives temporary relief. There is frequently a history of inadequate flea control. Concurrent tapeworm infestation is often reported.

Clinical Signs. The lesions of canine flea dermatitis are commonly distributed on the dorsal and caudal back, tail, and perineum. Lesions also frequently occur on the flanks and caudal ventral abdomen. In the cat, the lumbosacral and dorsal neck areas are most often associated with clinical signs. Flea excrement (dried blood), characterized by small, dark specks that look like dirt attached to the hair (Plate 4:A) is often observed with (Plate 4:B) or without fleas. The specks streak out with a reddish color when placed on damp white paper.

The primary morphologic lesions most frequently observed in dogs are erythematous papules on the ventral abdomen (Plate 4:C) and occasionally in the axillae. Diffuse erythema, scaling, hyperpigmentation, and hyperkeratosis are commonly seen on the caudal back, and perineal and tailhead regions (Plate 4:D,E). Alopecia varies from none to marked. The distribution may be only localized or may be generalized. Severe flea dermatitis, accompanied by marked pruritus and excoriation, may have a generalized distribution. In the dog, superficial pyoderma may be observed concurrently, especially on the ventral abdomen.

In the cat a miliary eczema-like syndrome, characterized by small adherent crusts on the dorsum (Plate 4:F), is common. Other lesions include focal excoriation and variable alopecia and inflammation (Plate 4:G).

Diagnosis. The history or observation of flea infestation (fleas or excrement) is the most important basis for a diagnosis of flea dermatitis. The distribution of clinical signs regionalized to the dorsum, perineum, and caudal ventral abdomen are suggestive, especially if other possible causes

for the clinical signs have been ruled out by skin scrapings, fungal cultures, diet testing, and ID skin testing. The most definitive diagnostic test for flea dermatitis is a therapeutic trial with topical parasiticides for all animals, and the use of parasiticides in the environment (Parasitic Disease Therapeutic Key, Appendix 2:8). A 100% clinical response to the flea control program is considered diagnostic for flea dermatitis. If the response is less than complete, concurrent problems must be considered.

Management. The basic control program for flea dermatitis must include two objectives: breaking the flea life cycle in the environment, and minimizing infestation of all animals in the environment.

The control of fleas in the indoor environment or closed kennel can be accomplished by fumigation by a commercial exterminator, or with insect fogger, thoroughly vacuuming the carpets and immediately removing the vacuum cleaner bag from the premises, removing all debris and old bedding, and disinfecting hard surfaces using lindane, delnav, or bioresmethrin. It is often necessary to repeat these procedures several times at intervals of 2 to 4 weeks. Methoprene is a new insect growth regulator that prevents the fourth instar larva from completing metamorphosis into adults. The residual action of foggers containing methoprene is reported to be 75 days. Methoprene should be used in conjunction with a fast-acting insecticide that kills the adults. Vacuuming should be done several times a week. Eliminating fleas in the outdoor environment is difficult. Periodic spraying of large areas of ground with lindane, chlordane, or malathion may be temporarily helpful. If possible, animals should be kept away from outdoor areas favorable for flea propagation, such as grass and damp, overgrown areas. All debris and old bedding should be removed from areas that are frequented by the animals.

Minimizing the flea infestation on the animals involves continuous flea control on all animals in the environment (see Appendix 2:8). Treatment should include the use of flea powders or sprays twice weekly, flea collars or medallions, insecticidal dips repeated every 7 to 14 days, and systemic insecticides. No single universal control measure can be recommended. In general, flea sprays are considered the least effective due to the difficulty of penetrating the hair. Flea powders on short-haired dogs and most cats may be effective and safe if worked well into the hair, but are often difficult to apply adequately to long-haired animals. Flea collars and medallions are not considered satisfactory in areas of moderate to heavy flea infestation or on the medium to large, long-haired dog. On small short-haired dogs and cats with minimal flea exposure, a flea collar is often satisfactory. Flea powder may be used concurrently with a collar to achieve better flea control in most animals without causing side effects. There are few reported problems of flea collar dermatitis with the advent of the new powder-impregnated collars. However, the owner should always be cautioned to look for signs of irritation for the first 2 weeks after a new collar is used. Insecticidal dips are often the most satisfactory method of continuous flea control on the medium to large or long-haired dog. Some insecticidal dips are approved for cats and are effective, but may be difficult to apply. Most dips have a residual, insecticidal effect for 7 to 14 days, but in hot climates, evaporation may decrease the effective time. Dips are impractical for dogs that are frequently wet. When a dip is recommended to an owner, the veterinarian must give explicit instructions as to its use. The client may confuse the dip with an insecticidal shampoo and rinse it off. Frequently, the client is advised to bathe the dog or cat first and then apply the dip while the animal is still damp, letting it air-dry. Most insecticidal shampoos do not have a residual effect, therefore, they should not be used for a continuous flea control program. One insecticidal shampoo containing resmethrin, which can be used on both dogs and cats, is reported to have a 5- to 7- day residual effect (see Appendix 2:8).

A systemic parasiticide, proban cythioate, may be used for dogs. It is reported to be effective if given as directed twice weekly. Generally, proban cythioate is practical on small dogs with minimal flea exposure. It should not be used if the dog is manifesting signs of fleabite allergic dermatitis, since the flea is not killed until it penetrates the skin and contacts the agent in the blood. It can be used concurrently with topical parasiticides that are not anticholinesterase inhibitors, such as resmethrins.

A potential problem of insecticides administered orally, or sprays and dips applied topically, is systemic absorption and storage of the insecticide in the body, which can lead to chronic toxicity, although this is seldom reported.

Development of resistance to insecticides is a major problem in endemic flea areas, with the most resistance observed to the carbamates. If there is a poor response to your routine control program, change types of insecticides, methods of application, or both.

All secondary or concurrent problems should be treated at the same time as the primary flea infestation. Often, flea control is sufficient to control pruritus. However, it is common to administer corticosteroids for 5 to 10 days while the flea control program is implemented to prevent continued self-trauma and to reduce inflammation. Antibiotics for a minimum of 10 to 14 days are also indicated when secondary superficial pyoderma is present.

SARCOPTIC MANGE

Sarcoptic mange or canine scabies is a commonly encountered parasitic disease of the dog caused by Sarcoptes scabiei var. canis. It transiently infests man causing pruritic, papular dermatitis.

Pathogenesis. The transmission of sarcoptic mites may be by direct or indirect contact with fomites or objects such as grooming instruments. The mites are more active and more likely to infect other animals at higher ambient temperatures. Other factors that favor mite infestation include a long, dirty haircoat and malnutrition. There is often a higher recovery from mite infestation in younger dogs than in older ones. It is postulated that the hypersensitivity reaction keeps the mite population lower, and at the same time is responsible for the generalized lesions in the adult dog.

The incubation period is variable, usually 4 to 6 weeks. If the infestation is heavy and the animal is in poor condition, visible lesions may appear within 2 weeks. Pruritus associated with infestation may be caused by a combination of factors including mechanical irritation of the mite, toxic materials produced by the mite, and the secretion of allergenic substances to which the host becomes sensitized.

Life Cycle. The adult sarcoptic mite lives for 3 to 4 weeks in the skin. Copulation occurs in the skin and 3 to 4 eggs are laid per day in the tunnels in the stratum corneum. The eggs hatch within 3 to 10 days into six-legged mobile larvae. Eight-legged nymphs represent the third stage of the life cycle before becoming adult mites. The entire life cycle, which takes place on the host, is 17 to 21 days with a longer survival time in a more humid environment.

History. Sarcoptic mange is characterized by marked pruritus and localized or generalized excoriation. There is no breed or sex predisposition. The distribution of lesions is often around the elbows and on the pinna margins. Infestation may occur at any age, although the highest incidence is in the young dog. There is often a drug history of poor response to anti-inflammatory dosage (0.5 to 1 mg/kg/day) of short-acting corticosteroids. There may be a history of recent exposure to other pruritic dogs, boarding, or recent acquisition from a pet store. Since human contagion is common, the owner may report a pruritic, papular skin eruption which occurred at the same time as the dog's clinical signs.

Clinical Signs.   Initially, the distribution of lesions is usually on the thin-haired areas of the dog, including ear margins and elbows (Plate 4:*I,J*). A predominantly ventral distribution or an entire trunkal distribution of lesions may be observed. Primary lesions include erythematous papules or pustules. The most common secondary and miscellanous lesions are crusts (Plate 4:*K*), excoriation, erythema, and alopecia (Plate 4:*L*). Secondary superficial bacterial infection and secondary seborrheic dermatitis are common. Although the clinical signs are suggestive, a definitive diagnosis of sarcoptic mange requires additional screening or definitive diagnostic tests.

Diagnosis.   A history of an intense pruritus, unresponsive to low-dose corticosteroids, is suggestive as are crusts and excoriations on the ear margins and elbows. Concurrent pruritic papular dermatitis in members of the family is also supportive. A relatively high incidence of peripheral eosinophilia is reported. Mites are occasionally observed during routine fecal examination.

Skin scrapings are the most widely used screening and definitive diagnostic tests, and a positive scraping for adults (Fig. 5–1), nymphs, larvae, or eggs (Fig. 5–2) is diagnostic. Fecal material is also suggestive (Fig. 5–2). Multiple negative scrapings, however, do not rule out sarcoptic mange. Two

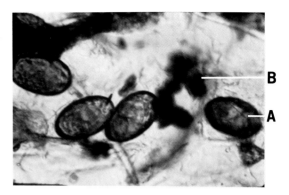

Fig. 5–2.   Sarcoptic mite eggs *(A)* and feces *(B)* in skin scraping (low power).

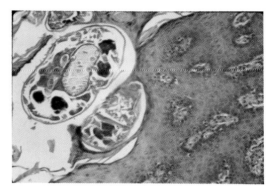

Fig. 5–3.   Sarcoptic mange: Microscopic section of canine footpad with cross sections of sarcoptic mites in the stratum corneum (low power). (Courtesy of S. Gilbertson.)

other methods described for identifying mites are the plastic box method and the centrifuge flotation method. The plastic box method involves placing a crust in a plastic box or petri dish and allowing it to set at room temperature for 12 hours. Close examination, by using a 4 × magnifying glass, may reveal mites on the floor of the dish. In the centrifuge flotation method, a large amount of material from scrapings is placed in a small tube or breaker. Then, 10% KOH is added, and the mixture is stirred and heated gently. This mixture is then added to a saturated sugar solution and centrifuged. A drop of the surface solution is examined for mites and eggs. The plastic box and centrifuge flotation methods should be reserved for those cases in which skin scrapings are negative. Occasionally, cross sections of mites will be observed in cutaneous biopsies (Fig. 5–3).

Treatment.   The environment should be thoroughly cleaned. The infected animal(s) should be isolated. Before specific treatment is started, long-haired dogs should be clipped. After the eyes are protected with a bland ophthalmic ointment, the

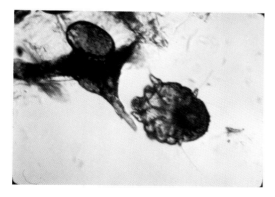

Fig. 5–1.   Sarcoptic mite (adult) and egg in skin scraping (low power).

dogs are bathed with an antiseborrheic shampoo to help remove the surface scale and crusts. While the dog is still wet, a miticide dip is applied, being careful to saturate all of the surface of the body, including the ear pinnae and face.

Amitraz (Miteban, Upjohn) is reported to be highly effective and safe. One or 2 treatments at 1- to 2-week intervals is usually required. Organophosphates have been routinely used on adult animals. Sulfurated lime is recommended for the dog less than 3-months old or for the debilitated dog (Parasitic Disease Therapeutic Key, Appendix 2:8). If there is a poor response after 3 or 4 insecticide dips, a different one should be tried since resistance to insecticides can occur. All asymptomatic dogs on the premises should be given 1 prophylactic dip with Amitraz or 2 to 3 prophylactic dips with organophosphates to prevent contagion. Corticosteroids can be used concurrently with parasiticides to help alleviate pruritus and self-trauma. They should be discontinued as soon as possible since immunosuppression may delay clinical response. Tranquilizers can be used to help control pruritus because of their sedative effect, but they are usually much less effective.

Prognosis. The prognosis for sarcoptic mange is good. Occasionally a dog will not respond as expected; however, sarcoptic mange should be considered a curable disease with minimal permanent side effects. Reinfection can occur if there is re-exposure to the mites.

NOTOEDRIC MANGE

Notoedric mange, or feline scabies, is an uncommon parasitic disease of cats caused by Notoedres cati, a sarcoptic mite. It can also affect rabbits, dogs, and humans.

The transmission and life cycle of N. cati is similar to that of Sarcoptes scabiei.

History. Notoedric mange is characterized by intense pruritus about the hed and neck. There is often a history of an epidemic among a litter of young kittens. Concurrent human contagion may be reported. There may be a poor response to low-dose corticosteroids.

Clinical Signs. Lesions often appear on the ear margins, and then spread to the rest of the ear, face, and neck (Plate 4:M). The feet (Plate 4:N) and perineum may also become involved. The lesions consist of crusts, scales, erythema, excoriation, alopecia, and in chronic disease, lichenification. In kittens the abdomen may be more severely involved than the head.

Diagnosis. A history of intense pruritus of the head and neck is suggestive, as are crusts and excoriation on the ear margins, face, and neck.

Prior to treatment, numerous mites are usually observed on skin scrapings. A good clinical response to a therapeutic trial with a parasiticide is also considered diagnostic.

Treatment. Infected animals should be isolated and the contaminated environment thoroughly cleaned. The cats should be clipped and crusts and debris removed by gentle washing. A weekly sulfurated lime solution should be applied as a total body dip (Parasitic Disease Therapeutic Key, Appendix 2:8). This should be continued until 2 weeks beyond clinical remission. Concurrent corticosteroids and antibiotics may be indicated to prevent self-trauma and secondary infection.

All other animals in the environment should be dipped at least twice at weekly intervals.

CHEYLETIELLA MANGE

Cheyletiella mange or cheyletiellosis is caused by Cheyletiella yasguri in the dog and by C. blakei in the cat.

Pathogenesis. Cheyletiella mites are transmitted by direct contact. Young puppies and kittens, 2- to 8- weeks-old, usually have the largest number of mites. Adult dogs and cats normally have a small number of mites even if there is direct contact with more heavily infested young animals, suggesting that an immune mechanism may be involved. The mites do not burrow into the skin, but live in the keratin layer of the epidermis and are not associated with hair follicles. The mites move rapidly in pseudotunnels in dermal debris. They periodically attach firmly to the epidermis, pierce the skin, and become engorged with a clear colorless fluid.

Life Cycle. The entire life cycle of the mite is spent on the host. Ova are laid and stick to the hair or surface debris. The incubation period is approximately 4 days, and the larval stage is approximately 7 days after which there are two nymphal stages each lasting 4 to 5 days. The adult has a short life of approximately 14 days. The larvae, nymphs, and adult males die within 48 hours after leaving the host. It has been reported that the adult females may live up to 10 days separated from the host if refrigerated, suggesting that the infestation may exist in cooler climates longer than in warmer ones.

History. Mild to marked dandruff on the dorsum of a puppy or kitten with no irritation and variable pruritus is often reported. Occasionally, there will be a report of family members developing a pruritic rash shortly after obtaining the dog or cat (Plate 4:O). There may be asymptomatic carrier animals associated with the human contagion. A drug history of clinical response to flea powders, shampoos, sprays, or dips is often elicited.

Clinical Signs. Puppies usually have a moderate to marked dandruff, which starts over the caudal back and then progresses anteriorly. However, dandruff may only be observed about the dorsal neck area. There is a notable absence of any primary morphologic lesions. Scales are often the only secondary lesions observed. Close examination may reveal "walking dandruff," especially if the hair is clipped. Some dogs are asymptomatic. Cats may have dandruff similar to puppies (Plate 4:P), a miliary eczema-like eruption of crusts and papules, or they may be asymptomatic carriers.

Diagnosis. A positive skin scraping at any stage of the mite is diagnostic (Fig. 5–4). In long-haired animals, it is helpful to clip the hair in the area to be scraped. The brush technique is an alternative method that yields a higher percentage of positive findings. A dry toothbrush or surgery scrub brush may be used to remove a local area of hair and scale and to transfer the debris to a slide for examination. If there are no suspicious focal areas, the entire dorsum of the animal may be brushed. Extensive brushing is usually reserved for those dogs and cats in which there are minimal to no clinical signs, a history of potential human contagion, and/or negative skin scrapings of a focal area. All stages of the mite may be found in the debris. Eggs are often attached to the hair. The adult Cheyletiella mite is identified by the hooks of the accessory mouth parts, and a typical saddle-shaped body (Fig. 5–5). C. yasguri is approximately twice the size of Sarcoptes scabiei. Occa-

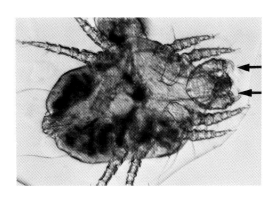

Fig. 5–5. Cheyletiella yasguri: Note the hooks on the accessory mouth parts (arrows). (Courtesy of G.S. Kedan.)

sionally, mites and/or eggs are found in fecal flotations.

Treatment. Most parasiticides are effective in controlling Cheyletiella mange (Parasitic Disease Therapeutic Key, Appendix 2:8). Pyrethrins, carbamates, organophosphates (dog only), and sulfurated lime are routinely used in the form of dusts, sprays, or dips. Treatment must be continued for several weeks to eliminate the infection. All animals on the premises must be treated, whether symptomatic or not. The premises should be kept clean and disinfected, especially the kennels or catteries. All new animals should be dusted, sprayed, or dipped prior to exposure to other animals.

Prognosis. The prognosis for Cheyletiellosis is good; however, reinfestation may occur whenever there is direct contact with the mites.

OTODECTIC OTITIS

Otodectic otitis or otodectic mange, the most commonly encountered parasitic disease of dogs and cats, is caused by Otodectes cynotis, a psoraptid ear mite.

Pathogenesis. O. cynotis is transmitted by direct contact. Pruritus associated with the infestation may be caused by a combination of factors, including mechanical irritation of the mite, toxic materials produced by the mite, and the secretion of allergenic substances to which the host becomes sensitized. The mites live on the surface of the skin and feed on epidermal debris. There is evidence that Type I and Type III hypersensitivity reactions may play a role in the pathogenesis of ear mite infestations.

Acute ear mite infestations are associated with hyperplasia of the ceruminous glands and a mild mononuclear cell infiltrate in the external auditory canal. In chronic otodectic otitis, the gross

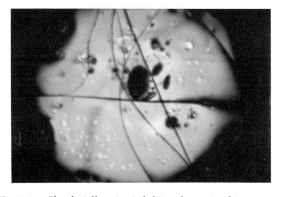

Fig. 5–4. Cheyletiella mite (adult) and eggs in skin scraping (scan power).

canal change is a crusted layer formed from dried serum, ceruminous secretions, and exfoliated epithelium. Microscopic findings include parakeratotic and acanthotic epithelium, squamous metaplasia of duct epithelium, hair follicle atrophy, and increased inflammatory infiltrate. Dilated venules and edema of subcutaneous tissue are also common.

Life Cycle. The adult O. cynotis may live for 2 months, laying eggs on the ceruminous substrate of the ear canal or skin. Larvae are hatched after 4 days of incubation. The larvae feed for 3 to 10 days, rest for 1 day, and then hatch to protonymphs. Following feeding for 3 to 10 days, and resting for another day, the protonymph molts to a deutonymph. Following another feeding and resting cycle, a male attaches to the deutonymph. If a female adult is hatched, copulation takes place immediately. The entire life cycle takes about 3 weeks.

History. Pruritus and head shaking are the most common clinical signs noted by the owner, or the primary complaint may be self-trauma about the head and neck. A dark waxy discharge is often observed at the external orifice of the ear canal. Dogs are frequently more sensitive to ear mite infestations than cats. The infestation may be associated with generalized multifocal dermatitis.

Clinical Signs. Otoscopic examination of the external ear canal reveals varying amounts of dark wax, usually with small white ear mites on the surface of the debris. The medial pinna may be normal, erythematous, or excoriated. Excoriation posterior to the base of the ear is common. The infestation and secondary trauma may be unilateral or bilateral. and there is commonly a secondary bacterial or yeast infection. Exudation is variable. Focal alopecic, erythemic and excoriated lesions may be observed on the head, neck, and lower back.

Diagnosis. The most common way to diagnose otodectic otitis is by visualizing the mites on otoscopic examination. Ear swabs and direct microscopic examination of the ear debris is sometimes necessary. Occasionally, it is necessary to flush the ears, and collect and examine the debris. Scrapings of the lesions on the head, neck, or trunk may reveal O. cynotis mites or eggs (Figs. 5–6 and 5-7).

A therapeutic trial with otic miticides and flea parasiticides resulting in 100% clinical response is suggestive of primary otodectic mange.

Treatment. The ear canals should be flushed and all wax and debris removed. An acaricidal preparation should be used either daily or 3-times weekly for at least 2 weeks. Antibiotics and corticosteroids may be indicated. Concurrent whole body treatment with a parasiticide must be done weekly. All animals in the environment must be treated.

CANINE DEMODECTIC MANGE

Canine demodectic mange (demodicosis, red mange, follicular mange) is caused by Demodex canis.

Pathogenesis. D. canis is a normal inhabitant of the skin. A large percentage (estimates vary from 30 to 80%) of the normal canine population are asymptomatic carriers of the mites. The pathogenesis of demodicosis is not completely understood. There is an apparent genetic predisposition in the dog. Puppies acquire the infection the first few days of life while nursing. If the puppies are delivered by cesarean section and not allowed to nurse, they will be free of demodectic mites, suggesting that the mites do not pass the placental barrier.

Immunologic factors have been demonstrated to

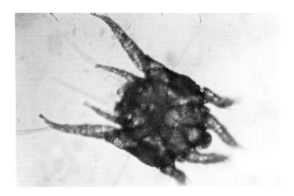

Fig. 5–6. Otodectes cynotis (ear mite) in skin scraping (low power).

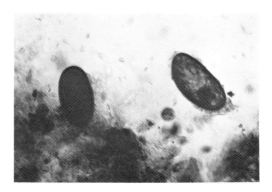

Fig. 5–7. Otodectes cynotis eggs in skin scraping (low power).

be involved with the course of canine demodectic mange. A serum factor is present which causes a suppression of T lymphocytes as measured by in vitro mitogenesis. Antilymphocyte serum precipitates the onset of demodicosis. A skin graft of the infected skin adjacent to normal skin on a puppy can produce localized disease; however, a generalized form is not observed. A spontaneous clinical remission is often observed in animals less than 1 year of age.

The mites apparently feed off the sebum in the hair follicles. Clinical disease is observed when the demodectic mites reproduce in sufficient numbers to cause alopecia. A mild microscopic follicular and perifollicular inflammatory response may be observed in the unruptured hair follicle. The specific factors causing this reaction have not been identified. If the hair follicle ruptures, there is a more severe intrafollicular and perifollicular inflammatory response most likely due to the mites or their metabolic products.

Life Cycle. The life cycle of D. canis is not completely understood. The mite spends the entire life cycle on the host. They are ingested during the neonatal period (within 2 to 3 days of birth) and migrate from the stomach to the regional lymph nodes, probably by way of the lymphatics. In 2 to 3 months the mites reach the hair follicles. The stages of mites observed in the hair follicles include fusiform eggs, six-legged larvae, eight-legged protonymphs and deutonymphs, and the eight-legged adult.

History. There appears to be an age predilection between 3 and 12 months for dogs. However, the mature dog (1 to 15 years) may be clinically infected. A breed predilection also exists in short-haired breeds including the Dachshund, Doberman Pinscher, Beagle, and Boston Terrier. Old English Sheepdogs are also commonly infected. However, demodicosis can be observed in any breed.

The distribution of lesions in the young animal is often localized to the head and feet. The owner usually observes focal, nonpruritic alopecic areas which may regress spontaneously without treatment. At times there is a history of focal lesions that progress to a more generalized distribution. There may be pruritus associated with superficial or deep pyoderma. The older dog is often examined for chronic interdigital pyoderma, which may be antibiotic-responsive and recurrent, or only partially antibiotic-responsive. Many of the generalized alopecic dogs with no secondary pyoderma have a drug history of poor response to

hormonal therapy. It is common to see an exacerbation of clinical signs following corticosteroid therapy. There is a higher incidence of relapse of clinical signs associated with estrus. With rare exceptions, there is no suggestion of contagion among dogs.

Clinical Signs. Two clinical forms of demodicosis are recognized. The localized or squamous form is characterized by a few (1 to 6) small, circumscribed erythematous, or hyperpigmented, scaly, nonpruritic, alopecic macules or patches, usually located periorbitally, facially (Plate 4:Q), or on the forelegs (Plate 4:R). Inflammation varies from none to moderate, and there may be an occasional papule or pustule. Alopecia varies from partial to complete, and from a macule to a patch.

The generalized form is characterized by large, multifocal areas of alopecia, erythema, hyperpigmentation, edema, and seborrhea (Plate 4:S,T). At times there is only alopecia and scaling without signs of acute inflammation. Superficial or deep secondary pyoderma is common. The ventral chin, face, and feet are the usual sites for the pyoderma (Plate 4:U,V,W). Peripheral lymphadenopathy is common. Occasionally a young dog is examined for signs of septicemia including fever and shock.

Diagnosis. Demodectic mange is often suspected on the basis of a history of focal, nonpruritic, alopecic areas on the face and forelimbs of a young dog. Chronic pyoderma of the feet or ventral chin, which is recurrent or only partially responsive to antibiotics, is also suggestive. Skin scraping is the screening and definitive diagnostic test. The area to be scraped should first be squeezed to force the mites out of the hair follicles. The scraping should be done on a small focal area and should be deep enough to draw a small amount of blood. Any or all stages of the demodectic mites may be observed (Figs. 5–8, 5–9, 5–10). If several lesions are present on physical examination, positive scrapings from multiple sites are diagnostic. If only

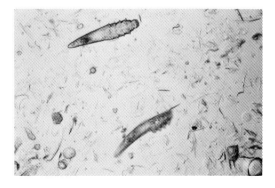

Fig. 5–8. Demodex canis adults in skin scraping (low power).

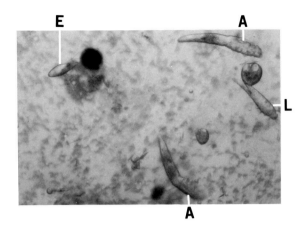

Fig. 5–9. Demodex canis adult (A), larva (L), and egg (E) in skin scraping (low power).

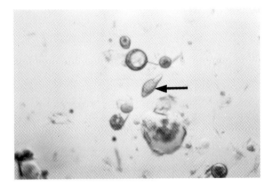

Fig. 5–10. Demodex canis egg in scraping (arrow) (low power).

one or two mites are found in scrapings from multiple areas, a diagnosis of active demodicosis must be questioned and scrapings should be repeated in 1 to 2 weeks.

The results of clinical laboratory testing including complete blood counts, differential counts, and biochemical testing are usually normal. If severe active pyoderma is present, there may be mild leukocytosis, elevated total protein, and elevated globulins. Some workers report a high degree of correlation between demodicosis and hypothyroidism based on baseline T_3 and T_4 or TSH stimulation tests. A direct cause-and-effect relationship has not been verified. These values usually return to normal after resolution of the demodicosis.

Demodicosis may also be diagnosed by means of a routine cutaneous biopsy. If demodectic mites have not been found on scrapings and are reported in biopsies, scrapings should be repeated. The pathologic findings include dilated hair follicles filled with keratin and mites (Fig. 5–11). The degree of inflammation associated with dilated hair

follicles varies from none to rupture of the follicle and total destruction (Fig. 5–12).

Treatment. Many young animals with either localized or generalized demodicosis have a spontaneous remission at maturity. Therefore, some consideration must be given to supportive treatment only until the animal is approximately 1-year-old. Local application of benzoyl peroxide or rotenone may have some beneficial effect. If pyoderma is present, antibiotics should be used. Antiseborrheic shampoos to remove the scale are indicated (Parasitic Disease Therapeutic Key, Appendix 2:8). It should be emphasized that any of the aforementioned supportive therapy will not prevent the localized type from changing to generalized demodectic mange.

A new drug, Amitraz (Upjohn) is the treatment

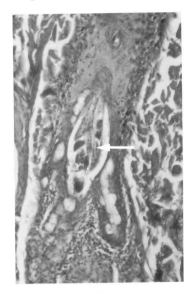

Fig. 5–11. Demodex canis: Microscopic section from demodicosis lesion with several mites within the intact hair follicle (arrow).

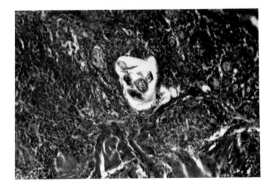

Fig. 5–12. Demodex canis: Microscopic section from demodicosis lesion with cross sections of mites in the dermis. Note granulomatous reaction surrounding the parasites following rupture of a hair follicle.

of choice (see Appendix 2:8). The use of Amitraz usually results in a good clinical response within 6 weeks in the majority of animals. The recommended frequency of Amitraz application is once every 2 weeks. Mites may still be recovered in small numbers in scrapings even though there is good resolution of the alopecia. In the past, the generalized form has responded best to a daily application of a 4% organophosphate (ronnel) in a propylene glycol vehicle (see Appendix 2:8). The use of 70% isopropyl alcohol in the solution is optional.

If there is a concurrent pyoderma, it must be treated vigorously and for a sufficient length of time with antibiotics and other supportive therapy when indicated (see Appendix 2:8). Avoid the application of organophosphate-propylene glycol solution to pyoderma lesions; wait until lesions are dry and crusting prior to application to avoid excessive absorption, toxicity, and irritation.

The course of the disease should be monitored by scraping the dog every 3 to 4 weeks and recording the ratio of the mature to the immature mites. If the disease is responding to treatment, there will be a gradual increase in the ratio of mature to immature mites. Then decreasing numbers of adult mites are observed. Treatment should be continued until there are multiple negative scrapings 2 to 3 weeks apart.

Several other factors should be considered when treating demodectic mange. All long-haired dogs and many short-haired dogs with a dense undercoat should have a total body clipping prior to initiating therapy.

Corticosteroids are contraindicated in the treatment of demodectic mange. If there is significant pruritus associated with secondary pyoderma, an ataraxoid (Atarax, Roerig) may be tried. Nonspecific immunostimulators such as levamisole have generally not resulted in a better or faster clinical response.

Ovariohysterectomy is recommended for two reasons. First, there is a potential for a higher incidence of relapse of clinical signs associated with estrus. Second, there is a hereditary predisposition associated with demodicosis.

Prognosis.   Reports indicate that 70 to 90% of dogs with generalized demodectic mange that are treated with organophosphate-propylene glycol solutions have a clinical recovery in 3 to 5 months. After an apparent clinical cure, which is based on multiple negative scrapings, there is a 10 to 15% relapse. There is generally a better prognosis for young animals, for those without secondary in-

fection, and for those dogs that have had a good clinical response within 4 to 6 weeks after initiating therapy; however, older dogs with interdigital pyoderma and demodicosis often respond as well as young dogs. Dogs that have a relapse often have a poorer response to repeat treatment than they did initially. The majority of dogs treated with Amitraz (Upjohn) have a marked improvement in clinical appearance, although a few mites may be found on scrapings. Periodic dips may be required to maintain good clinical control.

FELINE DEMODECTIC MANGE

Feline demodectic mange (demodicosis, follicular mange) is a rare disease caused by Demodex cati. The pathogenesis and life cycle of D. cati are assumed to be similar to that of D. canis. A new species (unnamed) of feline demodectic mite has recently been described (Conroy, 1982).

History.   There are no sex or breed predilections for this disease. Young cats are more commonly affected. The initial complaint is usually of focal alopecia with variable pruritus. There may be concurrent systemic disease.

Clinical Signs.   Clinical signs may be localized or generalized. The localized form is characterized by single or multiple areas of alopecia and erythema. Scaling, crusting, papules, and secondary pyoderma are variable. The localized form usually affects the head, ears, and neck. The generalized form is characterized by similar lesions, which are not localized to the head and neck. The disease has been associated with concurrent feline leukemia and diabetes mellitus. Ceruminous otitis may also be present.

Diagnosis.   Skin scraping is the definitive diagnostic test. The area to be scraped should first be squeezed, and multiple scrapings done. In cases of ceruminous otitis, the contents of the ear canal should be removed with an ear swab and examined microscopically for mites (see Figs. 5–8, 5–9, 5–10).

Treatment.   As in the dog, many young cats have spontaneous remission. Local application of rotenone and mineral oil has been used to treat ceruminous otitis associated with demodicosis. No successful treatment for generalized feline demodicosis has been reported.

TICKS

Based on taxonomic classifications, tick infestations are generally divided into two classes: hard (Ixodid) and soft (Argasid) ticks.

Hard Ticks (Ixodid)

The majority of ticks that cause clinical problems in dogs are ixodid or hard ticks. Ixodid tick infestations in cats are seldom reported. Several species are capable of infesting dogs and cats including Rhipicephalus sanguineus (brown dog tick), Dermacentor andersoni (Rocky Mountain wood tick), D. variabilis (American dog tick), Amblyomma maculatum (Gulf Coast tick), and A. americanum (Lone Star tick).

Incidence. The incidence of tick infestation is dependent on many factors including temperature, moisture, and availability of the hosts.

Pathogenesis. The tick attaches itself to the host, buries its mouth parts deeply into the tissues of the host to feed, and remains attached until it is engorged with blood. An inflammatory reaction occurs at the site of penetration. Crusting at the penetration site often follows removal of the tick.

Life Cycle and Diseases Transmitted. Rhipicephalus sanguineus is a three-host tick, but can complete its life cycle on one animal as a host. After engorgement, the tick drops off the host and moults on the ground. Because of its low moisture requirement, it is often found in kennels and houses.

The stages of the life cycle of ticks are listed in Table 5–1. Eggs are laid in sheltered spots such as under stones and in crevices of walls. The newly hatched larvae or seed ticks climb onto grass and shrubs and then attach to a host. Rhipicephalus sanguineus can transmit several viral, rickettsial, protozoan, and bacterial diseases (Table 5–2), and may cause tick paralysis.

Dermacentor andersoni and D. variabilis are three-host ticks. The stages and duration of the life cycle are listed in Table 5–1. The larvae and nymphs can attach to most small mammals, especially rodents. The unfed adults may live for 3 years, but engorged adults only live for a few weeks. D. variabilis is more sensitive to dryness, but resistant to cold. Diseases transmitted by Dermacentor spp. are listed in Table 5–2. They can also cause tick paralysis.

Amblyomma spp. have similar life cycles to the other ixodid ticks (Table 5–1). Diseases transmitted by this tick are listed in Table 5–2.

History. There is no age, breed, or sex predilection. The animal's exposure to tick-infested vegetation, or to rodents acting as hosts of tick larvae or nymphs are the major factors promoting infestation. During routine grooming or examination, ticks are usually observed on the dorsum, especially about the ears, head, and neck, or in the feet; however, they may found on any part of the body. Pruritus is usually minimal and localized to the site of the tick attachment.

Clinical Signs. Ticks in various stages of the life cycle can be observed attached to the skin.

TABLE 5–1. LIFE CYCLES OF TICKS

Tick	Stage	Activity	Duration
Rhipicephalus sanguineus	Adult female	Engorge; lays 2000–3900 eggs	6–21 days
	Adult male	Engorge	6 days to mo
	Adults	Nonengorge	Survive up to 19 mo
	Eggs	Hatch	17–30 days or longer
	Larvae	Engorge	2–6 days
		Moult	5–23 days
		Nonengorge	Survive up to 6 mo
	Nymphs	Engorge	4–9 days
		Moult	11–73 days
		Nonengorge	Survive up to 6 mo
Dermacentor spp.	Adult female	Engorge; lays 4000–6000 eggs	8–14 days
	Eggs	Hatch	15–57 days
	Larvae	Engorge	3–14 days
		Moult	6–87 days
	Nymphs	Engorge	3–9 days
		Moult	21 days
Otobius megnini	Adult female	Lays 500–600 eggs	
	Adult	Nonparasitic (do not feed)	
	Eggs	Hatch	10 days to 8 wk
	Larvae	Engorge	5–10 days after attaching to external ear canal
		Nonengorge	Survive for 2–4 mo
		Moult inside ears	
	Nymphs	Engorge	1–7 mo in ear
		Moult	Few days after dropping from host

TABLE 5–2.   DISEASES AND ORGANISMS TRANSMITTED BY IXODID TICKS

Disease or organism	Rhipicephalus sanguineus	Dermacentor andersoni	Dermacentor variabilis	Amblyomma americanum	Amblyomma maculatum
Babesia gibsoni	X				
B. canis		X			
Hepatozoon canis	X				
Coxiella burnetii	X	X			
Ehrlichia canis	X				
Pasteurella tularensis	X		X		
Rocky Mountain spotted fever		X	X	X	
Western equine encephalitis		X			
St. Louis equine encephalitis			X		
Leptospira pomona					X

Focal erythema of the skin adjacent to the attached tick is commonly seen (Plate 4:X). After the tick is removed, crusting and the development of a firm cutaneous nodule may follow. If pruritus has been present, mild excoriation and alopecia may be seen. The local lesions tend to persist for days to weeks, depending on the degree of local irritation present.

Diagnosis. The observation of ticks is diagnostic. A history of tick infestation, focal crusty lesions, or cutaneous nodules is suggestive.

Management. There are two objectives in the control of tick infestation: breaking the tick life cycle in the environment and minimizing infestation of all animals. Eliminating ticks from the indoor or kennel environment requires repeated spraying of the premises, including all cracks and crevices, with parasiticides (Parasitic Disease Therapeutic Key, Appendix 2:8). Infected animals should be isolated in areas that can be disinfected easily. In many endemic areas, repeated treatment at 2-week intervals is necessary. Eliminating ticks from the outdoor environment is difficult. An attempt should be made to eliminate or decrease the number of rodent hosts and to destroy or spray tick-infested vegetation. Avoidance of animal exposure to known infested vegetation is often helpful.

The control of ticks on animals is easier to accomplish than the environmental control. After soaking the tick with alcohol or ether, the tick should be mechanically removed with forceps by grasping it near the head. The dog or cat should then be dipped in an approved parasiticide to remove any ticks missed on physical examination. Tick control on all animals should be maintained by using powders, sprays, dips, or insecticide collars.

Soft Ticks (Argasid)

The only soft tick of clinical importance is the spinous ear tick, Otobius megnini, which is found only in warm, moist climates.

Pathogenesis. The larval and nymphal stages may be found in the ears of most mammals. The larvae feed on lymph while nymphs suck blood. Severe irritation and inflammation of the external ear canal occurs because of mechanical attachment and piercing of the mucosa.

Life Cycle. O. megnini is a one-host tick. Only the larvae and nymphal stages are parasitic (see Table 5–1).

History and Clinical Signs. The dog or cat may be examined for a history of head shaking, pain about the ears, and localized pruritus of the ear region. On physical examination, a waxy or oily exudate, together with larval and nymphal ticks, is usually found in the external ear canal. After removing the wax, acute otitis externa is observed. There are often excoriations at the base of the ears as a result of the pruritus.

Diagnosis. The observation of ticks during an otic examination confirms the diagnosis. A history of severe head shaking and pruritus around the ears is suggestive, especially if the animal lives in an endemic area.

Management. Ticks are mechanically removed with forceps, and tick powders or sprays are used on external surfaces (see Appendix 2:8). The otitis externa is treated locally with antibiotics and corticosteroids. Spraying the premises helps to control reinfestation.

LICE (Pediculosis)

Lice are wingless, dorsoventrally flattened insects that are host specific and spend their entire life cycle on the host. The incidence of pediculosis in the United States is low, and is more commonly associated with cool climates. The two types of lice that affect dogs are the biting and sucking types. The most common biting louse is Trichodectes canis. Heterodoxus spiniger is occasionally found in warm climates. The common sucking louse is Linognathus setosus (Fig. 5–13). Cats are only affected by biting lice, most commonly Felicola subrostratus. Trichodectes canis rarely affects kittens.

Pathogenesis. Lice can be transmitted directly by mechanical means (e.g., grooming tools). Biting lice cause an irritation at the attachment site. Sucking lice extract blood and thus can potentially cause anemia. Pruritus is caused by the release of proteolytic enzymes in the oral secretions of lice or following mechanical trauma associated with penetration of the tissue.

Life Cycle. Operculate eggs or nits are deposited and cemented to the hair. The eggs hatch into nymphs which moult three times prior to becoming adults. The entire life cycle lasts 2 to 3 weeks.

History and Clinical Signs. Owners may report observing lice. Often there is a complaint of mild pruritus. The most common clinical finding is white, glistening nits attached to the hair. Lice may be found incidentally following clipping in the absence of a history of infestation or pruritus. There may be mild to moderate alopecia in focal, densely haired areas with mild to moderate inflammation accompanied by scales, papules, or small crusts.

Treatment. Lice are susceptible to most parasiticides (Parasitic Disease Therapeutic Key, Appendix 2:8). It is necessary to treat all animals on the premises. All new dogs and cats should be dusted, sprayed, or dipped prior to exposure to other animals.

PELODERA DERMATITIS

Pelodera or rhabditic dermatitis is an uncommon disease of dogs caused by the larvae of the free-living nematode, Pelodera strongyloides. Parthenogenetic adult females may also be found in the hair follicles.

Pathogenesis. Pelodera dermatitis is associated with unsanitary conditions and damp bedding. Most lesions are secondary to pruritus. The larvae penetrate the skin causing microscopic subcutaneous inflammation. Previously injured skin may be predisposed to infection.

Life Cycle. The life cycle of P. strongyloides is direct. Adults live in damp soil or decaying organic matter. Female adults are parthenogenetic or oviparous.

History and Clinical Signs. Dogs with pelodera dermatitis are usually characterized by intense pruritus. There is often a history of exposure to damp bedding such as straw. Lesions are usually confined to the ventral contact parts of the body. The primary lesions are papules and pustules, which usually progress to secondary crusts and scales. Erythema may be intense. Alopecia is more variable depending on severity and duration of the pruritus.

Diagnosis. A history of intensely pruritic ventral dermatitis in a dog that sleeps on damp bedding is suggestive of pelodera dermatitis. A definitive diagnosis can be made by observing nematode larvae with a rhabditiform esophagus on scraping. Sections of larvae or adult females may be seen in cutaneous biopsy. Bedding may also be infested with larvae or adults.

Treatment. Complete removal and destruction of infested bedding is imperative. The premises should be washed and then disinfected with organophosphates or chlordane. The infected dog should be bathed with an antiseborrheic and antibacterial shampoo to remove crusts and surface infection and then dipped weekly for 3 weeks with a parasiticide (Parasitic Disease Therapeutic Key, Appendix 2:8).

TROMBICULIASIS

Canine and feline trombiculiasis is caused by the third-stage larvae of the North American chigger, Eutrombicula alfreddugesi.

Pathogenesis. Lesions follow attachment of the

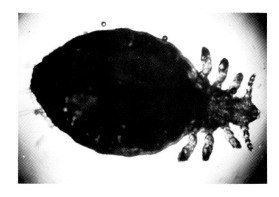

Fig. 5–13. Linognathus setosus (sucking louse) of dogs.

parasitic larvae to the skin. The mite injects saliva containing proteolytic enzymes, which hydrolyze the stratum corneum and allow the tissue fluids to be sucked up by the mite. The larvae stay attached for several hours and then drop off. Pruritus occurs within a few hours of the bite and may persist for several days. A hypersensitivity reaction to the components of the mite saliva is suspected.

Life Cycle.   Adult chiggers are free-living, or prey on other arthropods. The eggs are laid in the moist ground. The six-legged orange larvae hatch and usually parasitize hosts such as snakes, lizards, wild rodents, or birds. The larvae, however, parasitize dogs, cats, or man when there is direct contact with larvae-infected foliage in fields or forests. The larvae drop to the ground and develop into nymphs. The free-living adults live on decaying vegetable material. The life cycle is completed in 50 to 70 days; however, adult females may survive more than 1 year.

History and Clinical Signs.   Pruritus is the most common sign. Pinhead-sized, orange-red mites may be observed tightly adhered to the skin. There is local irritation characterized by erythematous papules, scaling, and alopecia. The most common distribution is on the head, neck, axillary regions, and feet. However, lesions of trombiculiasis may be generalized.

Diagnosis.   A history of a dog or cat having been exposed to an endemic chigger area lends support to the diagnosis. The definitive diagnostic test is identification of the six-legged larvae on examination of skin scrapings. A good response to a therapeutic trial with a parasiticidal shampoo or dip (Parasitic Disease Therapeutic Key, Appendix 2:8), is highly suggestive if the history and clinical signs are consistent with trombiculiasis.

Treatment.   If there is much scaling or crusting, a bath with an antiseborrheic shampoo should be given followed by a parasiticidal dip (see Appendix 2:8). In endemic areas, dips should be repeated every 10 to 14 days.

MYIASIS

Myiasis is caused by two families of flies: the calliphorids or blow flies, and the sarcophagids or flesh flies.

Pathogenesis.   Flies are attracted to moist, traumatized areas. The fly larvae cause marked destruction of the skin by secreting proteolytic enzymes. Secondary fly larvae infections may occur, causing more severe lesions. Deep tunnels may form in the subcutaneous tissue. Toxemia occa-

sionally is seen in dogs and cats with neglected myiasis, which is likely caused by metabolic breakdown products of the necrotic tissue.

Life Cycle. *Calliphorids.*   Calliphorid eggs are laid in clusters on moist skin lesions. The larvae hatch in 8 hours to 3 days. Within the next 2 to 19 days, 2 ecdyses follow. The larvae drop off the host and become pupae. The pupae persist for a minimum of 3 to 7 days before becoming adults, which live for 1 month or longer.

Sarcophagids.   The sarcophagids are larviparous; thus they deposit larvae rather than eggs on the skin. The rest of the life cycle is similar to that of the calliphorids.

History.   Myiasis usually occurs in a chronically neglected wound. There may or may not be a history of previous trauma or injury. The disease is more common in a sick or debilitated animal. There is often complaint of a foul odor from a large, open wound.

Clinical Signs.   Myiasis is characterized by the presence of a large number of fly larvae in solitary or multiply ulcerated lesions, which are often associated with marked tissue necrosis (Plate 4:Y,Z). It is common for the dog or cat to be in a state of toxemia, manifested by weakness and depression, if the myiasis has persisted for a long period of time.

Diagnosis.   The definitive diagnosis is based on finding larvae in a wound.

Treatment.   The wounds and surrounding area must be cleaned by clipping and scrubbing, and removing all larvae. It is best to use an iodine solution and hydrogen peroxide to clean the wound. Insecticide sprays may be absorbed too rapidly through the traumatized tissue, resulting in toxicity as well as potential local irritation. Insecticide sprays or powders should be used on the rest of the body for continuous fly control. Most animals with myiasis require local wound treatment as well as general supportive care.

HOOKWORM DERMATITIS

In the dog, hookworm dermatitis or ancylostomiasis is caused by the larvae of Ancylostoma caninum or Uncinaria stenocephala.

Pathogenesis.   The third-stage larvae enter the skin of the distal extremities. Local tissue inflammation occurs which results in intense pruritus. Clinical signs appear within 16 hours of the hookworm larvae penetration and may persist for 1 month. Microscopic examination of the resulting lesion suggest an immune-mediated reaction.

History.   There is intense pruritus and inflammation of all feet. A history of exposure to a hookworm endemic environment is generally reported.

Clinical Signs. There is moderate to severe erythema, and the feet are characterized by edema, pain, and heat. The pads are soft and spongy in the acute stage; if dermatitis is chronic, the footpads become hyperkeratotic, dry, and cracked. Paronychia is also reported.

Diagnosis. A presumptive diagnosis of hookworm dermatitis is based on history of exposure, concurrent intestinal hookworm parasitism based upon fecal examination, and pedal dermatitis. A therapeutic trial with a hookworm anthelmintic, which results in clinical improvement of the pedal dermatitis is further support for the diagnosis.

Treatment. Specific treatment involves appropriate anthelmintic therapy. The environment must be cleaned and the premises kept dry to minimize hookworm infestation in the soil. Borax should be applied to dirt or gravel runs.

CUTANEOUS DIROFILARIASIS

Cutaneous dirofilariasis in the dog is caused by the microfilariae of Dirofilaria immitis, the heartworm larvae.

Pathogenesis. The pathogenesis of lesions associated with microfilarial infection caused by D. immitis is not known; however, a hypersensitivity reaction is suspected.

History and Clinical Signs. Skin lesions are suggestive. The clinical signs associated with cutaneous dirofilariasis include erythematous and alopecic eruptions, or multiple ulcerating nodules on the head, neck, trunk, and proximal limbs. Pruritus is often associated with the nodules.

Diagnosis. A positive test for circulating microfilariae and a cutaneous biopsy of a lesion that reveals microfilariae within vessels surrounded by a pyogranulomatous infiltrate (Fig. 5–14) are diagnostic. A good clinical response following treatment for the heartworm infection supports the diagnosis of cutaneous dirofilariasis.

Treatment. The standard protocols for heartworm treatment including administration of the adulticide, thiacetarsamide, and the microfilarialcide, dithiazanine or levamisole are recommended.

SELECTED READINGS

Anderson, R.K.: Canine scabies. Compend. Cont. Ed. Pract. Vet. 1:687, 1979.

Baker, K.P.: Parasitic skin diseases of dogs and cats. Vet. Rec. 87:452, 1970.

Bledsoe, B., Fadok, V., and Bledsoe, M.E.: Current therapy and new developments in indoor flea control. J. Am. Anim. Hosp. Assoc. 18:415, 1982.

Bowen, P.M., and Caldwell, N.J.: Use of Cythioate to control external parasites on cats and dogs. Vet. Med. (Small Anim. Clin.) 77:79, 1982.

Buelke, D.L.: Hookworm dermatitis. J. Am. Vet. Med. Assoc. 158:735, 1971.

Bullmore, C.C., et al.: Feline trombiculiasis. Feline Pract. 6:36, 1976.

Carroll, H.F., and Theis, J.H.: Cheyletiella mite dermatitis: A review. J. Am. Anim. Hosp. Assoc. 9:573, 1973.

Conroy, J.D., Healey, M., and Bane, A.G.: New Demodex sp. infesting a cat : A case report. J. Am. Anim. Hosp. Assoc. 18:405, 1982.

Fadok, V.A.: Ectoparasites of the dog and cat. Compend. Cont. Ed. Pract. Vet. 2:292, 1981.

Fadok, V.A.: Miscellaneous parasites of the skin (Part I). Compend. Cont. Ed. Pract. Vet. 2:707, 1980.

———: Miscellaneous parasites of the skin (Part II). Compend. Cont. Ed. Pract. Vet. 2:782, 1980.

Foxx, T.S., and Ewing, S.A.: Morphologic features, behavior and life history of Cheyletiella yasguri. Am. J. Vet. Res. 30:269, 1969.

Gabbert, N., and Feldman, B.F.: Feline demodex. Feline Pract. 6:32, 1976.

Halliwell, R.E.W.: Flea bite dermatitis. Compend. Cont. Ed. Pract. Vet. 1:367, 1979.

Hardison, J.L.: A case of Eutrombicula alfreddugesi (chiggers) in a cat. Vet. Med. (Small Anim. Clin.) 72:47, 1977.

Krawiec, D.R., and Gaafar, S.M.: Studies on the immunology of canine demodicosis. J. Am. Vet. Med. Assoc. 16:669, 1980.

Lapage, G.: Monnigs Veterinary Helminthology and Entomology. 5th Ed. Baltimore, Williams & Wilkins, 1962.

Lennox, W.J.: Notoedric mange in cats (head mange). In Current Veterinary Therapy IV: Small Animal Practice. Edited by R.W. Kirk. Philadelphia, W.B. Saunders, 1971.

Miller, W.H.: Canine demodicosis. Compend. Cont. Ed. Pract. Vet. 2:334, 1980.

Nesbitt, G.H., and Schmitz, J.A.: Fleabite allergic dermatitis: A review and survey of 330 cases. J. Am. Vet. Med. Assoc. 173:282, 1978.

Pett, E.J.: Three ectoparasites of veterinary interest communicable to man (Sarcoptes, Cheyletiella, Trombicula). Med. Biol. Illus. 20:106, 1970.

Reedy, L.M.: Ectoparasites. In Current Veterinary Therapy VI: Small Animal Practice. Edited by R.W. Kirk. Philadelphia, W.B. Saunders, 1977.

Scott, D.W.: Parasitic disorders. J. Am. Anim. Hosp. Assoc. 6:365, 1980.

———: Nodular skin disease associated with Dirofilaria immitis in the dog. Cornell Vet. 69:233, 1979.

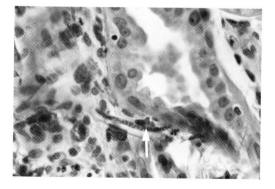

Fig. 5–14. Cutaneous dirofilariasis: Microscopic section from a dog with dirofilariasis. Note microfilaria in capillary (arrow). Lymphocytes and occasional mast cell are predominant inflammatory cells (high power).

———: Feline dermatology. Proceedings of the 43rd Annual Meeting of the American Animal Hospital Association, 1976.

Scott, D.W., Schultz, R.D., and Baker, E.: Further studies on the therapeutic and immunologic aspects of generalized demodectic mange in the dog. J. Am. Anim. Hosp. Assoc. 12:203, 1976.

Willers, W.B.: *Pelodera strongyloides* in association with canine dermatitis in Wisconsin. J. Am. Vet. Med. Assoc. 136:319, 1970.

6

Bacterial Diseases

Canine (Appendix 1:4) and Feline (Appendix 1:5) Bacterial Diagnostic Keys list the most pertinent historical and clinical findings and definitive diagnostic tests necessary to differentiate the common bacterial diseases.

CLASSIFICATION

Pyoderma is the term commonly used to denote bacterial infection of the skin. Such infection may be either primary or secondary bacterial disease. In dogs, infection is more commonly secondary to another dermatologic problem such as pruritus, abnormal keratinization, or parasitic infestation. Other than abscesses following bite wounds or scratches, bacterial disease is uncommon in cats.

Bacterial disease is divided into three types based on the depth of involvement of the skin: surface, superficial, and deep. Surface pyoderma is characterized by superficial overcolonization of the skin in an area where inflammation is the inciting cause. The infection is only as deep as the inflammation. Pyotraumatic dermatitis (acute moist dermatitis) and skin fold pyodermas are classified as surface pyodermas.

Superficial pyoderma is localized to the epidermis and manifests as subcorneal pustules or as a microabscess within the epithelium and lumen of an intact hair follicle. Impetigo, superficial folliculitis, and short-haired dog pyoderma are included in the superficial pyoderma classification.

Deep pyoderma is characterized by bacterial involvement of the dermis and subcutis, and includes the clinical entities of furunculosis, cellulitis, hidradenitis suppurativa, and cat abscesses. A miscellaneous group of bacterial diseases in the dog includes juvenile and dry pyoderma.

ETIOLOGIC FACTORS

The normal bacterial flora of canine and feline skin includes nonpathogenic Micrococcus spp., Corynebacterium spp., and Staphylococcus epidermidis. Clostridium spp. are frequently isolated anaerobically from canine skin. Staphylococcus aureus is the most common pathogen isolated from canine lesions. S. epidermidis (coagulase negative) is isolated with some frequency from dogs that have been treated either topically or systemically. Streptococcus spp., most commonly isolated at the same time as Staphylococcus aureus, may be an opportunist in some animals and may not contribute to the disease process. Proteus spp., and Pseudomonas spp. are infrequently isolated from canine skin lesions; these species cause a severe superficial ulcerative pyoderma, and are commonly associated with Staphylococcus aureus as secondary pathogenic opportunists. Pseudomonas spp. and Proteus spp. are the most common isolates from acute and chronic bacterial otitis externa lesions.

The most common organisms isolated from cat abscesses are Pasteurella multocida, beta hemo-

81

lytic streptococci, and Fusiformis spp., which are all normal flora of the oral cavity. Bacteria isolated from feline folliculitis lesions include beta hemolytic streptococci, Staphylococcus aureus, and Pasteurella multocida. Mycobacterium bovis is the most common cause of feline cutaneous tuberculosis. M. avium and M. microti are rarely isolated.

Several nontubercular mycobacteria including M. lepraemurium, M. xenopi, M. ulcerans, and M. fortuitum have been isolated from feline leprosy lesions.

PATHOGENESIS

There are three major factors involved in the pathogenesis of pyoderma: the pathogenic properties of the organism, the portal of entry, and the host response to microbial invasion. The important pathogenic properties of Staphylococcus aureus include the antiphagocytic properties of the capsule and protein, and the presence of a protease, leukocidin, which acts on the cytoplasmic membrane of neutrophils and macrophages to cause cell lysis, an alpha hemolysin (necrotizing toxin), which is highly toxic to macrophages and epithelial cells, and lipase and esterase, which permit the bacteria to survive the antibacterial action of lipids on the skin.

Although coagulase activity is associated with S. aureus, it is not considered essential that the bacteria be pathogenic. In man, some coagulase negative staphylococcal mutants appear to be fully virulent.

Bacteria may gain entrance into the skin by way of several routes; through the hair follicles, through the epidermal barrier on the surface of the skin, by focal penetration directly into the deeper layers of skin, or systemically by way of the blood or lymph vessels. Hyperkeratosis and follicular plugging, which are commonly observed in many chronic skin conditions, predispose to the entrance and colonization of bacteria in the follicles. The increased epidermal cell turnover time associated with abnormal keratinization, as seen in seborrheic syndromes and endocrine disease, increases the permeability of the epidermal barrier. The physical irritation of external parasites and the secretions of parasites and bacteria also alter the epidermal barrier. Direct penetration of the skin through the epidermis into the dermis and subcutis by way of bite wounds, trauma, or penetrating foreign bodies can cause tissue damage resulting in a more favorable environment for colonization of the bacteria in the deeper tissues. A

systemic origin of bacterial skin infections, such as cutaneous feline tuberculosis, is rare.

The host response to the invasion of bacteria appears to vary among individual dogs and cats. Both cellular and humoral factors are probably involved. It is generally accepted that alterations in cell-mediated immune mechanisms play a role in the development of generalized pyoderma; however, the specific changes have not been well documented.

CANINE BACTERIAL DISEASE

History

The history of a dog with pyoderma is variable and depends on primary and secondary etiologic factors, duration and distribution of lesions, and previous therapy. Historical data commonly obtained include: no systemic involvement excluding peripheral lymphadenopathy; mild to marked pruritus; partial to good response to antibacterial therapy, often with an exacerbation of signs following withdrawal; concurrent external parasites or allergic dermatitis, and offensive odor.

If the bacterial dermatitis is primary, pruritus will usually follow the onset of clinical signs. If the infection is secondary to parasites or allergic disease, pruritus will be observed prior to or concurrently with the signs of pyoderma. Deep pyoderma is usually persistent or recurrent.

There are some age and breed predispositions. Primary superficial folliculitis is most commonly observed in young animals less than 1 year of age; the breeds that are predisposed include the Doberman Pinscher, the Dachshund, and the English Bulldog. Impetigo is a disease of young puppies 2- to 8-weeks old, and is associated with crowding and unsatisfactory sanitary conditions. Skin fold pyoderma, which persists for a lifetime, is seen commonly in breeds such as the English Bulldog, the Pekingese, and the Pug. A history of systemic bacterial involvement associated with superficial pyoderma is rare.

Primary deep pyoderma is usually seen in middle-aged to older dogs. Callous pyoderma is found in the large or giant breed dog unless associated with generalized pyoderma. Primary interdigital pyoderma occurs most often in the larger breeds, which include the German Shepherd, the Doberman Pinscher, the Bull Mastiff, and the Great Dane. Deep generalized pyoderma may occur in any breed; however, it is observed most frequently in breeds of German Shepherd, Irish Setter, and Doberman Pinscher. Perianal pyoderma is common in the German Shepherd. Hidradenitis suppurativa is reported in the Collie and Shetland Sheepdog. Juvenile pyoderma (puppy strangles) is a disease of puppies less than 4-months old and is associated with lymphadenopathy and extensive facial swelling; there is a reported breed predilection for the Pointer and Dachshund.

Secondary superficial pyoderma is often associated with a history of pruritus caused by allergic disease or primary parasitic disease (Demodex, fleas).

Acute exacerbation of deep pyoderma may be associated with a history of anorexia and lethargy. Pain and lameness are more common in interdigital pyoderma.

Clinical Signs

The lesions associated with primary and secondary bacterial infection are variable. Primary morphologic lesions commonly observed with staphylococcal and streptococcal infections are papules, pustules, and macules; secondary lesions include scale, crust, excoriation, and hyperpigmentation; erythema and alopecia vary.

Most dogs with a primary bacterial skin infection have regionalized lymphadenopathy and a normal rectal temperature. There are seldom any other systemic signs. Edema of the extremities may be observed, especially with chronic deep pyoderma. Septicemia is uncommon, but will occur in puppies, most frequently secondary to demodicosis.

Pseudomonas and Proteus skin infections are associated with moist, diffuse, erosive lesions. Occasionally they may be generalized. These skin infections are commonly found in association with interdigital pyoderma, skin fold pyoderma, and, occasionally, pyotraumatic dermatitis.

Acute and chronic bacterial otitis externa are characterized by mucosal erythema and exudation; erosions are frequently found.

Surface Pyoderma. Pyotraumatic dermatitis (acute moist dermatitis) is a focal or multifocal eroded area with an erythematous moist surface (Plate 5:A), most commonly found on the caudal dorsal back, lateral thighs, or shoulder. The lesion is often matted with hair and associated with mild to severe pain. Concurrent evidence of flea infestation is common.

Skin fold pyoderma is associated with moisture, accumulation of debris in the skin folds, and a foul odor. The degree of epidermal damage varies. There may be some erythema and erosion, which are usually associated with lip, facial, vulvar, or tail fold pyoderma (Plate 5:B,C,D). Lesions, excoriation, hyperkeratosis, and hyperpigmentation are commonly observed around the involved skin folds as a result of pruritus.

Superficial Pyoderma. Most S. aureus infections associated with superficial pyoderma involve the hair follicles. The following sequence of clinical signs is characteristic of superficial folliculitis or impetigo (Plate 5:E to I): an erythematous papule with minimal peripheral erythema; a pustule; and a flattened crust, 5 to 10 mm in diameter. When the crust is removed, a moist erythemic lesion remains; when the crust loosens, the center falls off and a thin layer of epidermal tissue on the periphery of the lesion remains with an alopecic dry center. The final stage is a hyperpigmented macule. Frequently, all of the aforementioned stages are present at the same time. Papules and pustules are commonly observed on the abdomen or on other sparsely haired areas of the body, while the lesions that characterize the more mature stages, such as crusts and hyperpigmented macules, are found on the dorsal and lateral trunk as well as ventrally.

An acne-like lesion on the ventral chin may be secondarily infected and is characterized by follicular plugs or comedones, hemorrhagic bullae, or pustules (Plate 5:J).

Deep Pyoderma. Furunculosis is associated with a follicular rupture caused by a bacterial infection that extends to the dermis. The lesions may be focal (Plate 5:K), multiple, or generalized (Plate 5:L), and often occur on pressure points such as the lateral stifle, muzzle, and dorsum of the nose. Exudate can usually be expressed from the dermal tracts. In the acute stages, the surface is moist with crusts, alopecia, and erythema. Chronic deep pyoderma lesions are characterized by thickened skin, hyperpigmentation, hyperkeratosis, and frequent scarring (Plate 5:M). Generalized furunculosis of the extremities is often associated with marked distal edema.

Callous pyoderma is usually associated with marked proliferation of the callous surface. Persistent exudate, erosions, and crusting result from constant irritation and friction (Plate 5:N). Nasal pyoderma is characterized by erosions, ulceration, and crusting on the dorsum of the nose. In the chronic stages, scarring is common.

Interdigital pyoderma, a type of cellulitis, is characterized in the active stages by deep draining tracts of large, deep pustules in one or more interdigital spaces of one or more feet (Plate 5:O).

There are often pustules between the pads (Plate 5:*P*). The feet are usually moist and erythemic secondary to foot licking.

The lesions associated with hidradenitis suppurativa are usually confined to the groin and axilla and are characterized by well-demarcated ulcerations that subsequently scar.

Perianal pyoderma (perianal fistula) is characterized by ulcerations and deep, fistulous tracts (Plate 5:*Q*). Excoriation and trauma may occur secondary to biting and licking, or to accumulation of fecal material in the perianal area.

Miscellaneous Pyodermas. Juvenile pyoderma is associated with ulcerations, purulent discharges, and abscesses of the facial region, especially the periorbital and perioral areas. Erythema and crusts are usually present. Scarring may occur with the resolution of the lesions. Marked mandibular lymphadenopathy is always present.

Dry pyoderma (dry juvenile pyoderma) is characterized by large accumulations of tightly adhered crusts and scale on the face, extremities, and pressure points (elbows, hocks, chin, feet). A moist surface usually remains after a crust is removed. No primary lesions are observed in dry pyoderma.

FELINE BACTERIAL DISEASE

History and Clinical Findings

Surface and Superficial Pyoderma. Surface pyoderma, associated with "mouthing" by the queen, has been observed in young kittens. Lesions are characterized by alopecia, papules, and crusts on the dorsal neck, occasionally progressing caudally on the trunk. Systemic signs are unusual.

There is no breed, sex, or age predilection for feline folliculitis, which is commonly observed on the chin and associated with feline acne (Plate 5:*R*). The clinical signs vary depending on the depth of skin involvement. Alopecia, erosions, ulcers, crusts, and occasionally fistulous tracts and cellulitis have been reported. Pain and pruritus are variable. Peripheral lymphadenopathy may be observed in cats with deep folliculitis.

Deep Pyoderma. Most bacterial infections are associated with a history of cat scratches or bites that result in abscesses or cellulitis.The highest incidence occurs in intact males with no breed or age predilection. Lesions are most commonly associated on the extremities, face (Plate 5:*S*), dorsal tail, and back. The history is variable; acute pain, fever, anorexia, and lameness may be noted. In some cats, focal or diffuse soft-tissue swelling or a ruptured abscess is the first sign observed by the

pet owner. Physical examination may reveal varying degrees of focal erythema and swelling, and evidence of a puncture wound may be observed. If an abscess has not ruptured, a thick white to reddish brown odorous exudate is seen on aspiration or drainage.

Cellulitis is characterized by diffuse soft-tissue swelling, which usually occurs on one limb. There may be heat, pain, and erythema, and the animal's hair may epilate easily. Fever and peripheral lymphadenopathy may be observed. Pyothorax, osteomyelitis, septic arthritis, and septicemia may be sequelae to cat abscesses and cellulitis; leukocytosis and neutrophilia are also common findings.

Miscellaneous Pyodermas. Feline cutaneous tuberculosis is a disease of young adult cats (average age, 2 years) living in geographic areas of the world in which tuberculosis is endemic in cattle. Feline tuberculosis is frequently asymptomatic without signs or outward evidence of disease. Cutaneous lesions are characterized by single or multiple ulcers, abscesses, plaques, and nodules; thick, yellow to green exudate can usually be discharged from the lesions; lesions are most commonly distributed on the head, neck, and extremities. Regional lymphadenopathy and pyrexia may also be present.

Feline leprosy (atypical mycobacterial granuloma) is a disease with no age, breed, or sex predilection. Solitary and occasionally multiple subcutaneous nodules or abscesses with or without draining tracts are the lesions most commonly seen. If the nodule is at the dermoepidermal junction, ulceration is observed. The head, neck, and limbs are most frequently involved.

DEFINITIVE DIAGNOSTIC TESTS

Bacterial culture is the definitive diagnostic test of choice for most bacterial disease. Cultures are not routinely recommended for mild or first occurrence surface or superficial pyodermas; however, they are indicated for all dogs and cats with chronic or frequently recurring pyodermas or deep pyodermas, and for animals with a history of poor or partial response to antibiotics. The sampling techniques for bacterial cultures are described in Table 2–10. The techniques for bacterial culture and in vitro antibiotic sensitivity testing are described in Chapter 2.

Valid results may be obtained when the animal is still undergoing treatment if there is bacterial resistance to the antibiotic being used. All bacteria that grows on the culture medium should be identified since it is common to have both pathogenic and nonpathogenic bacteria in a mixed culture. Gram-negative bacteria (Pseudomonas or Proteus) should be suspected as a primary opportunistic pathogen when the surface of superficial pyoderma is unresponsive to antibiotics with a gram-positive spectrum.

In vitro antibiotic sensitivity testing is routinely performed on all bacteria isolates. Tests should be run on individual isolates, inasmuch as testing performed on a mixed culture is not valid due to overgrowth of one of the bacteria. The antibiotic discs should include both bacteriostatic and bactericidal antibiotics, including some of the less commonly used gram-positive and gram-negative antibiotics.

Cutaneous biopsies are sometimes definitive and often supportive of a diagnosis of bacterial dermatitis. They are necessary to determine the depth and extent of dermal and adnexal involvement, data which are useful for establishing treatment protocols and prognosis.

The microscopic findings of a surface bacterial lesion mainly involve the upper epidermis. Erosion of the stratum corneum is observed in pyotraumatic dermatitis and many skin fold pyodermas (Fig. 6–1). In superficial pyoderma the surface is often intact. Epidermal changes include hyperkeratosis, variable acanthosis, spongiosis (Fig. 6–2), and microabscesses (Figs. 6–3 and 6–4) with neutrophils traversing the stratum spinosum (diapedesis). The dermal changes are limited to the adnexa and upper dermis (dermoepidermal) junction. There often is mild hyperkeratosis and edema of the follicular epithelium. Perifollicular or periglandular involvement can include a mixed

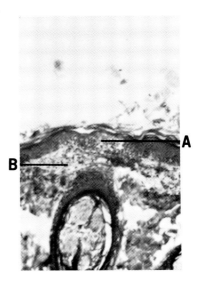

Fig. 6–2. Superficial folliculitis: Microscopic section with spongiosis *(A)* and edema at dermoepidermal junction *(B)* (low power).

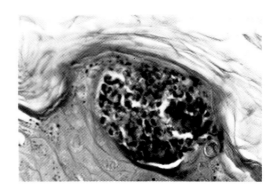

Fig. 6–3. Superficial pyoderma: Microscopic section of a pustule with a subcorneal microabscess (high power).

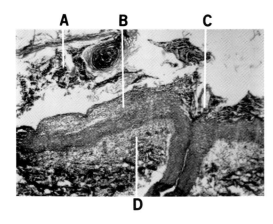

Fig. 6–1. Surface pyoderma: Microscopic section with crusts *(A)* and epidermal erosion *(B)*, follicular infundibulum plugging *(C)*, and a cellular infiltration at the dermoepidermal junction *(D)* (low power).

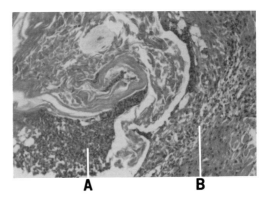

Fig. 6–4. Superficial folliculitis: Microscopic section with an intrafollicular microabscess *(A)* and perifollicular mixed inflammatory cell infiltrate *(B)* (low power).

inflammatory cell infiltrate (Fig. 6–4), and edema. The upper dermal infiltrate that consists of a variable number of mixed inflammatory cells is most often focal or perivascular, but it may be diffuse.

Chronic superficial pyoderma is characterized by hyperkeratosis, variable hypergranulosis, acanthosis, and a mild to moderate mononuclear cell infiltrate at the dermoepidermal junction. The perifollicular and periadnexal changes include a minimal to moderate number of mononuclear leukocytes and variable fibrosis (Fig. 6–5). There may be proliferation of upper dermal blood vessels.

The epidermal changes in a deep pyoderma are similar to those of severe superficial pyoderma. Usually moderate to severe crusting is observed. The dermal changes may involve all of the dermis (Fig. 6–6), and sometimes extend into the pan-

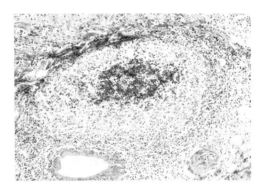

Fig. 6–7. Deep pyoderma: Microscopic section with a pyogranuloma in the dermis. The hair follicle has been destroyed (low power).

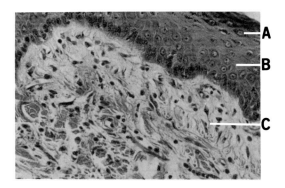

Fig. 6–5. Chronic superficial folliculitis: Microscopic section with mild hypergranulosis *(A)*, acanthosis *(B)*, and fibrosis at dermoepidermal junction *(C)* and an occasional mononuclear cell in the upper dermis (low power).

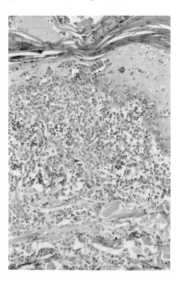

Fig. 6–6. Deep pyoderma: Microscopic section with hyperkeratosis and parakeratosis, diffuse dermal edema, and mixed dermal inflammatory cell infiltrate. The hair follicle has been destroyed (low power).

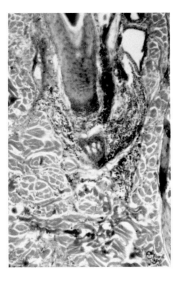

Fig. 6–8. Deep pyoderma: Microscopic section with edema and dense perifollicular inflammatory cell infiltrate (low power).

niculus. Frequently there is a focal to diffuse mixed inflammatory infiltrate. As the lesion becomes chronic, fibroplasia increases. In many microscopic sections, multifocal pyogranulomatous lesions are observed in the dermis, characterized by a central core of mixed inflammatory infiltrate surrounded by histiocytes (Fig. 6–7) and an occasional multinucleated giant cell. Follicular and perifollicular involvement varies (Fig. 6–8). Often there is partial to total destruction of the follicle and replacement with fibrous tissue. The adnexal glands are usually few in number and apocrine gland ducts may be dilated.

Microscopic lesions of feline tuberculosis and feline leprosy are granulomas with acid-fast organisms identified by using special stains (Plate 5:T).

DIRECT SMEARS

Direct smears are helpful in differentiating superficial bacterial disease from nonbacterial bullous disease. A direct smear of the contents of a pustule stained with Wright's or Giesma stain will reveal a predominance of neutrophils (Fig. 6–9). The number of free or phagocytized bacteria observed varies from none to many. Almost all bacteria seen will be cocci since Pseudomonas and Proteus spp. seldom manifest as isolated pustules.

DIAGNOSIS

The subjective or definitive confirmation of bacterial dermatitis is based on several factors including history (response to antibiotics), clinical signs (pustules), and diagnostic tests (direct smears, cultures, biopsy). The major challenge is to interpret the diagnostic findings in order to formulate therapeutic protocols and to improve the prognostic acumen. Interpretation should include determination of primary or secondary bacterial disease, depth of infection (surface, superficial, or deep), and chronicity.

TREATMENT

The Bacterial Disease Therapeutic Key (Appendix 2:9) lists drugs and their indications for most bacterial skin diseases. Several guidelines should be kept in mind when selecting the treatment protocol to be used. First, the proper antibiotic should be selected. In general, bacteriostatic antibiotics, such as erythromycin and lincomycin, are effective in treating most mild superficial pyodermas. In treating first-occurrence superficial pyoderma, most antibiotics are effective including penicillin derivatives and chloramphenicol. For deep or chronic pyoderma and frequently recurring superficial pyoderma, bactericidal antibiotics should be used initially.

The second general guideline should be the use of therapeutic dosages of the drug(s) for a minimum of 7 to 10 days *after* there is a complete clinical response. This often results in a treatment time of 3 to 6 weeks. If there is minimal response to a specific antibiotic after 5 to 7 days of therapy, a different antibiotic should be tried. If long-term administration of antibiotics is required, it may be advantageous to use more than one antibiotic during the course of the treatment.

Third, topical therapy using antibacterial and antiseborrheic shampoo or water soaks is indicated for most pyodermas. Removing crusts, debris, and excess sebum from the skin surface reduces the surface bacterial population, helps prevent follicular plugging, and helps restore normal keratinization. Clipping the hair and local cleansing, soaking, or washing with an antibacterial solution is helpful when there are lesions of deep pyoderma. Astringents are indicated for use in areas that remain persistently moist, such as skin folds and between digits.

Fourth, concurrent problems such as primary allergic or parasitic diseases must be treated symptomatically or specifically at the same time as the pyoderma. If there is marked pruritus causing exacerbation of clinical signs, an ataraxic drug (e.g., Atarax, Roerig) may be effective.

Biologic management is indicated in chronic or recurrent pyoderma and in deep pyoderma in the dog. The products currently available are nonspecific immune stimulators (see Appendix 2:9). Clinical response is variable. These drugs should be considered as adjunct therapy to be used concurrently with antibiotics initially, and then continued as prophylactic therapy.

Feline bacterial infections often respond to penicillin, amoxicillin, ampicillin, and hetacillin. All abscesses must be drained. Flushing with hydrogen peroxide and antibacterial agents is also recommended. Castration of intact male cats is an effective preventative measure. The use of progestational compounds is also recommended as a behavioral modifier.

SELECTED READINGS

Halliwell, R.E.W.: Antibiotic therapy in canine skin disease. Bi-weekly Small Animal Vet. Med. Update Series. Princeton, N.J., Veterinary Publications, 12:1, 1978.

Ihrke, P.J.: Antibiotic therapy in canine skin disease: Dermatologic therapy, Part III. Compend. Cont. Ed. Pract. Vet. 2:177, 1980.

Ihrke, P.J., Halliwell, R.E.W., and Deubler, M.J.: Canine pyoderma. In Current Veterinary Therapy VI: Small Animal Practice. Edited by R.W. Kirk. Philadelphia, W.B. Saunders, 1977.

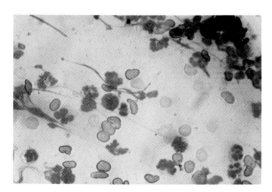

Fig. 6–9. Direct smear of exudate with neutrophils and fibrin (Giemsa stain).

Jennings, A.B.: The distribution of tuberculous lesions in the dog and cat, with reference to the pathogenesis. Vet. Rec. 61:380, 1949.

Joshua, J.O.: Abscesses and their sequelae in cats, Part I. Feline Pract. 1:9, 1971.

Kunkle, G.A.: Canine pyoderma. Compend. Cont. Ed. Pract. Vet. 1:7, 1979.

Nesbitt, G.H., and Schmitz, J.A.: Chronic bacterial dermatitis and otitis: A review of 196 cases. J. Am. Anim. Hosp. Assoc. 13:442, 1977.

Scott, D.W.: Bacterial disorders. J. Am. Anim. Hosp. Assoc. 16:340, 1980.

Snider, W.R.: Tuberculosis in canine and feline populations. Review of the literature. Am. Rev. Respir. Dis. 104:877, 1971.

Wilkinson, G.T.: Feline leprosy. In Current Veterinary Therapy VI: Small Animal Practice. Edited by R.W. Kirk. Philadelphia, W.B. Saunders, 1977.

7

Fungal Diseases

Fungal diseases of the dog and cat can be divided into three major groups: superficial or dermatomycosis, subcutaneous, and systemic. The Fungal Diagnostic Key (Appendix 1:6) lists the most pertinent historical and clinical findings and diagnostic tests necessary to differentiate the common etiologic factors of canine and feline fungal disease.

DERMATOMYCOSES

Dermatomycosis (dermatophytosis) denotes the superficial fungal infections that remain localized to the cornified parts of the skin.

Etiologic Factors. Three dermatophytes commonly cause infection in dogs and cats: Microsporum canis, M. gypseum, and Trichophyton mentagrophytes. T. rubrum, the common human athlete's foot fungus, is occasionally isolated from dogs and cats.

The relative incidence of each fungus varies in different geographic areas. Microsporum canis is the most common isolate according to incidence surveys of all feline and most canine dermatomycoses. Warm, moist climates are more favorable for a high incidence of dermatomycosis; cold, dry climates are less favorable.

Classification. M. canis is classified as a zoophilic fungus; the cat is the natural host. M. gypseum is geophilic since the soil is the natural habitat. Trichophyton mentagrophytes is a zoophilic fungus and rodents are the natural host. There is

also an anthropophilic form of T. mentagrophytes for which man is the natural host.

Pathogenesis. Dermatophytes normally do not invade, nor can they survive in living tissue. They only parasitize keratinized structures, which include the horny layer (stratum corneum) of the epidermis, the hair, and the nails. Dermatophytes invade hair only in the anagen or growing stage.

When a dermatophyte contacts the skin of an animal, one of several alternatives will ensue. The fungus may be removed mechanically, but may be prevented from invading the skin due to host resistance; or it may invade the skin, but not produce disease; or the fungus may invade the skin and produce disease.

Several factors are involved in the production of dermatomycosis. The fungus invades the hair shaft and weakens it, which makes the hair shaft susceptible to breakage. During the downward growth of the fungus on the hair shaft or follicular epithelium, metabolic products are produced. When these soluble, irritant toxins or allergens reach the dermal vasculature, they cause an inflammatory response which is detrimental to the fungal growth. If an irritant reaction to the metabolic products occurs, a mild, irritant contact dermatitis is manifested with erythema and scaling. If an allergic reaction occurs, there is inflammation with edema, suppuration, and necrosis. The inflammatory reaction to the fungal growth causes hypertrophy of the corneal layer of the hair follicle and surface of the epidermis (hyperkeratosis), resulting in increased scale formation and the plugging of the hair follicle. If bacteria are trapped in the follicle, bacterial folliculitis may develop. The fungus must grow downward at a rate equal to normal desquamation of the epidermis, or the organism will be shed. The hairs in the telogen stage will be shed without fungal invasion and growth.

Young or debilitated animals appear to be more susceptible to fungal infections. This may be the result of differences in structure and physiology of the skin at different ages, including differences relative to nutritional, immunologic, and hormonal factors. There is some evidence that vitamin A deficiency predisposes the skin to susceptibility to dermatophyte infection. A resistance to recurrent dermatophytosis develops in some animals following initial infection.

History. Young dogs and cats are often seen with a history of a slowly progressive focal or multifocal alopecic, proliferative skin disease. Pruritus is absent to minimal in most dermatophyte infections in young animals.

The history for older dogs and cats with dermatomycosis varies. Most older animals have a chronic skin disease with variable degrees of alopecia, inflammation, and pruritus. Frequently these animals are characterized by a poor response to antibiotics and corticosteroids. A poor clinical response to an inadequate griseofulvin trial is often reported. Some animals have a drug history of long-term immunosuppressive therapy with corticosteroids or chemotherapeutic agents prior to the onset of the fungal disease.

There may be a history of contagion between animals or between animals and man for all three species of common dermatophytes. In some households, there may be a history of human dermatophyte infection while all animals in the same household are asymptomatic.

Clinical Signs. The lesions of dermatomycosis vary; the most common are circular or irregular alopecic patches with variable degrees of inflammation. There may be erythemic plaques as well as heavy scales and crust. In general, T. mentagrophytes causes the most severe inflammatory response on both dogs and cats. Large areas of the body are frequently involved with erythema and scale or crust (Plate 6:A). Microsporum gypseum is usually characterized by proliferative hyperkeratotic lesions, mainly about the face and feet (Plate 6:B). Lesions caused by M. canis infection in dogs and cats vary from a mild, alopecic, slightly

erythemic focal lesion to marked generalized scaling or severe crusting (Plate 6:C to F). Dermatomycosis of the nails (onychomycosis), observed mostly in dogs, is manifested by distorted claws that break easily and grow improperly; they may fall off. The nail bed is often inflamed, and painful when palpated. Many cats and a few dogs are asymptomatic carriers of dermatophytes, most commonly M. canis.

A less common clinical presentation of dermatomycosis is a papulopustular form with no significant scaling. Staphylococcal infection is frequently superimposed on this form. A kerion is occasionally seen, which is characterized by a sharply demarcated, raised, erythematous, hairless nodule (Plate 6:G). Draining suppurative tracts may be associated with the kerion.

Diagnosis. There are three routine methods used for diagnosing dermatomycosis. The Wood's light (Fig. 7–1), if used properly in a totally darkened room, detects approximately 50% of M. canis infections. A tryptophane metabolite is the fluorescing material. The direct microscopic examination, using KOH-DMSO to identify fungal hyphae or spores, requires an experienced technician in order to achieve a high degree of success. The most reliable definitive diagnostic test for superficial fungal infection is a culture using DTM (Plate 6:H,I), or Sabouraud's medium and subsequent identification of the fungus by microscopic examination of microconidia and macroconidia (Figs. 7–2 to 7–6). The procedures for these three diagnostic tests are discussed in Chapter 2. Specific identification of the dermatophyte grown on the culture should always be made. This is especially important if human contagion is suspected, since it may aid in identifying the source of the human infection.

Cutaneous biopsy is sometimes used to diagnose dermatomycosis. Biopsy is indicated if a fungal infection is suspected but no pathogenic growth

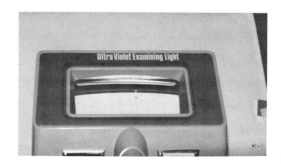

Fig. 7–1. Wood's lamp (ultraviolet lamp) used as a screening diagnostic test for Microsporum canis infection.

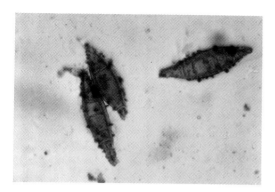

Fig. 7–2. Microsporum canis: Macroconidia with a thick wall and more than six cells.

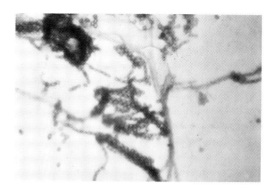

Fig. 7–5. Penicillium spp.: Small, round conidia in un-branched chains giving "paint brush" appearance.

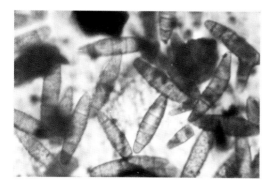

Fig. 7–3. Microsporum gypseum: Macroconidia with a thin wall and six or less cells.

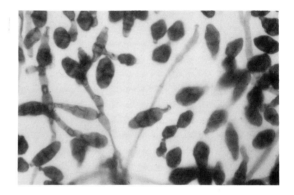

Fig. 7–6. Alternaria spp.: Macroconidia with longitudinal and transverse divisions.

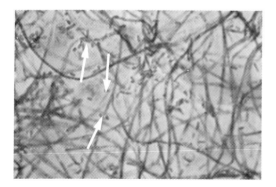

Fig. 7–4 Trichophyton mentagrophytes: Tear-drop shaped microconidia (arrows).

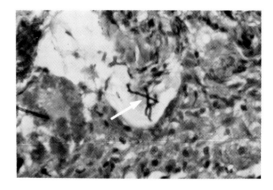

Fig. 7–7. Dermatomycosis: Microscopic section with fungal hyphae (arrow) in stratum corneum (high power).

is obtained on fungal culture, or if a skin condition has been unresponsive to antibiotics and corti-costeroids. Most pathologists can identify fungal hyphae (Fig. 7–7) and spores (Fig. 7–8) on routine hematoxylin and eosin (H & E) stains, or with special stains such as periodic acid-schiff (PAS).

Treatment. There are four therapeutic principles to consider when treating dermatomycosis. These include disinfecting the environment, preventing recontamination of the environment, and

using topical and systemic fungicides (Fungal Disease Therapeutic Key, Appendix 2:10).

The environment may be disinfected by using tamed iodine or hypochlorite solutions on all washable surfaces. Furniture and carpets should be vacuumed well, washable bedding should be laundered, and thorough cleaning is recommended.

Preventing recontamination of the environment can be partially achieved by frequent vacuuming

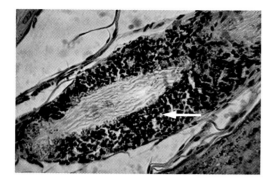

Fig. 7–8. Dermatomycosis: Microscopic section with numerous fungal spores around hair shaft (arrow) (high power).

and disinfecting the environment, by isolating the animals(s) to an area with a washable surface, and by using topical fungicidal agents. Routinely clipping the hair from local lesions and totally clipping the body of dogs and long-haired cats with generalized lesions will help reduce contamination of the environment.

Bathing weekly with a tamed iodine, sulfurated lime, captan, or chlorhexidine solution is recommended to prevent reinfecting the dog or cat as well as recontaminating the environment. Topical fungicidal agents such as miconazole nitrate, clotrimazol, cuprimyxin, and thiobendazole are helpful for treating localized dermatomycosis. Refer to the Fungal Disease Therapeutic Key (Appendix 2:10) for the specific protocols.

Griseofulvin (Fulvicin-U/F, Schering), a fungistatic drug, is the systemic treatment of choice for dermatomycosis. Better intestinal absorption of the drug is achieved with the addition of fat to the diet. There is a wide dosage range although doses ranging from 90 to 132 mg/kg/day PO usually result in the fastest clinical response. An ultramicrosize form of griseofulvin (Gris-PEG, Dorsey), requires one half the dosage and is absorbed without additional dietary fat supplementation. All treatments with griseofulvin should be given daily and continued for at least 2 weeks beyond apparent clinical recovery, resulting in a minimum treatment time of 6 weeks in most dogs and cats. Griseofulvin is teratogenic, therefore, it should never be given to a pregnant animal.

Ketoconazole is reported to be an efficacious drug in human dermatophytosis. Experience with ketoconazole in animals is limited. A suggested dose is 11 mg/kg bid or tid. This drug is not approved for use in dogs and cats.

Daily therapeutic doses of griseofulvin and weekly antifungal baths for 2 weeks are recommended as a prophylactic treatment for asymptomatic animals in an infected household. One massive dose of griseofulvin (200 to 220 mg/kg) is also reported to be an effective preventative for exposed, asymptomatic animals. Refer to the Fungal Disease Therapeutic Key (Appendix 2:10) for specific protocols.

Prognosis. The prognosis for dermatomycosis in dogs and cats is variable; treatment may be necessary for weeks to years. Generally there is a better prognosis for rapid and complete recovery in young dogs and cats. The poorest prognosis must be given for older animals with long-standing dermatomycosis and for any animal with onychomycosis, recurrent dermatophytosis, or concurrent debilitating and/or immunosuppressive disease or therapy.

SUBCUTANEOUS (INTERMEDIATE) MYCOSES

Sporotrichosis

Sporotrichosis is caused by a dimorphic soil saprophyte, Sporothrix schenckii. The saprophytic form exists in nature and the parasitic form is an oval or elongated budding yeast in the tissues.

Pathogenesis. The fungus usually penetrates the skin following a traumatic injury that breaks the epidermal barrier. There also have been reports of infection caused by inhalation or ingestion of the fungus. The saprophytic form lives in the soil, on plants, in water, and on small insects. It is commonly found in warm, moist climates.

Following entrance of the organism, tissue invasion occurs with penetration into the subcutis and often into the lymphatic vessels, with subsequent penetration into the regional lymph nodes. There may be further spread by way of the lymphatics from the regional lymph nodes to most organs of the body. The fungus elicits a chronic inflammatory response with shallow cutaneous ulcers, nodules, and granulomas.

Clinical Signs. Sporotrichosis is characterized by three distribution patterns: cutaneous, cutaneolymphatic, and disseminated. The skin lesions include firm, round, tender nodules and crusted ulcers in the subcutis associated with a traumatized site (Plate 5:J,K). A thick, brownish-red exudate may be present. Often the nodules are found along the lymphatics. The regional lymph nodes may be swollen and ulcerative. In both dogs and cats the disseminated form may be seen with involvement of many organs, especially the lungs and liver.

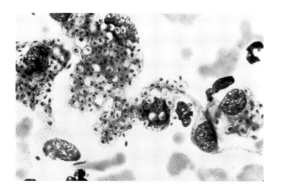

Diagnosis. Fungal culture of aspirated exudate or affected tissue on Sabouraud's medium is the diagnostic test of choice. The yeast phase may be observed in direct smears of exudate (Fig. 7–9), impression smears of tissue (Fig. 7–10), or in microscopic sections from biopsy specimens using special fungal stains.

Treatment. The treatment of choice is administration of 20% sodium iodide. A good response from animals with the cutaneolymphatic form of sporotrichosis is expected within 30 days; however, to prevent relapse, therapy should be continued for an additional 3 to 4 weeks. Cats treated with sodium iodide may manifest iodine toxicity characterized by vomiting, anorexia, depression, muscular twitching, cardiovascular collapse, and death. Animals with the disseminated form of sporotrichosis do not respond well to sodium iodide therapy. Amphotericin B is the drug of choice for animals with this form of disease (Fungal Disease Therapeutic Key, Appendix 2:10).

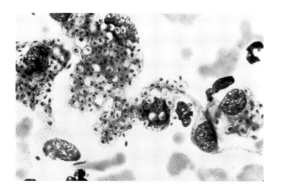

Fig. 7–9. Sporothrix schenckii: Direct smear of exudate from sporotrichosis lesion with numerous phagocytized yeast bodies (high power). (Courtesy of Nita Gulbas.)

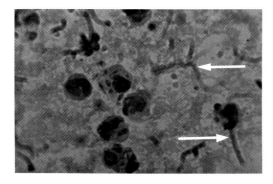

Fig. 7–10. Sporothrix schenckii: Impression smear of surface of sporotrichosis lesion with septate hyphae (arrows) (high power). (Courtesy of Nita Gulbas.)

Zygomycosis

Zygomycosis, formerly known as phycomycosis, is caused by several fungi of the class Zygomycetes. Members of the genera Mucor, Rhizopus, Absidia, Hyphomyces, Entomophthora, and Basidiobolus have been isolated from lesions.

Pathogenesis. Zygomycetes are usually associated with soil, water, or decaying vegetation. They are opportunistic organisms that gain entrance into the skin following a traumatic injury. The most common form of zygomycosis in dogs is gastrointestinal, in which infection occurs following ingestion. In the cutaneous form the organism elicits a granulomatous response in the subcutaneous tissue.

History. There appears to be a breed predilection for German Shepherd dogs. Age of occurrence is usually 2 to 4 years. Zygomycosis is observed primarily in warm, moist climates such as the southeastern region of the United States. Most affected dogs have some history associated with swimming. There is usually a drug history of poor response to therapy, which includes antibiotics and surgical excision.

Clinical Signs. The subcutaneous form of zygomycosis is characterized by raised, granulomatous lesions often accompanied by fistulous tracts and a thick exudate, usually on the extremities or near the base of the tail. There may be ulcerations and necrosis of the oral cavity with the gastrointestinal form. Physical examination may reveal abdominal masses.

Diagnosis. Wet mounts of exudate should be examined in 10 to 20% KOH for wide, nonseptate hyphae. Staining the preparation with India ink may be helpful. Aspirated exudate from an unopened lesion should be cultured on Sabouraud's medium. A biopsy of the granuloma often reveals broad, nonseptate hyphae involved in the lesion.

Treatment. The treatment of choice is complete surgical excision of the lesions. Cryotherapy and intravenous administration of amphotericin B have been suggested as adjunctive therapy.

Prognosis. Prognosis for zygomycosis is poor since there is usually recurrence following therapy.

Mycetoma

Etiologic Factors Mycetoma is caused by two groups of fungi. Actinomycotic agents include Actinomyces, Nocardia, Actinomadura, and Streptomyces. Eumycotic agents include Allescheria boydii, Curvularia geniculata, and Madurella spp.

Pathogenesis. The normal habitat of the fungi

is soil or plants. Penetration of the skin usually follows traumatic injury to the extremities. Once the fungi penetrate the subcutaneous tissue, they elicit an inflammatory reaction characterized by swelling, abscessation, and fistulous tracts. The fungi can invade deeper into the periosteum.

History and Clinical Signs. Animals with mycetoma generally do not respond well to the administration of nonsulfa antibiotics. The classical signs include swelling and fistulous tracts. Ulcerations of the involved area can occur. Lesions are usually found on the extremities, especially on the feet.

Diagnosis. Wet mounts of crushed granules examined in 10 to 20% KOH reveal hyphae and chlamydospores if the cause is a eumycotic fungus. The granules should be washed several times in sterile saline solution, crushed and streaked onto Sabouraud's medium and blood agar. A biopsy of the lesions may reveal a pyogranulomatous reaction with mycelial elements (Fig. 7–11).

Treatment. Eumycotic mycetoma is best treated by radical surgical excision. Actinomycotic mycetoma is most commonly treated with a combination of surgical excision and antibiotics. Penicillin or ampicillin combined with trimethoprim and sulfadiazine has been recommended (Fungal Disease Therapeutic Key, Appendix 2:10).

Aspergillosis

Etiologic Factors. Aspergillus fumigatus and A. flavus are species most frequently isolated. They are commonly found in most environments, both on and off animals. Feline aspergillosis is rarely seen.

Pathogenesis. The respiratory tract is the most common site of Aspergillus spp. infection. Other areas of involvement include the eyes and gas-

trointestinal tract. Involvement of the skin is usually a manifestation of generalized aspergillosis.

Skin infection can occur following immune suppression caused by disease, drugs, or other causes of debilitation. Such infections are the result of direct contact with the fungus spores. The specific mechanisms involved with the production of lesions vary and depend on predisposing factors such as immune status, integrity of epidermal barrier, and concurrent disease.

History and Clinical Signs. A dog with aspergillosis is generally examined for a history of sneezing for several weeks, usually accompanied by a nasal discharge. Neurologic signs, weight loss, diarrhea, conjunctivitis, and blepharitis may be seen on physical examination. A generalized or focal chronic skin lesion, which does not respond well to antibiotics and corticosteroids, may be present. The gross appearance of skin lesions caused by Aspergillus spp. varies from ulcers to granulomas.

Diagnosis. The finding of septate hyphae and characteristic conidiophores on examination of direct smears of lesions in KOH preparations supports the diagnosis, but association with the disease process must be demonstrated. A combination of fungal cultures and biopsy, in which tissue invasion and resultant inflammatory reaction associated with septate hyphae are observed, are necessary to establish a diagnosis of cutaneous aspergillosis. Specimens for culture must be obtained as aseptically as possible.

Treatment. There is no satisfactory treatment for generalized cutaneous aspergillosis. Focal lesions may be surgically excised. The nasal form is treated with surgery and amphotericin B. Alternative therapy includes administration of potassium iodide, 5–fluorouracil, and thiabendazole (Fungal Disease Therapeutic Key, Appendix 2:10).

SYSTEMIC MYCOSES

Systemic mycoses are characterized by primary pulmonary infection with subsequent dissemination to other organs. The pulmonary infection may be subclinical and resolve without clinical signs. Inhalation is the route of most infections. There is no known contagion of systemic mycoses between animals or between animals and man.

Blastomycosis

Etiologic Factors. Blastomycosis is caused by Blastomyces dermatitidis, a dimorphic fungus. It is endemic in the eastern United States and parts

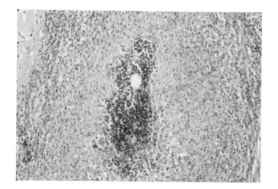

Fig. 7–11. Fungal granuloma: Microscopic section from a cutaneous nodule from which Nocardia spp. was cultured. Note dermal granulomatous reaction. No fungal organisms are observed (high power).

of southern Canada. Areas drained by rivers have the highest incidence.

Pathogenesis. In nature the fungus is in the mycelial or saprophytic phase. Growth of the saprophytic stage requires high humidity. Pulmonary infection occurs following inhalation of spores and dissemination to the skin, eyes, and bone may occur by way of the blood or lymphatic vessels. Altered immune function, especially cell-mediated, appears to predispose to dissemination of the disease. On microscopic examination of tissue, B. dermatitidis appears as a large, thick-walled budding yeast of 8 to 20 μm in diameter. The yeast phase elicits a tissue inflammatory response manifested by suppuration and granulomatous reactions.

History and Clinical Signs. Animals with the disseminated form of blastomycosis are affected with a chronic debilitating disease beginning with respiratory signs which are followed by eye and skin lesions. Clinical signs include pyrexia, emaciation, lethargy, coughing, dyspnea, and anorexia. Peripheral lymph nodes are frequently enlarged and often draining. Skin lesions seen most frequently include cutaneous and subcutaneous abscesses, ulcers, draining tracts, and granulomas (Plate 6:L,M).

Diagnosis. History of concurrent respiratory, skin, and eye lesions in an endemic blastomycosis area is suggestive. Specific diagnostic tests include direct smears of lesions demonstrating the large, thick-walled budding yeasts with double-contoured walls and cutaneous biopsy showing a pyogranulomatous reaction associated with the budding yeast (Fig. 7–12). Isolation of the fungus performed by a reference laboratory is diagnostic, but growth may be slow or nonexistent. Serologic diagnosis using the complement fixation test is supportive, but cross-reactions do occur between histoplasmosis and blastomycosis.

Treatment. Intravenous administration of amphotericin B is the standard treatment for blastomycosis. 5–Fluorouracil may be used. There are some reports of better results using combination therapy with amphotericin B and tetracycline in dogs (Fungal Disease Therapeutic Key, Appendix 2:10).

Histoplasmosis

Etiologic Factors. Histoplasmosis is caused by Histoplasma capsulatum, a dimorphic fungus. It is endemic in the Great Lakes region, Appalachian Mountains, and the Mississippi, Ohio, and St. Lawrence river valleys of the United States. Histoplasmosis has been found in most areas of the world.

Pathogenesis. Histoplasmosis is found in nature in the mycelial or saprophytic form. It is often associated with soil contaminated by bird or bat feces. Infection occurs when small microaleuriospores are inhaled into the alveolar spaces of the lung. In the tissue the fungus transforms into tiny, intracellular oval bodies measuring 2 to 4 μm in diameter and can be found in the reticuloendothelial cells. Dissemination from the lungs is uncommon, but when it does occur the intestinal tract is usually involved. Occasionally dissemination to the skin occurs by way of the lymphatic or blood vessels. Tissue reaction to the yeast is that of suppuration and granuloma formation.

History and Clinical Signs. The history is usually that of an animal with chronic respiratory disease with subsequent enteritis and the development of focal skin lesions that do not respond to antibiotics and steroids. The clinical signs include chronic cough, gradual weight loss, persistent or intermittent diarrhea, lethargy, and anorexia. The skin lesions include granulomas, ulcers, abscesses, or fistulous tracts.

Diagnosis. The diagnosis of histoplasmosis is based on identifying the yeast within reticuloendothelial cells from lymph nodes (Fig. 7–13), cutaneous biopsy specimens and from isolating the organism on Sabouraud's medium. The diagnosis is supported by complement fixation tests. Cross-reactions do occur with blastomycosis and coccidioidomycosis.

Treatment. Histoplasmosis is treated with intravenous administration of amphotericin B (Fungal Disease Therapeutic Key, Appendix 2:10).

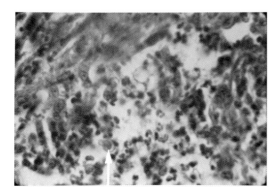

Fig. 7–12. Blastomycosis: Microscopic section with budding yeasts of Blastomyces dermatitidis in a dermal granuloma (arrow) (high power). (Courtesy of J. MacDonald.)

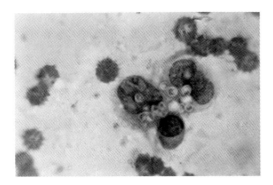

Fig. 7–13. Histoplasmosis: Yeast phase of Histoplasma capsulatum phagocytized by macrophages in aspiration biopsy of a lymph node (high power). (Courtesy of Robert Wilkins.)

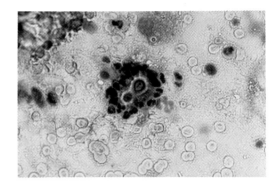

Fig. 7–14. Cryptococcosis: Budding yeast of Cryptococcosus neoformans in a direct smear of exudate (high power). (Courtesy of Robert Wilkins.)

Cryptococcosis

Etiologic Factors. Cryptococcosis is caused by a soilborne fungus, Cryptococcus neoformans, which has a worldwide distribution. The fungus is associated with soil contaminated by excreta of bats, pigeons, and other birds.

Pathogenesis. The yeast form of C. neoformans is found in nature as well as in the tissue. It is 4 to 7 μm in diameter and surrounded by a polysaccharide capsule. The pulmonary system is the primary site of infection, which occurs by inhaling the fungus. Most of the lesions are localized to the head area; included are the oral, nasal, and pharyngeal mucosae; the skin is occasionally affected. The central nervous system (CNS), bone (especially nasal turbinates), facial sinuses, and lymph nodes may be involved. The means of dissemination is primarily by the blood and lymphatic vessels. Direct extension from the oropharynx has been suggested. Animals with an altered immune system may predisposed to disseminated cryptococcosis.

History and Clinical Signs. The history often includes a chronic course of multiple facial lesions that are unresponsive to antibiotics and corticosteroids. The clinical signs are variable. There may be oral, pharyngeal, or nasal mucosal ulcerations, involvement of the nasal turbinates, facial sinuses, facial bones, and CNS signs such as incoordination or blindness. The skin lesions consist of ulcerations, granulomas (Plate 6:N), and occasionally abscesses containing a mucoid exudate.

Diagnosis. Diagnosis of cryptococcosis is based on demonstration of the encapsulated budding yeast by means of a direct smear of the exudate (Fig. 7–14) or in tissue biopsy.

Treatment. Intravenous amphotericin B is used to treat cryptococcosis. The use of miconazole and

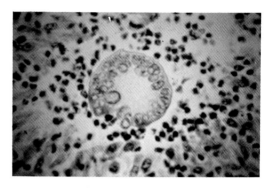

Fig. 7–15. Coccidioidomycosis: Coccidioides immitis spherules with endospores in an aspiration biopsy of a lymph node (high power). (Courtesy of Robert Wilkins.)

5-fluorouracil has also been recommended (Fungal Disease Therapeutic Key, Appendix 2:10).

Coccidioidomycosis

Etiologic Factors. Coccidioidomycosis is caused by a dimorphic fungus, Coccidioides immitis, which is endemic to the arid southwestern United States and northern Mexico.

Pathogenesis. Coccidioides immitis exists in nature in the mycelial form. In tissue it is a thick-walled spherule, 20 to 60 μm in diameter, with endospores. The mycelial form is often associated with rodent burrows. The organism grows in the soil during periods of rainfall. Infection occurs by inhalation of spores associated with dust and other fomites especially during dry periods of the year.

Often the disease remains localized to the respiratory system, and is sometimes asymptomatic. There is occasional dissemination to bones and skin. Altered cellular immunity is believed to be a predisposing factor to dissemination of coccidioidomycosis.

History and Clinical Signs. The age of onset

of canine coccidiodomycosis is usually less than 2 years; there is no age predilection in felines. Intermittent respiratory signs are usually observed prior to evidence of lesions. Episodes of coughing and intermittent pyrexia, anorexia, dyspnea, listlessness, weight loss, and lymphadenopathy with drainage of the lymph nodes are often reported. Lameness is common in the disseminated form. There is a history of poor clinical response to systemic treatment.

Skin lesions associated with coccidioidomycosis in dogs include granulomas, subcutaneous abscesses, indolent ulcers, and fistulous tracts. Abscesses are the most common lesions in cats with the disease.

Diagnosis. Supportive evidence of coccidioidomycosis is obtained with history of exposure to an endemic area, radiographic evidence of lung and bone lesions, and positive precipitin and complement fixation tests. Demonstration of the thick-walled refractile spherules containing endospores can be made by means of a direct smear of lymph node aspirates (Fig. 7–15), or by identifying endospores in tissue biopsy.

Treatment. Coccidioidomycosis is treated with intravenous amphotericin B (Fungal Disease Therapeutic Key, Appendix 2:10).

SELECTED READINGS

Adler, P.C.: Phycomycosis in fifteen dogs and two cats. J. Am. Vet. Med. Assoc. 174:1216, 1979.

Attleberger, M.: Cutaneous manifestation of mycotic disease in dogs. Gaines Vet. Symp. October, 1979.

Barbee, W.C., et al.: Sporotrichosis in the domestic cat. Am. J. Pathol. 86:281, 1977.

Barrett R.E., and Scott, D.W.: Treatment of feline cryptococcosis: Literature review and case report. J. Am. Anim. Hosp. Assoc. 11:511, 1975.

Blakemore, J.C.: Diagnosis of dermatophyte infection. Part II. Pract. Vet. 47:8, 1975.

————: Diagnosis of dermatophyte infection. Part I. Pract. Vet. 46:15, 1974.

Campbell, K.L., Humphrey, J.A., and Ramsey, G.H.: Cutaneous blastomycosis. Feline Pract. 10:28, 1980.

Chester, D.K.: Superficial fungal infection of the skin. Compend. Cont. Ed. Pract. Vet. 1:910, 1979.

Fadok, V.A.: Dermatologic manifestations of the subcutaneous and deep mycoses. Compend. Cont. Ed. Pract. Vet. 2:506, 1980.

Ford, R.B.: Canine histoplasmosis. Compend. Cont. Ed. Pract. Vet. 2:637, 1980.

Greer, D.L.: Agents of zygomycosis (phycomycosis). In Manual of Clinical Microbiology, 3rd Ed. Edited by E.H. Lennette, et al. Washington D.C., American Society for Microbiology, 1980.

Lewis, G.E., Jr, et al.: Mycetoma in a cat. J. Am. Vet. Med. Assoc. 161:500, 1972.

Jasmin, A.M., et al.: Systemic blastomycosis in Siamese cats. Vet. Med./Small Anim. Clin. 64:33, 1969.

Mahaffey, E., et al.: Disseminated histoplasmosis in three cats. J. Am. Anim. Hosp. Assoc. 13:46, 1977.

Padhye, A.A., and Ajello, L.: Fungi causing eumycotic mycetomas. In Manual of Clinical Microbiology, 3rd Ed. Edited by E.H. Lennette, et al. Washington, D.C., American Society for Microbiology, 1980.

Pyle, R.L., et al.: Canine blastomycosis. Compend. Cont. Ed. Pract. Vet. 3:963, 1981.

Reedy, L.M.: Feline miliary dermatitis with emphasis on dermatomycosis. Compend. Cont. Ed. Pract. Vet. 2:833, 1980.

Scott, D.W.: Fungal disorders. J. Am. Anim. Hosp. Assoc. 16:349, 1980.

Scott, D.W., Bentinck-Smith, J., and Haggerty, G.F.: Sporotrichosis in three dogs. Cornell Vet. 64:416, 1974.

Werner, R.E., et al.: Sporotrichosis in a cat. J. Am. Vet. Med. Assoc. 159:407, 1971.

8

Endocrine Diseases

Endocrine disorders are relatively common in the dog and uncommon in the cat. The Endocrine Diagnostic Key (Appendix 1:7) lists the most pertinent historical and clinical findings and diagnostic tests necessary to differentiate the common canine and feline endocrine dermatoses.

HYPOTHYROIDISM

Canine hypothyroidism is characterized by a decreased level of circulating thyroid hormone. Clinical feline hypothyroidism has been rarely reported. Decreased circulating concentrations of thyroid hormone have not been reported in the cat.

Etiologic Factors. There are several pathophysiologic mechanisms that may lead to hypothyroidism. The most common cause of primary hypothyroidism in the dog is atrophy of the thyroid gland, usually associated with lymphocytic thyroiditis. Other causes are classified as idiopathic atrophy. Congenital thyroid agenesis is rare. Secondary hypothyroidism is caused by a lack of thyroid-stimulating hormone (TSH). This may be the result of either congenital hypopituitarism or an acquired disorder associated with pituitary neoplasia. Other potential causes of hypothyroidism include iodine deficiency, dyshormonogenesis (an intrinsic defect in synthesis of thyroid hormone), a defect in the transport of thyroid hormone, a peripheral defect in the conversion of thyroxine (T_4) to triiodothyronine (T_3), and

inappropriate deiodination of T_4 associated with an excess of reverse T_3. All of these conditions are uncommon. Dietary insufficiency of iodine leading to atrophy of the thyroid gland has been reported in the cat.

Thyroid Physiology. The canine thyroid gland secretes two hormones, T_4 and T_3, in a ratio of 20:1. The large majority of both hormones are bound to plasma proteins. The unbound or free thyroid hormones are those available for the tissues. The binding affinity of plasma proteins for T_4 is lower in dogs than in man. Thus the total T_4 concentration is lower, the unbound or free T_4 is higher, and the hormone turnover is more rapid in dogs than in man. Approximately 40% of the extrathyroidal T_4 is in the plasma; the majority of the remaining portion is taken up by the liver where conversion to T_3 occurs. Although there is controversy concerning the biologic activity of T_4 and T_3, it is generally agreed that T_3 is the most biologically active. However, there is some evidence that T_4 also has intrinsic biologic activity. Although diurnal oscillations of thyroid hormone plasma levels occur, they do not seem to be clinically significant.

Extrathyroidal T_4 is metabolized two ways—45% by deiodination and 55% by fecal excretion. Approximately 70% of T_3 is metabolized by deiodination and 30% by fecal excretion. Fecal excretion contributes to the inefficiency of hormone utilization and raises the level of tolerance to exogenous thyroid hormone.

The half-life of T_4 is 24 hours; the peak plasma or serum level occurs 4 to 12 hours following thyroid replacement. The half-life of T_3 is approximately 3 to 4 hours, with a peak blood level occurring approximately 3 hours after administering the hormone.

Serum or plasma thyroid hormone levels are lowered by the administration of several drugs including glucocorticoids, phenytoin, phenobarbital, and phenylbutazone. Levels of T_3 are more susceptible to the influence of corticosteroids than T_4; thus, stress conditions can result in a rather sudden and sustained decrease in T_3 concentrations. Long-term corticosteroid influence, either endogenous or exogenous in origin, results in a marked decrease of both T_3 and T_4.

There are several important actions of thyroid hormones which correlate with the clinical signs observed in a hypothyroid animal. The most pronounced action of both T_3 and T_4 is the stimulation of metabolism in the tissues resulting in an increased oxygen consumption. These thyroid hormones activate the enzyme systems which are responsible for oxidation processes. These hormones also promote growth and development of tissue, regulate lipid metabolism, increase the absorption of carbohydrates from the intestine, and influence function of the CNS.

The major modulator of thyroid-hormone production is thought to be TSH, which is secreted by the anterior pituitary gland. TSH is regulated at the level of the anterior pituitary by the antagonistic effects of thyroid hormone and TSH-releasing hormone (TRH), which is released by the hypothalamus.

History. The historical findings in dogs with hypothyroidism are variable. There is a reported breed predilection for the English Bulldog, Golden Retriever, Irish Setter, Basenji, and Great Dane. The breeds of Doberman Pinscher, Poodle, Dachshund, Schnauzer, and Boxer have also been identified as having a higher incidence of hypothyroidism than the general population. The age of onset of clinical signs associated with hypothyroidism is usually 2 to 5 years, although the disease has been reported in younger dogs. The two most common owner observations are diminished physical activity denoted by fatigue, lethargy, and increased sleeping time and hair coat changes. Slow regrowth of hair after clipping for a routine procedure may be the primary complaint. There may be a history of sensitivity to cold manifested

by the avoidance of cold areas and the seeking out of warm areas such as heat vents or radiators.

Clinical Signs. Clinical signs are variable. In an untreated dog they tend to increase in number and severity with age. However, the primary problem in one dog may remain a minor problem or be nonexistent in another dog. Many owners do not recognize the signs of hypothyroidism since there is minimal opportunity for dogs living in cities or densely populated suburban areas to exercise, and the signs are generally characterized by minimal changes over a prolonged period of time.

Often a dog is examined for one or more changes in the hair coat. These changes include dryness, dullness, coarseness, and sparseness. Alopecia on pressure points or wear areas such as the posterior thighs and the neck beneath a collar is common (Plate 7:A,B). Alopecic patterns may be small, multifocal areas (Plate 7:C) or occasionally total alopecia (Plate 7:D). Changes in the skin can include hyperpigmentation, thickened skin, scaling, and variable degrees of seborrheic dermatitis. Some edema of the facial folds and periorbital skin may cause a tragic expression. Superficial pyoderma is commonly associated with hypothyroidism. Large breed dogs tend to have more skin and hair coat changes on the extremities starting at an earlier age; in small- and medium-sized dogs, trunkal signs predominate.

Obesity is variable, although the majority of hypothyroid dogs are near normal in weight. Subtle changes in cardiac function may be manifested by a slow heart rate, weak apex beat and pulse, and low voltage on an electrocardiogram. Abnormal sexual activity may be noted in intact animals: females may have a shortened estrus or prolonged anestrus and infertility, and males may show a lack of libido. Clinical laboratory findings may include borderline normocytic, normochromic anemia, hypercholesterolemia, and elevated serum creatinine phosphokinase. Studies have not shown any correlation between clinical signs and the class of hypothyroidism based on low T_3, T_4, or combined low serum levels.

Signs of protracted dietary insufficiency of iodine causing thyroid gland atrophy in the cat include stunted growth, short, sparse coats, thickened skin, and edema of the tissues of the head. Other signs associated with feline hypothyroidism are bilateral symmetric alopecia, dry, easily epilated hair coat, obesity, lethargy, and bradycardia.

Diagnosis. The diagnosis of canine hypothyroidism is based on history, clinical signs, quantitation of baseline serum or plasma thyroid hormone levels, results of TSH-response testing, and therapeutic trials. Thyroid biopsy has been used as a satisfactory diagnostic test for secondary hypothyroidism in veterinary clinics in Europe. Results of skin biopsy showing hyperkeratosis and epidermal and sebaceous gland atrophy are consistent with endocrine dermatoses, but not diagnostic for hypothyroidism (Fig. 8–1).

Quantitation is predominantly based on radioimmunoassay (RIA) of T_4 and T_3 blood levels. Although veterinary reference laboratories vary in regard to normal values, a T_4 level value of <1.5 μg/dl is generally considered low and a T_3 serum or plasma value of <50 ng/dl is low; however, values between 50 and 70 ng/dl are considered low by some laboratories. Human reference laboratories must make an adjustment in technique to accurately detect the low T_3 and T_4 values of canine blood.

The finding of low baseline T_4 and T_3 values constitutes a good screening test for hypothyroidism, although it is not possible to distinguish between primary, secondary, or drug-induced hypothyroidism in this way. The TSH-response test is used to identify primary hypothyroidism. The technique involves obtaining a baseline T_4 value, injecting 0.5 IU of TSH/kg of body weight intravenously, and determining a 4-hour poststimulation T_4 value; T_3 values associated with TSH stimulation are not diagnostic. In primary hypothyroidism there is minimal response following TSH stimulation. In both secondary and drug-induced hypothyroidism, the stimulation of 2 to 3

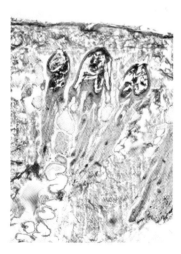

Fig. 8–1. Hypothyroidism: Microscopic section with follicular plugging and atrophy of the epidermis and sebaceous glands (scan power).

times the baseline approximates the stimulation in the normal dog even though the baseline is lower; thus a definitive diagnosis of hypothyroidism is not obtained. Thyroid biopsy is the most conclusive diagnostic test to confirm secondary hypothyroidism.

A therapeutic trial is one of the most practical and economical diagnostic tests for hypothyroidism. It is an alternative to the TSH-response test, which establishes the clinical significance of a borderline or low T_4 blood level. A treatment trial is initiated with L-thyroxine at 20 to 22 μg/kg of body weight once or twice a day. If primary or secondary hypothyroidism is the problem, there should be some clinical response within 4 to 6 weeks, and a good response within 2 to 3 months in most animals. If there is drug-induced hypothyroidism or hyperadrenocorticism, there will be a minimal response to the therapeutic trial.

Some effort has been made to distinguish between T_4 hypothyroidism (low T_4, normal T_3), T_3 hypothyroidism (low T_3, normal T_4,) and T_3-T_4 hypothyroidism (low T_3, low T_4). Thus far a good correlation between clinical signs or treatment response based on the above subclassification has not been found. True T_3 hypothyroidism may represent a "euthyroid sick" category resulting from chronic systemic disease. A peripheral conversion problem of T_4 to T_3 may also be considered.

Treatment. There are several satisfactory treatment protocols for canine hypothyroidism. L-thyroxine is the most widely used replacement hormone; it is given once or twice daily. Triiodothyronine and combination T_3-T_4 products have been used with good clinical results (Endocrine Disease Therapeutic Key, Appendix 2:11). Treatment should be continued for a minimum of 3 to 4 months since treatment response time is variable. There is usually an increase in activity within 1 to 2 weeks if lethargy has been a problem. Hair coat and skin changes may require treatment for 1 to 4 months before a satisfactory clinical response is obtained. Lifetime therapy is usually required, although the dosage may be decreased in some dogs.

Post-Treatment Monitoring. Indications for therapeutic monitoring include an excessive or inadequate response to the standard recommended dosage of thyroid replacement, a change in the type or dosage of thyroid replacement, or the development of thyrotoxicosis. Several factors must be considered when using post-treatment serum or plasma T_3 and T_4 values to monitor therapeutic response or to decide on changes in therapy. The best time to monitor T_3 and T_4 concentrations after treatment is dependent on the half-life of these hormones in the circulation. The maximal increase from baseline values occurs in approximately 3 hours for T_3 and 4 to 12 hours for T_4 following treatment with L-thyroxine. Peak blood levels for T_3 following triiodothyronine replacement are more variable and have not been determined accurately. If the dog is on T_3 replacement, the T_4 values will be depressed and of no interpretive value due to a negative feedback effect; thus, the monitoring of T_4 levels would not be indicated. The single most important criterion for therapeutic monitoring is the response to thyroid replacement based on physical examination and history. Post-treatment monitoring of serum thyroid hormones is most valuable when a poor response to replacement therapy is observed in the absence of other identifiable causes for the clinical signs.

A suggested protocol for the diagnosis, treatment, and monitoring of a dog with suspected hypothyroidism is outlined in Table 8–1.

HYPERADRENOCORTICISM

The terms hyperadrenocorticism, hypercortisolism, and Cushing's syndrome all refer to a general disease state resulting from a chronic excess of plasma cortisol. Hyperadrenocorticism is the second most common endocrine dermatosis in the dog and is rare in the cat.

Etiologic Factors. The most common cause (85 to 90%) of excessive cortisol levels is bilateral adrenocortical hyperplasia, which results from an excessive secretion of ACTH by the pituitary gland. This is classified as pituitary-dependent hyperadrenocorticism. Functional neoplasms of the adrenal cortex are found in 10 to 15% of dogs with Cushing's syndrome. These neoplasms secrete cortisol independent of pituitary control. Long-term exogenous corticosteroid administration can cause iatrogenic Cushing's syndrome.

Pathogenesis. Cortisol influences the function of most body systems. An excess of cortisol causes atrophy of the hair follicles and sebaceous glands, which leads to the development of alopecia. Inhibition of fibroblast activity results in atrophy of the collagen and fibroelastic tissue in the dermis. This leads to loss of the primary support of the skin, which results in thin skin and a pendulous abdomen.

Excess glycogen is accumulated within hepatocytes leading to impaired liver function and hepatomegaly. The catabolic action of cortisol causes rearrangement of the molecular structure

TABLE 8–1. PROTOCOL FOR THE DIAGNOSIS, TREATMENT, AND MONITORING OF A DOG WITH SUSPECTED HYPOTHYROIDISM

I. Diagnosis
  A. Obtain a good history
  B. Perform a thorough physical examination to rule out concurrent disease
  C. Determine pretreatment T_4 radioimmunoassay (RIA) serum or plasma concentration
  D. Determine pretreatment T_3 RIA serum or plasma concentration if economical or if baseline T_4 is not diagnostic
  E. TSH-response test may be done initially if economically feasible

II. Treatment
  A. Indications
    1. T_4 is < 1.5 µg/dl
    2. Poor response to TSH-stimulation test
    3. Low baseline T_3 (< 50 ng/dl) and T_4 (< 1.5 µg/dl)
  B. Drug and dosage
    Use thyroxine (T_4) at a dosage of 22 µg/kg BID for a minimum of 6 to 8 weeks before changing drug or dosage

III. Initial therapeutic monitoring
  A. If there is a good clinical response, decrease frequency of T_4 replacement to once daily
  B. If there is a poor or minimal clinical response, recheck T_4 concentrations at 4 hours post-T_4 treatment; if practical, recheck T_3 concentrations

IV. Action based on initial monitoring
  A. If T_4 concentrations are low, increase dosage of T_4 replacement
  B. If T_4 concentrations are normal, continue initial dosage and look for another cause for clinical signs
  C. If T_3 and T_4 concentrations are markedly low, consider changing to a combination T_3 and T_4 replacement therapy and look for concurrent problems (e.g., hyperadrenocorticism)
  D. If T_4 concentrations are normal or high, T_3 concentrations are < 30 ng/dl, and there is no concurrent stress or drug-induced hypothyroidism, initiate T_3 replacement alone or in combination with T_4

V. Further therapeutic monitoring
  A. Allow 2 to 3 months for a clinical response
  B. If a good clinical response is achieved, maintain dog on the lowest possible dose, adjusting as necessary
  C. If there is continued poor response to T_4 therapy, and no concurrent disease has been identified, recheck T_3 and T_4 serum or plasma values 4-hours post-treatment; if blood levels are adequate, look for another cause for clinical signs
  D. If there is continued poor response to T_3 therapy or combination T_3 and T_4 therapy, recheck T_3 serum levels 3- to 4-hours post-treatment; if blood levels are adequate, look for another cause for clinical signs

of collagen and elastic tissue, which leads to the dystrophic binding of calcium to the altered protein matrix. This manifests clinically as calcinosis cutis. The anti-inflammatory and immunosuppressive effects of cortisol excess result in secondary superficial pyoderma and systemic infection. Cortisol excess causes a collagen defect in vessel walls, which predisposes to an abnormal hemostatic reaction between collagen, platelets, and coagulation factors, leading to bruising and ecchymoses.

Anestrus and testicular atrophy are believed to result from the inhibition of gonadotrophin release by cortisol. The mechanisms of action of cortisol that lead to polydipsia, polyuria, polyphagia, and hyperpigmentation are not completely known.

History. The classical history associated with hyperadrenocorticism includes the signs of polydipsia, polyuria, and polyphagia in a middle-aged to older dog and in the few cats in which it has been reported. There is a breed predilection in Poodle, Dachshund, and Terrier breeds. Often there is a gradual, progressive, trunkal thinning of hair with the legs and head spared. A drug history of chronic corticosteroid therapy is not unusual. There may be prolonged anestrus in the female or lack of libido and infertility in the male. There may also be a history of pruritus and excoriation associated with focal proliferative lesions.

Clinical Findings. Physical examination of the dog with hyperadrenocorticism usually reveals hepatomegaly, and some distention of the abdomen, and various degrees of trunkal alopecia (Plate 7:E,F). This is often slowly progressive over a 6- to 12-month period from the time the hair coat starts thinning. A thin skin, often with comedone formation and prominent veins, is commonly found together with a distended abdomen (Plate 7:G). Mild to moderate hyperpigmentation may be observed in the alopecic areas. Hyperpigmentation occurs noticeably less in dogs with hyperadrenocorticism than in most dogs with hypothyroidism or gonadal dermatosis. Testicular and temporal muscle atrophy are observed in the longstanding disease. Cats with hyperadrenocorticism have pendulous abdomens, bilateral symmetric alopecia, and scaly, hyperpigmented skin.

Superficial pyoderma and urinary and respiratory tract infections are relatively common findings. There may be evidence of ecchymoses, especially following venipuncture (Plate 7:H). In a small percentage (10%) of dogs, calcinosis cutis is present. This is manifested by focal areas of proliferation of a silver-white, firm plaque, often found over the dorsal shoulder area. Tissue reaction to dermal calcium deposits varies from none (Plate 7:I) to marked (Plate 7:J).

Diagnosis. A tentative diagnosis of hyperadrenocorticism is based on the history and clinical findings. Screening clinical laboratory tests include a hemogram, total eosinophil count, blood chemistry, urinalysis, and thoracic and abdominal radiographs. Results of a hemogram usually reveal mild to moderate leukocytosis, neutrophilia, and mild lymphopenia (< 1000 lymphocytes/m³), and a total eosinophil count of < 200 cell/m³. Mild polycythemia is also common. An elevated alkaline phosphatase concentration occurs in most dogs with Cushing's syndrome. Mild to marked elevation of alanine aminotransferase (ALT, GPT) may occur, especially in disease of long duration.

Of dogs with hyperadrenocorticism, 15 to 20% have concurrent diabetes mellitus associated with an elevated blood glucose. Resting T_4 and T_3 levels are often low, but the TSH-response test is normal. Urinalysis reveals low specific gravity in most dogs unless glycosuria is a complication. White blood cells and casts are found in urinary sediment in conjunction with urinary tract infection. Radiographs of the chest and abdomen reveal mineralization involving the skin, tracheobronchial tree (Fig. 8–2), vasculature, skeletal muscles, kidney, and occasionally the adrenal gland (Fig. 8–3). Hepatomegaly is the most common radiographic finding and osteoporosis may also be seen. Cutaneous biopsy may reveal epidermal and sebaceous gland atrophy (Fig. 8–4) or dermal mineralization (Fig. 8–5) associated with collagen degeneration.

The definitive diagnostic test for hyperadrenocorticism is the measurement of plasma cortisol levels in conjunction with ACTH administration. See Table 8–2 for the ACTH-response test protocol. Normal values for baseline and post-ACTH stimulation cortisol vary among veterinary reference laboratories. Most normal resting cortisol values range from 0.8 to 3.0 μg/dl. The mean resting cortisol value in a dog with naturally occurring hyperadrenocorticism is approximately 5.5. μg/dl (range, 2 to 15 μg/dl). The normal post-ACTH stimulation cortisol values range from 5 to 12.5 μg/dl.

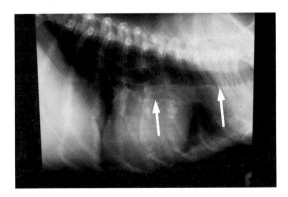

Fig. 8–2. Hyperadrenocorticism: Thoracic radiograph with calcification of the tracheobronchial tree (arrows). (Courtesy of Robert Sikes.)

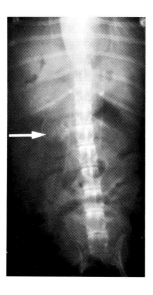

Fig. 8–3. Hyperadrenocorticism: Abdominal radiograph with calcification of the left adrenal gland (arrow). (Courtesy of Robert Sikes.)

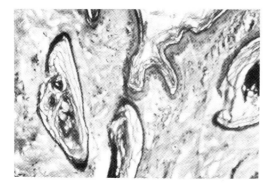

Fig. 8–4. Hyperadrenocorticism: Microscopic section with mild hyperkeratosis, follicular plugging, epidermal atrophy, and an absence of sebaceous glands (low power).

In most cushingoid dogs, the poststimulation cortisol values range from 15 to 50 µg/dl. Dogs with iatrogenic hyperadrenocorticism usually have low to normal resting cortisol values and none to minimal response following ACTH administration. The ACTH-response test does not differentiate between pituitary-dependent bilateral adrenal hyperplasia and an independently secreting adrenal gland tumor.

The low-dose dexamethasone-suppression test is used to verify hyperadrenocorticism if results of the ACTH-response test are borderline or questionable. In the normal dog, a low dose of dexamethasone given intramuscularly (0.015 mg/kg) inhibits the release of pituitary ACTH, which results in a decrease of plasma cortisol compared to

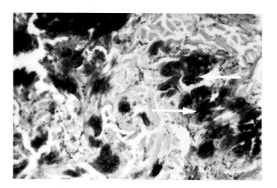

Fig. 8–5. Hyperadrenocorticism: Microscopic section of dermis with multifocal areas of calcium deposition (arrows) among disrupted collagen fibers.

the resting value. A low dose of dexamethasone will not suppress the plasma cortisol level in a dog with hyperadrenocorticism of any origin. See Table 8–3 for the diagnostic protocol.

A high-dose dexamethasone-suppression test is used to differentiate between pituitary-dependent adrenal hyperplasia and adrenal tumor. See Table 8–3 for the diagnostic protocol. In dogs with functional adrenal tumors, a high dose of dexamethasone (1 mg/kg) should not suppress the plasma cortisol level, since it is only acting by suppressing ACTH secretion. With pituitary-dependent hyperadrenocorticism there will be suppression of the plasma cortisol compared to the baseline.

Treatment. *Adrenal Tumors.* Unilateral adrenalectomy is the treatment of choice for an independently secreting adrenal tumor in dogs and cats. Glucocorticoid supplementation is necessary until the opposite adrenal gland regains its normal function. There is usually a poor response to the corticolytic drug, o,p'-DDD (Lysodren, Bristol).

Pituitary-Dependent Bilateral Adrenal Hyperplasia. Both medical and surgical treatment have been advocated for pituitary-dependent Cushing's syndrome in dogs. Most dogs with hyperadrenocorticism due to adrenal hyperplasia are treated medically with o,p'-DDD, a chlorinated hydrocarbon. This drug causes selective necrosis of the adrenal zona reticularis and fasciculata, sparing the mineralocorticoid-producing zona glomerulosa. A loading dose of 50 mg/kg is given daily for 10 days or until polydipsia stops. Glucocorticoids are given concurrently and are continued for 3 to 5 days after discontinuing the loading dose of o,p'-DDD (Endocrine Disease Therapeutic Key, Appendix 2:11). Once the polydipsia has stopped, a maintenance dosage of o,p'-DDD is given weekly,

TABLE 8-2. PROTOCOL AND INTERPRETATION OF ACTH-RESPONSE TEST

Step	Normal Response	Hyperadrenocorticism	
		Average	Range
1. Collect baseline (pre) plasma cortisol sample*	0.8 to 3.0 μg/dl	5.5 μg/dl	2.0–15 μg/dl
2. Administer 20 IU ACTH gel IM			
3. Collect post-ACTH plasma cortisol sample in 2 hours*	5.0 to 12.5 μg/dl	28.6 μg/dl	15.0–60.0 μg/dl†

*All plasma samples should be immediately separated and frozen until assayed.
†Poststimulation plasma cortisol values of 15 to 20 μg/dl are considered to be in the questionable range and should be repeated or a low-dose dexamethasone suppression test should be performed.

TABLE 8-3. PROTOCOL AND INTERPRETATION OF DEXAMETHASONE-SUPPRESSION TESTS FOR THE DIAGNOSIS OF SPONTANEOUS CANINE HYPERADRENOCORTICISM

I. Low-dose dexamethasone-suppression test

Hour	Procedure	Interpretation
0 (early AM)	Collect baseline plasma cortisol*	Baseline
0	Give 0.015 mg/kg dexamethasone IV or IM	
6–8 hours	Collect postdexamethasone plasma cortisol*	Suppression → normal
		No suppression → hyperadrenocorticism

II. High-dose dexamethasone-suppression test

Hour	Procedure	Interpretation
0 (early AM)	Collect baseline plasma cortisol*	Baseline
0	Administer 1.0 mg/kg dexamethasone IV or IM	
6–8 hours	Collect postdexamethasone plasma cortisol*	Suppression → pituitary-dependent adrenal hyperplasia
		No suppression → adrenal tumor

*All plasma samples should be immediately separated and frozen until assayed.

or divided twice weekly. In dogs with eosinopenia and lymphopenia, hemograms should be performed periodically. The eosinophil count returns to normal prior to the lymphocyte count. If economically feasible, an ACTH-response test should be performed within 3 to 4 days after discontinuing the daily loading dosage of o,p'-DDD. If the dog remains symptomatic, or retains the ability to hyper-respond to the ACTH, daily therapy should be continued until the symptoms abate or until there is no hyper-responsiveness to ACTH.

Toxicity from o,p'-DDD is common. Gastrointestinal signs of vomiting, diarrhea, and associated anorexia are the most common, although weakness, lethargy, and depression are frequently observed. These latter signs are usually associated with hypoadrenocorticism and respond well to glucocorticoid supplementation if treated immediately. Occasionally, neurologic signs of weakness, head pressing, and ataxia may be observed in dogs that have been on long-term o,p'-DDD therapy. These direct neurotoxic signs are most often

observed on the day of medication and resolve within 12 to 24 hours. Permanent neurologic signs, such as blindness, circling, and seizures may result from the growth of a pituitary tumor (Nelson's Syndrome). The treatment of choice for feline pituitary-dependent hyperadrenocorticism has not been defined. Bilateral adrenalectomy may be the best treatment. Since most chlorinated hydrocarbons are toxic for cats, o,p'-DDD may not be satisfactory therapy.

Although the overall prognosis improves with therapy, death due to the compressive effects of a pituitary tumor, metastasis of an adrenal carcinoma, or hypoadrenocortisol crisis may occur at any time.

THERAPEUTIC MONITORING. Complete therapeutic monitoring of a dog being treated with o,p'-DDD improves the long-term prognosis by allowing for the detection of toxicity or rising plasma cortisol levels while they are still reversible. However, this is time-consuming and expensive; therefore, good client education is an important part of a treatment and monitoring program. A suggested monitoring program is outlined in Table 8–4.

SURGICAL TREATMENT. Surgical treatment with bilateral adrenalectomy was the treatment of choice for canine pituitary-dependent hyperadrenocorticism prior to the advent of o,p'-DDD therapy. This procedure is still used successfully. Lifetime maintenance therapy with desoxycorticosterone acetate (DOCA) is necessary following adrenalectomy. Also, sodium chloride should be added to the diet daily.

Hypophysectomy is a satisfactory method of treatment for pituitary-dependent spontaneous hyperadrenocorticism. Lifetime maintenance therapy following hypophysectomy includes cortisone, 1 mg/kg divided q12h and L-thyroxine, 15 µg/kg to 20 µg/kg daily. There is usually a temporary increase in scaling of the skin, and regrowth of the hair coat is usually darker than before surgery. Occasionally, diabetes insipidus develops and requires antidiuretic hormone (ADH) therapy.

Prognosis. The prognosis for untreated spontaneous hyperadrenocorticism is poor, with death usually occurring within 6 to 24 months due to septicemia, ketoacidotic diabetes mellitus, or congestive heart failure. After initiation of treatment, complete remission of all clinical signs may take 3 to 5 months. There is a high percentage of relapse, most likely due to the development of resistance to o,p'-DDD or to the growth of the pituitary tumor. Diabetes mellitus may precede or develop following the diagnosis of hyperadrenocorticism. Some dogs with hyperadrenocorticism are in a ketoacidotic state at the time of initial examination.

TABLE 8–4. SUGGESTED THERAPEUTIC MONITORING PROTOCOL FOR DOGS TREATED WITH o,p'-DDD (LYSODREN, BRISTOL)

Daily
Water consumption

Weekly until clinical signs subside (optional)
Total eosinophil count
Absolute lymphocyte count

ACTH-Response Test
1. During the o,p'-DDD loading period if signs suggestive of toxicity occur.
2. Following the o,p'-DDD loading regimen (should be minimal stimulation)*
3. Every 6 months on maintenance therapy
4. Whenever the clinical condition varies and the dosage of o,p'-DDD needs adjusting

*The poststimulation plasma cortisol value should be in the range of 1.5 to 2.0 µg/dl.

CANINE OVARIAN IMBALANCES

Two uncommon syndromes involving the canine skin have been attributed to ovarian imbalance. The specific pathomechanisms involved in these syndromes are unknown. The etiologic association with the ovaries is based on clinical response to treatment.

Ovarian Imbalance Type I

History. A middle-aged to older intact female dog is usually examined for a history of pseudocyesis or anestrus. Chronic, slowly progressive skin changes are observed in the ventral caudal abdomen, flank, and perineal regions.

Clinical Findings. The initial lesions are alopecia, hyperpigmentation and hyperkeratosis of the flanks, perigenital area, and perineum (Plate 7:K,L). Lichenification is prominent in the advanced stages. The axilla may also become involved with similar lesions. Other common findings include vulvar hyperplasia, crusting, and enlargement of the nipples. In the advancing stages of the syndrome, generalized seborrhea and ceruminous otitis are observed.

Diagnosis. Diagnosis of ovarian imbalance type I is based on the history, clinical signs and response to ovariohysterectomy.

Treatment. Ovariohysterectomy results in near-total reversal of clinical signs in most dogs several months following surgery. If seborrhea is present, antiseborrheic shampoos are helpful (see Appendix 2:1).

Ovarian Imbalance Type II

History. A middle-aged to older female dog that has had an ovariohysterectomy at a young age is examined for a history of immature coat and progressive alopecia around the perineum, ventral abdomen, neck, and ears. Occasionally urinary incontinence is present.

Clinical Findings. The skin is soft, pliable, and smooth. Alopecia is noted on the perineum, ventral abdomen, neck, and head (Plate 7:M,N). The hair coat is fine and silky. The vulva and nipples often appear juvenile. All biochemical and hematologic parameters are normal.

Diagnosis. The history and clinical findings are suggestive of ovarian imbalance type II. Normal thyroid serum levels and cortisol function tests further support the diagnosis. The most definitive diagnostic test is a therapeutic trial with estrogen replacement.

Treatment. Replacement therapy with 1 mg diethylstilbestrol, 2 to 3 times weekly, usually results in reversal of clinical signs within 2 to 4 months. Other forms of estrogen replacement must be used with caution. In most dogs this therapy must be continued for a lifetime, since relapses often occur. If long-term maintenance therapy is required, potential bone marrow depression and platelet dysfunction may occur.

CANINE TESTICULAR ABNORMALITIES

Canine Sertoli Cell Tumor

Sertoli cell tumors are estrogen-secreting and often cause signs of a feminizing endocrine dermatosis and prostatic hyperplasia.

Incidence. Sertoli cell tumors are the most common canine testicular tumors and represent about 4% of all canine tumors reported. There is a much higher incidence in cryptorchid testes (53%) compared to scrotal testes (10.2%).

History. Breeds reported to have a high incidence of Sertoli cell tumor include the Chihuahua, Pomeranian, Miniature Schnauzer, Miniature and Standard Poodle, Shetland Sheepdog, Siberian Husky, Boxer, and Yorkshire Terrier.

The age of onset is usually greater than 7 years. Sertoli cell tumors occur in cryptorchid testes of animals that are younger than those with tumors in the scrotal testes.

Owners are often unaware of the presence of a Sertoli cell tumor until it is revealed by physical examination. There may be a history of slowly progressive symmetric alopecia and hyperpigmentation of the perineal and periscrotal regions. Attraction of male dogs and decreased libido may be reported. In advanced cases, lethargy and systemic illness may also be observed. Pruritus is variable, but occurs more frequently in dogs with advanced clinical signs.

Clinical Signs. Palpation of the testes reveals one enlarged testis, either scrotal or, more commonly, extrascrotal. The other testis, if descended, is usually smaller and softer.

Most dogs show signs of skin change. Symmetric alopecia, starting in the periscrotal and perineal areas and on the posterolateral thighs and slowly advancing craniad along the sides of the dog, is observed (Plate 7:O). The hair is dry and epilates easily. Common findings are marked hyperpigmentation of the alopecic areas and an apparent thinning of the skin. In advanced cases of Sertoli cell tumor, there may be more hyperkeratosis and lichenification in the perineal and periscrotal areas (Plate 7:P) as well as near-total trunkal alopecia.

A pendulous and edematous prepuce may be observed (Plate 7:Q). Gynecomastia is reported in about 25% of affected dogs.

Concurrent palpable prostatic hyperplasia is frequently observed. Systemic signs associated with metastasis may occur, although the incidence is low. Signs of thrombocytopenic purpura rarely are seen.

Diagnosis. The history and clinical findings are suggestive of Sertoli cell tumor. Screening diagnostic procedures should include abdominal radiography if there is an intra-abdominal testicle. Estrogen and testosterone serum levels may be measured. Although results vary, an intact male dog with history and clinical findings of Sertoli cell tumor, elevated serum estrogen, and low serum testosterone is highly suspect.

The only definitive diagnostic test is a biopsy of the testes and the identification of neoplastic Sertoli cells.

Treatment. Removal of the testes is required. Some dogs need exogenous testosterone replacement for 1 to 2 months following castration to bring about reversal of clinical signs (see Appendix 2:11).

Prognosis. The prognosis for most dogs with Sertoli cell tumor is good since the incidence of metastasis is low and clinical signs of feminization are usually reversible.

Seminoma

Seminoma is a benign testicular tumor arising from the germinal epithelum of the seminiferous tubules which occasionally causes signs of endocrine dermatosis.

Incidence. The incidence of seminoma in dogs is reported to be about one third that of Sertoli cell tumor. Seminoma occurs most frequently in cryptorchid testes with the highest incidence found in retained inguinal testes. Skin lesions are only occasionally associated with seminoma.

Pathogenesis. The specific biologic mechanisms associated with seminoma are not known. There is some suggestion that the tumor cells are estrogen-secreting since associated prostatic disease, perineal hernias, and perianal gland tumors are reported with seminomas.

History. The cryptorchid dog more than 7 years of age is predisposed, although seminoma may occur in the younger dog, especially if an inguinal testis is present. Since skin lesions are uncommon, most owners are not aware of the presence of a seminoma until it is revealed by physical examination.

History of mild alopecia of the perineum, ventral abdomen, and posterolateral trunk may be reported. Results of thyroid-function tests are normal.

Clinical Signs. Palpation usually reveals one testis larger than the other, usually associated with cryptorchid testis if present. The scrotal testis may be softer and smaller.

The skin lesions associated with seminoma are usually limited to mild alopecia of the perineum, ventral abdomen, and posterolateral trunk. There is minimal hyperpigmentation (Plate 7:R). Mild prostatic hyperplasia, perianal gland tumor, and perineal hernia may be present.

Diagnosis. The history and clinical findings are suggestive of testicular tumor. Abdominal radiographs should be taken if the cryptorchid testis is intra-abdominal. Estrogen and testosterone serum evaluations have not been diagnostic.

Biopsy of the testicles and subsequent identification of neoplastic germinal epithelial cells of the seminiferous tubules is the definitive diagnostic test.

Prognosis. Prognosis for seminoma is good since it is benign and the skin changes reverse following castration.

Male Feminizing Syndrome

Male feminizing syndrome is an uncommon clinical entity of unknown etiology that occurs in intact male dogs and results in gynecomastia and hyperestrogenism.

History. A middle-aged to older intact male dog is examined for chronic, progressive skin changes. Clinical signs may have been partially responsive to corticosteroids at anti-inflammatory dosages.

Clinical Signs. Hyperpigmentation, hyperkeratosis, and lichenification are observed in the perigenital region and on the posterior thighs and flanks. Other findings include gynecomastia and ceruminous otitis. Seborrhea oleosa may be present. Both descended testes either palpate normally or are atrophied.

Diagnosis. A history of feminizing signs in a dog with normal testes is suggestive of male feminizing syndrome. Normal plasma estradiol and testosterone levels and histologic confirmation that there is no neoplastic process in the testes also lend diagnostic support. Response to castration is the most definitive diagnostic test, although some dogs do not respond to surgery alone.

Treatment. If the history, clinical signs, and results of clinical laboratory testing are consistent with a diagnosis of male feminizing syndrome, castration is the treatment of choice. In some cases chronic systemic corticosteroid therapy is required. Antiseborrheic shampoos are indicated (see Appendix 2:1) as are medications for ceruminous otitis.

Feline Endocrine Alopecia

Feline endocrine alopecia (FEA) is the most common hormonal dermatosis in the cat.

Etiologic Factor. The specific cause of feline endocrine alopecia is unknown; however, it is classified as a hormonal disorder on the basis of therapeutic response to sex hormones.

History. Feline endocrine alopecia is observed most often in male cats neutered at a premature age. About 10% of those cats affected are spayed females. There is no breed predilection. Feline endocrine alopecia is most common in the middle-aged cat; the reported age range is 2 to 12 years.

The owner usually observes a slowly progressive, symmetric thinning of the haircoat or total alopecia in the perineal and ventral abdominal areas. Pruritus or excessive licking is usually not a feature of feline endocrine alopecia.

Clinical Signs. There is bilateral symmetric alopecia beginning in the perineal and ventral posterior trunk, thorax, and forelimbs (Plate 7:S,T,U). Inflammation is not usually seen. Hair epilates easily in the involved areas.

Diagnosis. History and clinical signs are suggestive of feline endocrine alopecia. Results of biochemical testing are normal. Sex hormone assays have not been diagnostic. Histopathologic findings including thin skin (epidermal and dermal atrophy) with inactive hair follicles and minimal dermal cellular infiltration are not specific for feline endocrine alopecia (Fig. 8–6).

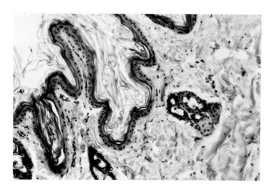

Fig. 8–6. Feline endocrine alopecia: Microscopic section with hyperkeratosis and atrophy of the epidermis, hair follicles, and sebaceous glands (low power).

The most definitive diagnostic test is a therapeutic trial with sex hormones, bearing in mind that other feline dermatoses may also respond to sex hormone replacement therapy, especially progestational compounds.

Treatment. Feline endocrine alopecia is reported to respond to several different treatment protocols. Combined injections of a repositol form of testosterone and stilbestrol are given intramuscularly to all cats with feline endocrine alopecia regardless of sex, and repeated in 6 weeks if there has not been good regrowth of hair (see Appendix 2:11). Stilbestrol is difficult to obtain in the United States. Testosterone (repositol form) has been used in male cats and stilbestrol in female cats, but these single hormone protocols are generally less effective than the combined therapy. The infrequent transient side effects of androgen-estrogen therapy are signs of estrus in females and aggressiveness and/or urine spraying in males. An overdose of either hormone can result in hepatobiliary disease and death.

A second common form of treatment for feline endocrine alopecia is administration of progestational compounds. A repositol form of progesterone or medroxyprogesterone acetate is given intramuscularly and repeated in 6 weeks if needed. Megestrol acetate is an effective treatment in many cats (see Appendix 2:11).

Relapse of clinical signs is common with all forms of therapy. The clinician must know that none of the aforementioned recommended hormones are approved for use in cats in the United States.

PITUITARY DWARFISM

Pituitary dwarfism is a congenital disease occasionally observed in the German Shepherd or German Shepherd cross.

Etiologic Factors. The cause of pituitary dwarfism is reported to be a congenital cystic distention of Rathke's pouch.

History. The most common observation made by the owner is a marked difference in the size of the dog compared with its littermates; an affected dog is often 50% shorter and lighter than its littermates at 1 year of age. At 2 to 4 months of age, the pituitary dwarf shows a lack of normal hair coat development. As the dog matures, the owner notes a retention of secondary hairs; when the dog is between 9 and 12 months of age, trunkal alopecia is observed. The adult dog has a variable history depending on which endocrine functions are impaired. The most common history is lethargy, heat seeking, and anestrus or infertility attributable to hypothyroidism. The dog may be polyuric, polydipsic, and polyphagic, symptoms associated with Cushing's syndrome.

Clinical Signs. Clinical signs vary depending on the age of the dog and the severity of disease. Hair coat change is the most obvious abnormal finding in the 3- to 6-month-old puppy. There is persistence of secondary hairs (puppy coat) with a lack of development of the primary or guard hairs. Pituitary dwarfism is usually suspected if the dog is smaller than normal for the breed by 6 months of age. Thinning of the hair coat and partial alopecia, especially in areas of wear or friction, become apparent between 9 to 12 months of age (Plate 7:V). The color of the hair may be lighter than that of littermates. Hyperpigmentation usually appears in the alopecic area of the skin. There is lack of development of the genital organs including the testes and vulva; the penile sheath is usually flaccid. In the adult dog, scales, progressive alopecia, and hyperpigmentation may develop. These skin changes can occur at a young age or may not become generalized for several years.

Diagnosis. The difference in size of the affected dog and its littermates and concurrent skin and hair coat changes are the most suggestive clinical findings associated with pituitary dwarfism. Thyroid-function tests in the adult dog usually reveal hypothyroidism. Occasionally, ACTH-response tests are abnormally elevated. The only definitive diagnostic test is the demonstration of a cystic pituitary gland on necropsy.

Treatment. Treatment consists of specific therapy for the endocrinopathies identified including thyroid replacement and o,p'-DDD or surgery if there is hyperadrenocorticism. Antiseborrheic shampoos are helpful to control dandruff (see Appendix 2:1). Growth hormone replacement may be of value in the young dog (Endocrine Disease Therapeutic Key, Appendix 2:11).

GROWTH HORMONE RESPONSIVE DERMATOSIS–ADULT ONSET

Growth hormone responsive dermatosis of adult onset is a recently recognized syndrome based on therapeutic response to growth hormone replacement. Specific etiologic factors and pathogenesis of this syndrome are not known.

History. There appears to be a breed predilection in the Keeshond, Chow Chow, Pomeranian, and Poodle. A sex predilection for males is reported. The owner observes initial alopecic lesions at 1 to 2 years of age. The dog shows no systemic signs. Evaluations of thyroid and adrenal gland function are normal. There may be a history of poor clinical response to thyroid hormone replacement and castration.

Clinical Signs. Focal alopecic and hyperpigmented areas of skin are observed on the dorsal neck, trunk, and medial thighs (Plate 7:*W,X,Y*). Areas of mild trauma on biopsy sites often subsequently grow new tufts of hair.

Diagnosis. All hematologic and biochemical parameters are normal, including thyroid and cortisol function tests and sex hormone serum levels. Growth hormone stimulation tests using xylazine hydrochloride may prove to be diagnostically valuable.

A biopsy of alopecic areas reveals changes consistent with endocrine dermatosis including hyperkeratosis, a thin epidermis, atrophy of hair follicles, and follicular plugging with keratin. Dogs with hyposomatotropism have less structured and fewer elastin fibers compared with the normal site- and age-matched controls. These findings support a presumptive diagnosis as will normal thyroid and cortisol function tests.

The most definitive diagnostic test at this time is a therapeutic trial with growth hormone.

Treatment. Porcine or bovine growth hormone has been used (see Appendix 2:11); however, relapses have been observed within 5 months following treatment in some dogs. Growth hormone is difficult to obtain commercially.

SELECTED READINGS

Anderson, R.K.: Canine hypothyroidism. Compend. Cont. Ed. Pract. Vet. 1:103, 1979.

Catchin, E.: Testicular neoplasms in dogs. J. Comp. Pathol. 70:232, 1960.

Eigenmann, J.E.: Diagnosis and treatment of dwarfism in a German Shepherd dog. J. Am. Anim. Hosp. Assoc. 17:798, 1981.

Joshua, J.O.: Some conditions seen in feline practice attributable to hormonal causes. Vet. Rec. 88:511, 1971.

Lipowitz, A.J., et al.: Testicular neoplasia and concomitant clinical changes in the dog. J. Am. Vet. Med. Assoc. 163:1364, 1973.

Lorenz, M.D.: Canine hyperadrenocorticism: Diagnosis and treatment. Compend. Cont. Ed. Pract. Vet. 1:315, 1979.

Lorenz, M.D., and Stiff, M.E.: Serum thyroxine content before and after thyrotropin stimulation in dogs with suspected hypothyroidism. J. Am. Vet. Med. Assoc. 177:78, 1980.

Milne, K.L., and Hayes, H.M.: Epidemiologic features of canine hypothyroidism. Cornell Vet. 71:3, 1981.

Nachreiner, R.F.: Laboratory diagnosis of endocrine diseases. Proceedings of the 48th Annual Meeting of the American Animal Hospital Association, 1981.

Nesbitt, G.H., et al.: Canine hypothyroidism: A retrospective study of 108 cases. J. Am. Vet. Med. Assoc. 177:1117, 1980.

Parker, W.M., and Scott, D.W.: Growth hormone responsive alopecia in the mature dog: A discussion of 13 cases. J. Am. Anim. Hosp. Assoc. 16:824, 1980.

Peterson, M.E.: Canine Cushing's syndrome. Proceedings of the 48th Annual Meeting of the American Animal Hospital Association, 1981.

Peterson, M.E., Nesbitt, G.H., and Schaer, M.: Diagnosis and management of concurrent diabetes mellitus and hyperadrenocorticism in thirty dogs. J. Am. Vet. Med. Assoc. 178:66, 1980.

Priester, W.A.: Epidemiology. In Veterinary Cancer Medicine. Edited by G.H. Theilen and B.R. Madewell. Philadelphia, Lea & Febiger, 1979.

Reap, M., et al.: Thyroxine and triiodothyronine levels in ten species of animals. Southwest Vet. 31:31, 1978.

Reimers, T.J.: Radioimmunoassays and diagnostic tests for thyroid and adrenal disorders. Compend. Cont. Ed. Pract. Vet. 4:65, 1982.

Scott, D.W.: Hormonal and metabolic disorders. J. Am. Anim. Hosp. Assoc. 16:390, 1980.

Scott, D.W., et al.: Clinicopathological findings in a German Shepherd with pituitary dwarfism. J. Am. Anim. Hosp. Assoc. 14:183, 1978.

Scott, P.P., Greaves, J.P., and Scott, M.G.: Nutrition of the cat: Calcium and iodine deficiency on a meat diet. Br. J. Nutr. 15:73, 1961.

Siegel, E.T., et al.: An estrogen study in the feminized dog with testicular neoplasia. Endocrinology 80:272, 1967.

Theilen, G.H., and Madewell, B.R.: Tumors of the urogenital tract. In Veterinary Cancer Medicine. Edited by G.H. Theilen and B.R. Madewell. Philadelphia, Lea & Febiger, 1979.

9

Seborrheic Syndrome

In veterinary dermatology, the term seborrhea denotes any abnormality in sebum production and/ or any abnormality in the process of normal desquamation leading to the formation of visible scale. The Seborrheic Syndrome Key (Appendix 1:8) lists the most pertinent historical and clinical findings and diagnostic tests associated with seborrhea.

ETIOLOGIC FACTORS

The etiologic classification of canine and feline seborrhea is given in Table 9–1. It is estimated that in at least 90% of the cases of seborrheic syndrome in the dog the condition is secondary. The most common primary problems associated with the syndrome are ectoparasites and allergies. Hypothyroidism is the most common cause of primary metabolic seborrhea; a smaller percentage is included in the fat-deficient, lipid-related category of primary metabolic seborrhea. In idiopathic primary seborrhea, neither external nor internal causes can be determined, but hereditary factors play a role in predisposition.

The Schnauzer comedo syndrome and tail gland hyperplasia are two specific syndromes in the dog of unknown cause characterized by clinical signs of seborrhea.

Most feline seborrheic conditions are associated with ectoparasites, endoparasites, dermatophytes, systemic diseases, or dry skin resulting from high environmental temperatures and low humidity.

Stud tail and feline acne are syndromes of unknown cause that fall under the classification of seborrhea.

PATHOGENESIS

The processes of keratinization, desquamation, and sebum production are discussed in Chapter 1. In seborrheic dogs, the content of the sebum changes, with an increase in the percentage of total labile fatty acids and total cholesterol, and a decrease in the percentage of diester waxes. As the cutaneous lipids are altered, the cutaneous microflora also change. Corynebacterium spp., micrococci, and Clostridium spp. constitute the normal cutaneous flora with a combined average population of 100 to 200 colonies/cm^2 of skin. In a dog with either seborrhea oleosa or seborrhea sicca, there is a marked increase in the bacterial count to an average of 16,000 colonies/cm^2 of skin. The species of flora change from nonpathogenic bacteria to predominantly pathogenic Staphylococcus aureus.

PRIMARY AND SECONDARY SEBORRHEA

History. There is breed predisposition for all forms of primary canine seborrhea. Doberman Pinschers and Irish Setters are predisposed to hypothyroid primary seborrhea. Reportedly, a higher incidence of gonadal related cyclic seborrhea occurs in Golden Retrievers, Afghan Hounds, and

111

TABLE 9–1. CLASSIFICATION OF CANINE AND FELINE SEBORRHEA

I. Etiologic classification
  A. Primary seborrhea (canine)
    a. Idiopathic seborrhea
    b. Generalized metabolic seborrhea
      1. Endocrine related
        (a) Hypothyroidism
        (b) Gonadal malfunction
      2. Lipid related
        (a) Fat deficiency
        (b) Malabsorption/maldigestion
        (c) Liver disease
    c. Focal metabolic seborrhea (keratin factor deficiencies)
      1. Zinc
      2. Vitamin A
  B. Secondary seborrhea—focal and generalized (canine and feline)
    a. Ectoparasites
    b. Allergy
    c. Fungal infection
    d. Bacterial hypersensitivity
    e. Bullous diseases
    f. Neoplasia (systemic or cutaneous)
    g. Dry skin—environmental predisposition
    h. Other systemic diseases
  C. Seborrheic syndromes of unknown origin
    a. Canine
      1. Schnauzer comedo syndrome
      2. Tail gland hyperplasia
    b. Feline
      1. Stud tail
      2. Acne
II. Clinical classification—(canine and feline)
  A. Seborrhea sicca
  B. Seborrhea oleosa
  C. Seborrheic dermatitis

Borzois. Siberian Huskies are predisposed to zinc-responsive, focal facial seborrhea. German Shepherds, Cocker Spaniels, Irish Setters, Doberman Pinschers, and Labrador Retrievers are prone to idiopathic seborrhea. Any breed predisposition to secondary seborrhea is related to predisposition to the primary disease.

Cocker Spaniels, Springer Spaniels, and Basset Hounds are predisposed to an oily coat (seborrhea oleosa). There is a higher incidence of dry seborrhea (seborrhea sicca) in Labrador Retrievers and Dachshunds.

With primary seborrhea, there is usually a history of slowly progressive scaling and alopecia starting at about 1 year of age. Exception to this occurs with seborrhea caused by liver or pancreatic disease, which normally affects older dogs. Age predilection for secondary seborrhea is variable, depending on the primary cause. Signs of seborrhea may develop more rapidly with secondary than with primary seborrhea. Often the owner's primary complaint is that the animal emits a strong, persistent odor, especially when oily seborrhea or ceruminous otitis is present.

Pruritus of varying intensity is frequently associated with primary idiopathic or secondary seborrhea.

Variable histories are associated with feline seborrhea, depending on the primary cause. As in dogs, clinical signs may appear rapidly following the onset of the primary disease.

Clinical Findings. Scaling, crusting, and alopecia are present on most dogs with seborrhea. Variable degrees of inflammation are observed. Some dogs have a dry, waxy debris or dandruff (seborrhea sicca) (Plate 8:A) that is easily shed from the hair and skin. Other dogs have a greasy or oily debris (seborrhea oleosa) (Plate 8:B) which causes matting of the hair and some crusting on the skin. Multifocal areas of inflammation are often associated with the crusts characterized by seborrheic dermatitis (Plate 8:C).

Primary canine seborrhea is often characterized by generalized dorsal scaling, ceruminous otitis, and involvement of the tail gland. The distribution of seborrheic lesions due to secondary causes varies; see the appropriate chapters for the specific diseases.

The most common clinical signs associated with feline seborrhea are generalized dry skin and hair coat with excessive scaling (seborrhea sicca) (Plate 8:D). Signs of excessive oiliness or seborrhea oleosa (Plate 8:E) are rare in the cat, but when present are usually associated with systemic signs of feline leukemia, liver disease, neoplasia, or bullous diseases.

SEBORRHEIC SYNDROMES OF UNKNOWN ORIGIN—CANINE

History and Clinical Signs. Two specific clinical syndromes in dogs have been classified as seborrheic disease. The first, Schnauzer comedo syndrome, affects the dorsum of Miniature Schnauzers. The owner observes small crusts on the back, often at the time of grooming, which generally cause little or no discomfort to the dog. The lesions are well-demarcated, crusted papules associated with the individual hair follicles on the entire dorsum of the back from the shoulder to the tail. Soft, waxy comedones rather than crusting may also be observed.

The pet owner also observes the second specific seborrheic entity, tail gland hyperplasia, because of a swollen, alopecic area on the dorsum of the tail, approximately 2 inches from the anus (Plate 8:F). At times the dog may start chewing the area.

The owner may report periodic changes in the size of the swelling as well as the degree of alopecia. Following trauma, the area may become irritated and secondarily infected.

SEBORRHEIC SYNDROMES OF UNKNOWN ORIGIN—FELINE

History and Clinical Signs. Two specific clinical syndromes in cats have been classified as seborrheic disease.

The first, feline stud tail, occurs most frequently in intact males, although it has been observed in castrated males and both intact and altered females. There is a higher incidence in Siamese, Persian, and Rex cats. There is usually no pain or pruritus. The clinical signs include comedones and a yellow to black waxy accumulation on the hair and skin of the dorsal proximal tail; variable alopecia is also observed.

The second, feline acne, has no age, sex, or breed predilection. The lesions are characterized by comedones on the chin and lower lips (Plate 8:G). These lesions are usually not associated with any other clinical signs. Occasionally, pain and pruritus are observed in association with a secondary bacterial infection. Papules, pustules, and edema are also seen on the chin and lips.

DIAGNOSIS OF SEBORRHEIC SYNDROMES

The history and distribution of clinical signs are helpful in differentiating primary and secondary seborrhea. Multiple skin scrapings are always indicated to rule out external parasites. Therapeutic trials with parasiticides also help with the diagnosis. Fungal cultures should be performed since dermatophytes routinely cause scaling and are sometimes associated with crusting. If allergies are

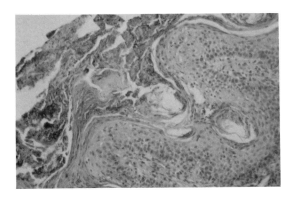

Fig. 9–1. Seborrheic syndrome: Microscopic section with crusts, hyperkeratosis, parakeratosis, acanthosis, and a cellular infiltrate at the dermoepidermal junction (low power).

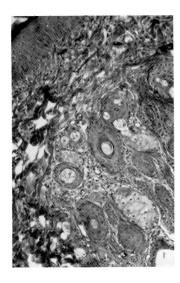

Fig. 9–2. Seborrheic syndrome: Microscopic section with a mild mixed inflammatory cell infiltrate at the dermoepidermal junction and perifollicular. Edema in the upper dermis is observed (low power).

suspected, diet testing or intradermal skin testing is indicated. Thyroid-function tests should be performed if an endocrine-related primary seborrhea is suspected, and therapeutic trials with animal fat and vegetable oil are recommended if fatty acid deficiencies are suspected.

Cutaneous biopsy is often useful in ruling out specific entities such as immune-mediated disease, primary bacterial dermatitis, dermatomycosis, and neoplasia. The microscopic findings of idiopathic seborrhea are nonspecific, but may include crusts, hyperkeratosis, acanthosis, spongiosis, and often parakeratosis (Fig. 9–1). Usually there is a mild to moderate mixed, upper dermal cellular infiltrate (Fig. 9–2); keratin plugging of hair follicles (Fig. 9–3) and sebaceous gland hyperplasia (Fig. 9–4) are commonly observed.

The diagnostic workup for a dog with seborrhea first involves ruling out the specific causes of primary and secondary seborrhea; only then should a diagnosis of idiopathic seborrhea be made.

Schnauzer comedo syndrome is associated with concurrent hypothyroidism in approximately 25% of the animals; therefore, a thyroid-function test should always be performed. The diagnosis is based on breed and clinical signs. A presumptive diagnosis of canine tail gland hyperplasia and feline stud tail is based on the history and location of lesions. Microscopic findings of tail gland lesions include hypertrophy and hyperplasia of the sebaceous glands.

Feline acne is suspected on the basis of history, clinical signs, and location of lesions. Pasteurella

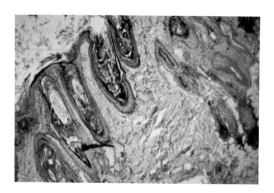

Fig. 9–3. Seborrheic syndrome: Microscopic section with hyperkeratosis and marked keratin plugging of hair follicles (low power).

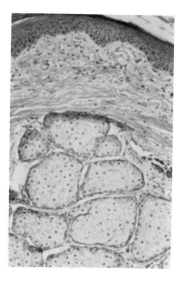

Fig. 9–4. Seborrheic syndrome: Microscopic section with hypertrophied sebaceous glands, mild dermoepidermal junction cellular infiltrate, and mild acanthosis (low power).

multocida or β-hemolytic streptococci are often isolated from secondarily infected acne lesions. Dermatophytes may be cultured most often from lesions refractory to routine treatment.

TREATMENT OF SEBORRHEIC SYNDROMES

The treatment of seborrhea should be based on diagnostic tests, and should be as specific as possible.

Primary hypothyroid-related seborrhea is treated with thyroid replacement. The most satisfactory method of treating cyclic gonadal-related seborrhea is ovariohysterectomy. For a seborrheic male dog with abnormally aggressive behavior, castration may be indicated. Owners should be cautioned that an operation may not elicit the clinical response desired, since the diagnosis is based on

history and the exclusion of other differential diagnoses.

Animals with fat-deficient seborrhea should be fed a balanced, commercial diet of dry and canned food in a ratio of 3:1; polyunsaturated vegetable oil (peanut, corn, safflower) and saturated animal fat (pork, beef, chicken) should also be given by gradually adding 1 to 4 teaspoons (depending on the size of the dog) of oil and fat to the daily diet.

Animals with all primary and secondary types of seborrhea benefit from the frequent use of keratolytic, keratoplastic shampoo. As the clinical signs are controlled, the frequency of bathing should be reduced. Emollient rinses are helpful in the dry, scaling types of seborrhea. A therapeutic trial with fat supplementation is routinely used for idiopathic seborrhea. Antibiotics are often used to reduce signs attributable to bacterial infection. Specific treatment for primary causes of secondary seborrhea must be pursued.

Schnauzer comedo syndrome is treated with antiseborrheic shampoo; continued bathing every 2 to 4 weeks may help prevent recurrence. Antibiotics may contribute to a faster clinical response. Thyroid replacement should be administered if indicated. Alcohol rubs twice weekly are helpful in preventing a recurrence of lesions.

Tail gland hyperplasia usually does not require specific treatment; however, if infection is present, the area should be kept clean with antibacterial soap and ointment. Corticosteroid cream helps reduce swelling if infection is not present. Surgically removing part of the glandular mass has been suggested if there is a persistent cosmetic or medical problem.

Specific treatment for feline stud tail is often unnecessary, unless requested by the owner for aesthetic reasons. Antiseborrheic shampoos often keep the surface of the lesion clean and progestational compounds, such as megestrol acetate, help to control the clinical signs.

Feline acne requires minimal treatment. Manually evacuating comedones, gently washing with a keratolytic shampoo, and applying a topical keratolytic agent are usually all that are required. If the acne becomes infected, treatment includes gently clipping and cleansing the area followed by an application of hot packs and the administration of systemic antibiotics.

Specific drugs and treatment protocols for the seborrheic diseases are noted in the Seborrheic Syndrome Therapeutic Key (Appendix 2:12).

CLIENT EDUCATION

Client education is important in the management of seborrheic syndrome. The client must realize that all primary seborrheas and seborrheic syndromes of unknown origin can never be totally cured. In addition, many secondary forms of seborrhea can be controlled but never completely eliminated. Most seborrheic dogs and cats require lifetime therapy, the nature of which must be thoroughly understood by the client.

SELECTED READINGS

Austin, V.H.: Common skin problems in cats. Mod. Vet. Pract. 56:541, 1975.

Baker, K.P.: The treatment of skin diseases in cats. Irish Vet. J. 28:173, 1974.

Doering, G.G.: Feline dermatology. Vet. Clin. North Am. 6:463, 1976.

————: "Stud tail" in cats. Feline Pract. 4:28, 1976.

Halliwell, R.E.W.: Seborrhea in the dog. Compend. Cont. Ed. Pract. Vet. 1:227, 1979.

Horowitz, L.N., and Ihrke, P.J.: Canine seborrhea. In Current Veterinary Therapy VI: Small Animal Practice. Edited by R.W. Kirk. Philadelphia, W.B. Saunders, 1977.

Ihrke, P.J., et al.: Microbiology of normal and seborrheic canine skin. Am. J. Vet. Res. 39:1487, 1978.

Muller, G.H.: Acne. In Current Veterinary Therapy V: Small Animal Practice. Edited by R.W. Kirk. Philadelphia, W.B. Saunders, 1974.

Scott, D.W.: Disorders of unknown or multiple origin. J. Am. Anim. Hosp. Assoc. 16:412, 1980.

————: Feline dermatology. In Proceedings of the 43rd Annual Meeting of the American Animal Hospital Association. 1976.

10

Bullous Diseases

Bullous skin diseases in the dog and cat are classified on the basis of the etiologic factors and microscopic appearance of the bullae. This group of diseases is the least common of the nine general dermatologic disease classifications. The etiologic factors are varied and the pathogenesis is poorly understood. The Canine and Feline Bullous Disease Keys (Appendices 1:9 and 1:10) list the most pertinent historical and clinical findings and diagnostic tests to aid in the differentiation of these diseases.

AUTOIMMUNE BULLOUS DISEASES

Incidence. Pemphigus foliaceus is the most common autoimmune bullous disease in the dog. Systemic lupus erythematosus (SLE), pemphigus vulgaris, and bullous pemphigoid are less common. Discoid lupus erythematosus (DLE), pemphigus erythematosus, and pemphigus vegetans have only recently been described in the dog. Inasmuch as autoimmune disorders in the cat have just recently been recognized, the incidence of the various diseases has not yet been established.

Etiologic Factors. The autoimmune diseases are characterized by circulating and tissue-bound autoantibodies. The immune response is characterized by the presence of autoantibodies and may or may not be associated with autoimmune disease. Pemphigus vegetans is thought to be a benign variant form of pemphigus vulgaris. Pemphigus

erythematosus may be a benign or abortive form of pemphigus foliaceus.

Pathogenesis. Autoimmune response as a cause of disease still remains hypothetical. Three hypotheses have been proposed to explain the mechanism and manifestations of autoimmune disease. These include (1) the forbidden-clone theory, (2) the sequestered-antigen theory, and (3) the immunologic-deficiency concept. The reader is referred to immunologic texts listed in the "Selected Readings" at the end of this chapter for in-depth discussion of these hypotheses. Two recently proposed factors suggest predisposition to the production of autoantibodies. First, the cell tissue may be antigenically changed by chemical or physical means so as to induce an immune response which cross-reacts with the original unaltered tissue. Second, the suppressor T-cell function may be abnormal, causing the aberrant immune response to go unchecked.

History. Patients with autoimmune bullous diseases have a drug history of poor response to low-dose corticosteroids and antibiotics. They may respond partially or totally to a therapeutic corticosteroid trial using a high dosage (2.2 to 4.4 mg/ kg daily). The onset of the autoimmune disease may be sudden or gradual and the course may be acute or chronic. The latter is more common. There may be a history of systemic involvement manifested by anorexia, weight loss, and fever. This would be more commonly observed in SLE, or in pemphigus vulgaris complicated by bacterial infection. The age of onset in dogs is variable, but is usually over 2 years. Cats are usually affected when 5 or more years old. No breed predilection has been identified. Many autoimmune bullous diseases may be aggravated by sunlight. Pruritus and pain are variable.

Clinical Signs. Most autoimmune bullous diseases of dogs and cats are characterized initially by facial distribution. The distribution and type of lesions are often helpful in differentiating the specific autoimmune bullous skin diseases. Pemphigus vulgaris is characterized by ulcerations and crusting at mucocutaneous junctions and on mucous membranes (Plate 9:A,B). Bullae may occasionally be seen prior to rupture. The oral mucosa, prepuce, anus, and vulva are the common sites of lesions in the dog. Sloughing of the toe nails and trunkal lesions are occasionally seen. Signs of systemic illness due to septicemia are commonly associated with untreated pemphigus vulgaris. In the cat, the distribution of pemphigus vulgaris lesions includes the oral cavity, nose, ear margins, lips, and feet (Plate 9:C).

Pemphigus vegetans in the dog is characterized by a proliferative dermatitis with scaling and/or crusting. There is no involvement of the mucosal surfaces and the mucocutaneous junctions are seldom involved. Erosions, pustules, erythematous crusts, scale, and alopecia are frequently observed. The face, ears, and footpads are the common sites of lesions; however, a generalized or multifocal trunkal distribution may also occur. There are seldom any systemic signs.

It is difficult to distinguish between pemphigus erythematosus and pemphigus foliaceus on the basis of initial clinical signs. However, the lesions of pemphigus erythematosus remain localized to the facial region, while those of pemphigus foliaceus may become more generalized. Pemphigus foliaceus and pemphigus erythematosus are both proliferative diseases characterized by alopecia and moderate to severe crusting in the involved regions of the skin (Plate 9:D). Ulcerations may be observed associated with pruritus. In a few dogs with less severe signs, scales rather than crusts are present. In some dogs, the lesions of pemphigus foliaceus are confined to the footpads and characterized by marked hyperkeratosis (Plate 9:E).

The type and distribution of lesions in canine bullous pemphigoid are identical to those of pemphigus vulgaris. The oral mucosa (Plate 9:F), perioral and periocular tissues, ears (Plate 9:G), and other mucocutaneous junctions are affected with vesiculopustular lesions, ulcerations, and crusting. Trunkal lesions are less commonly observed.

Canine SLE is a multisystemic disease; skin manifestations are seen in up to 33% of affected dogs. The lesions vary in distribution and type and are more commonly associated with light-exposed areas such as the muzzle and ears. Papules, ulcerations, and crusting are observed. Secondary bacterial infection can vary from none to severe. Alopecic, scarred lesions are more common in SLE than in the pemphigus diseases.

Cats with SLE may be examined for a generalized chronic dermatitis with gross morphologic lesions similar to those seen in cats with pemphigus foliaceus. Mucocutaneous junctions of the nares and nail beds have been affected. Fever and peripheral lymphadenopathy may also be observed.

DLE is facial dermatitis that begins with erythema and depigmentation of the anterior nares and nasal planum (Plate 9:H). These lesions then extend proximally to the bridge of the nose. Crusting and erosions or ulcerations may be accompanied by alopecia.

Diagnosis. The history and clinical findings usually support a diagnosis of autoimmune bullous disease. The demonstration of acantholytic keratinocytes in impression smears (Plate 9:I) or aspiration biopsies is suggestive. The definitive diagnosis is based on histopathologic and immunologic studies. Multiple cutaneous biopsies from the margins of lesions are obtained for both routine staining with H and E and immunofluorescent studies (Plate 9:J and 9:K). If possible, two adjacent biopsy specimens, 4 to 6 mm in size, are taken from each area. If bullae or vesicles are present they should be carefully and completely excised. If there is a ruptured bulla, a biopsy should be performed on the margin. One of the sections is then placed in 10% buffered formalin, and the other is quick frozen in N-butyl alcohol or liquid nitrogen and stored at −70°C until sectioned; or a fresh biopsy specimen can be immediately placed in Michel's transport medium.[1] This transport medium will preserve a specimen for the purposes of immunofluorescent studies for up to 1 week.

The biopsy specimens are processed and examined for the presence of characteristic microscopic and immunofluorescent findings. These findings are summarized in Table 10–1 and vis-

---

[1]Michel's medium is marketed commercially as Tissue Fixative and Wash Solution by Lews Scientific Inc., P.O. Box 38, Raritan, N.J. 08869.

TABLE 10–1. CLASSIFICATION OF CANINE AND FELINE BULLOUS SKIN DISEASES BY KNOWN OR SUSPECTED ETIOLOGIC FACTORS AND THE CORRESPONDING HISTOPATHOLOGIC AND IMMUNOLOGIC FINDINGS

Etiologic Classification	Disease	Histopathologic Findings			Immunofluorescence	
		Location of Bullae	Acantho-lysis	Other	Direct	Indirect
Autoimmune	Pemphigus foliaceus	Subcorneal	+		+ ICC*	±
	Pemphigus erythematosus	Subcorneal	+		+ ICC + DEJ‡	±
	Pemphigus vulgaris	Suprabasilar	+		+ ICC	±
	Pemphigus vegetans	Suprabasilar	+		+ ICC	±
	Bullous pemphigoid	Subepidermal	−		+ BMZ†	±
	Systemic lupus erythematosus (SLE)	Subepidermal Subcorneal	− ±	Liquefaction necrosis of basal layer	+ DEJ	−
	Discoid lupus erythematosus (DLE)	Subepidermal	−	Same as above	+ DEJ	−
Immune-mediated	Dermatitis herpetiformis	Subepidermal	−	Microabscess in dermal papilla	−	−
	Toxic epidermal necrolysis	Subepidermal	−	Total epidermal necrosis	−	−
	Drug eruption	Subepidermal	−	Liquefaction necrosis of basal layer	−	−
Hereditary	Epidermal bullosa simplex	Subepidermal	−	Liquefaction necrosis of basal layer	−	−
Idiopathic	Subcorneal pustular dermatosis	Subcorneal	±	Neutrophilic abscess	−	−

*ICC = Intercellular cement substance
†BMZ = Basement membrane zone
‡DEJ = Dermoepidermal junction

ualized in Figures 10–1 through 10–4 and Plates 9:J and 9:K. Serum samples from suspected pemphigus or bullous pemphigoid dogs can be evaluated for indirect immunofluorescent pemphigus titers. It should be remembered that although a positive immunofluorescent finding is diagnostic, a negative finding does not rule out autoimmune bullous disease. Most dogs and cats are reported to have negative indirect pemphigus titers.

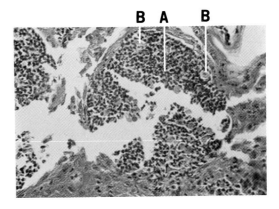

Fig. 10–2. Pemphigus foliaceus: Large subcorneal bulla filled with neutrophils *(A)* and some acantholytic keratinocytes *(B)*.

Dogs and cats with suspected SLE should have a positive antinuclear antibody (ANA) titer; dogs with other autoimmune bullous diseases usually have a negative ANA titer. The exception is pemphigus erythematosus, which is reported to have a positive ANA titer up to 50% of the time.

Treatment. The routine treatment for all of the autoimmune bullous skin diseases in dogs and cats

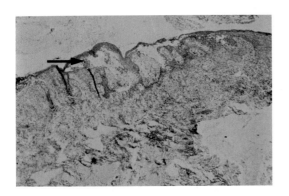

Fig. 10–1. Pemphigus vulagris: Large suprabasilar bullae. Note tombstone appearance (arrow) (low power).

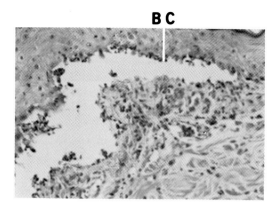

Fig. 10–3. Bullous pemphigoid: Subepidermal bulla with moderate upper dermal cellular infiltrate. Note intact basal cell layer (B,C) (low power).

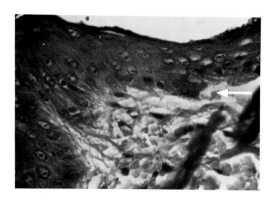

Fig. 10–4. Discoid lupus erythematosus: Liquefaction necrosis of the basal cell layer (arrow) and edema at dermoepidermal junction (low power).

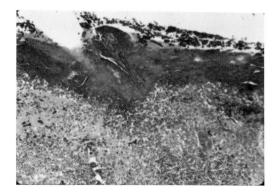

Fig. 10–5. Toxic epidermal necrolysis: Full-thickness necrosis of epidermis with loss of all cellular architecture. Collagen necrosis is observed in the upper dermis (low power).

is the administration of immunosuppressive doses (2.0 to 4.0 mg/kg bid) of corticosteroids. Due to the side effects of long-term corticosteroids in dogs, however, other methods of therapy have been used. These methods include combined corticosteroids and chemotherapy with cyclophosphamide, methotrexate, azathioprine, or chlorambucil. Chryso-

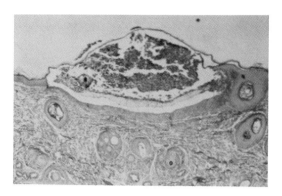

Fig. 10–6. Subcorneal pustular dermatosis: Large subcorneal pustule filled with neutrophils (scan power).

therapy, using aurothioglucose (gold salts), has been reported to be efficacious in both the dog and cat. Vitamin E has recently been used with some success, especially in the treatment of DLE. Refer to the Bullous Disease Therapeutic Key (Appendix 2:13) for specific treatment protocols.

The side effects of the various medications must be discussed with the owners prior to treatment. Cyclophosphamide, methotrexate, and azathioprine may cause leukopenia, thrombocytopenia, immunosuppression, and gastrointestinal signs. A serious side effect of cyclophosphamide is hemorrhagic cystitis, which can lead to irreversible fibrosis of the bladder. Chlorambucil occasionally will be associated with leukopenia. In a limited number of therapeutic trials with aurothioglucose in dogs, few side effects were observed. Thrombocytopenia and hemorrhage were reported to be associated with gold salt therapy in one dog. In man, cutaneous and mucous membrane reactions to aurothioglucose are relatively common. The drug is contraindicated in people with SLE. Long-term corticosteroid therapy commonly leads to cushingoid signs and occasionally to sepsis secondary to immunosuppression.

Prognosis. Pemphigus vulgaris is the most severe of the autoimmune skin diseases. Most dogs and cats require high dosages of immunosuppressive drugs to control the signs that often lead to secondary sepsis. Relapses due to drug resistance are also common. Animals with bullous pemphigoid and pemphigus foliaceus also frequently require large dosages of immunosuppressive drugs to control signs; the long-term therapeutic response is variable. A few dogs are reported to have periods of remission with therapy, although most dogs and cats require some continuous therapeutic method of treatment.

DLE is often a milder disease that can be controlled with alternate-day corticosteroid therapy, topical steroidal creams, and megadoses of vitamin E after initial remission; relapses may occur. The response to SLE therapy is variable. A number of animals can be maintained clinically normal with administration of alternate-day corticosteroids and a few have long-term remission without therapy.

IMMUNE-MEDIATED BULLOUS DISEASES

The immune-mediated bullous diseases are associated with known or suspected immunologic abnormalities without the presence of demonstrable autoantibodies. The three diseases in this group, dermatitis herpetiformis (DH), toxic epidermal necrolysis (TEN), and drug eruption, have a low-reported incidence in dogs. The only immune-mediated bullous disease reported in the cat is TEN. The specific etiologic factors and pathogenic mechanisms have not been verified.

History and Clinical Findings. DH is characterized by unresponsiveness to antibiotics and high-dose corticosteroids. Pruritus is often prominent in the reported history. The lesions are vesicles, papules, and pustules of varying size. Irregular scaling and erythema are associated with the lesions. The lesions are distributed on the feet, the nose, the head, the ears, and the dorsolateral aspect of the trunk. The flank and groin are usually spared. Primary pyoderma is the major differential diagnosis.

TEN is characterized by large, painful ulcerative areas on any part of the body. There may be a mucocutaneous distribution. In the dog, the disease is always associated with some predisposing disease such as a staphylococcal infection or systemic neoplasia. In the cat, the disease has been associated with the administration of feline leukemia virus (FeLV), anticaprine antiserum, and hetacillin. The gross lesion is a diffuse, slow-healing deep ulceration (Plate 9:L).

Drug eruption is characterized by a history of cutaneous eruptions following the administration of a specific drug. The clinical lesions and distribution are variable and mimic many other bullous and nonbullous skin diseases.

Diagnosis. The history and clinical signs support a diagnosis of one of the immune-mediated bullous diseases. A cutaneous biopsy is necessary for making a definitive diagnosis of DH and TEN. DH is characterized by eosinophilic and neutrophilic microabscesses at the dermal papilla. There is an associated subepidermal vesicle formation.

In man, DH is characterized by IgA deposition at the dermal papilla, but this has not been demonstrated in dogs.

TEN is characterized microscopically by necrosis of the entire thickness of the epidermis and by subepidermal vesicles (see Fig. 10–5).

Drug eruptions vary in their histologic characteristics. A drug eruption can cause liquefaction necrosis of the basal cells, subepidermal vesicles, and epidermal necrosis.

Treatment. DH is usually responsive only to dapsone (Avlosulfon, Ayerst), but occasionally the disease responds to sulfapyridine. Lifetime maintenance therapy may be required. Side effects of dapsone include leukopenia, anemia, and liver disease.

TEN is treated with low-dose corticosteroids following a higher loading dose. Supportive topical therapy with astringents and systemic antibiotics is usually indicated. The primary disease must also be treated concurrently.

The treatment of choice for a drug eruption is discontinuing and avoiding further use of the drug that caused the eruption. Corticosteroids are indicated on a short-term basis to decrease the immune-mediated reaction. Refer to the Bullous Disease Therapeutic Key (Appendix 2:13) for specific drugs and dosages for the treatment of immune-mediated diseases discussed in this chapter.

HEREDITARY BULLOUS DISEASE

Epidermolysis bullosa simplex is the only documented hereditary bullous disease in the dog. It has been reported in two breeds of dog (Collie and Shetland Sheepdog) and has never been reported in cats. The disease has been classified as a mechanobullous disease since mild friction or trauma over predisposed pressure points results in subepidermal vesicle formation. Pathogenesis of the disease is unknown. In man, epidermolysis bullosa simplex is transmitted as an autosomal dominant trait.

History. Clinical signs of epidermolysis bullosa are usually seen in the puppy under 6 months of age. The history may indicate a temporary, partial, or total response to corticosteroid therapy. There may be an exacerbation of clinical signs associated with warm weather. Pruritus may be mild or absent.

Clinical Signs. Lesions are found on the dorsal muzzle, tip of the tail, ear margins, and bony prominences such as the digits, carpi, tarsi, and elbows. There is usually periorbital alopecia and alopecia on the dorsum of the nose. The lesions are variable and include vesicles, erosions, ulcers, erythema, plaques, alopecia, scaling, or crusting. Some evidence of scarring (Plate 9:*M*) or atrophy of the skin may be observed.

Diagnosis. The history and clinical signs suggest epidermal bullosa simplex. Cutaneous biopsy reveals degeneration of the basal cell layer and subepidermal vesicle formation. The most definitive diagnostic test is to clip a small area of normal skin over a bony prominence and apply mild trauma with an eraser or thumbnail for approximately 1 minute. A biopsy should be performed at the newly traumatized site within 3 to 5 minutes and the pathologist should look for subepidermal vesicle formation.

Treatment The treatment of choice for controlling the disease is the administration of corticosteroids. However, relapses are common, and lifetime maintenance therapy is often required.

IDIOPATHIC BULLOUS SKIN DISEASE

Canine subcorneal pustular dermatosis (SPD) is the only disease presently classified as an idiopathic disease.

History. The classical history is that of pustular dermatitis that does not respond to antibiotics or corticosteroids. The majority of bacterial cultures of the lesions are sterile. The age of onset varies, but the disease commonly occurs when the animal is 3- to 4-years-old. Pruritus, frequently a primary complaint of the owner, is of variable intensity. The course of the disease is chronic with some dogs exhibiting alternating acute exacerbations and partial to total remissions. There is a reported breed predilection in Miniature Schnauzers, although the disease has been seen in many breeds.

Clinical Signs. Generalized trunkal lesions are

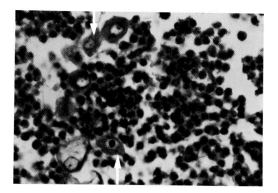

Fig. 10–7. Subcorneal pustular dermatosis: Neutrophils and acantholytic keratinocytes (arrows) in subcorneal pustule (high power).

the most common signs, but the head and medial thighs may also be involved. The lesions begin as erythematous macules, progressing to papules or pustules (Plate 9:*N*) within 36 to 48 hours. These subsequently rupture and form crusts (Plate 9:*O*). The healing stages include annular scaling with an erythemic border followed by a hyperpigmented alopecic lesion that persists for 8 to 10 weeks.

Diagnosis. The history and clinical signs suggest subcorneal pustular dermatosis. Cutaneous biopsy reveals subcorneal pustules with minimal dermal inflammation (Figs. 10–6 and 10–7). A therapeutic trial with dapsone is the most definitive diagnostic test used to differentiate SPD from other bullous diseases characterized by subcorneal bullae.

Treatment. The treatment of choice for SPD is dapsone. Refer to the Bullous Disease Therapeutic Key (Appendix 2:13). The side effects of this drug in dogs include anemia, leukopenia, hepatic toxicosis, and thrombocytopenia. In some dogs the medication can be discontinued during periods of complete remission.

SELECTED READINGS

Bellanti, J.A.: Immunology II. Philadelphia, W.B. Saunders, 1978.

Brown, N., and Hurvitz, A.I.: A mucocutaneous disease in a cat resembling human pemphigus. J. Am. Anim. Hosp. Assoc. 15:25, 1979.

Drazner, F.H.: Systemic lupus erythematosus in the dog. Compend. Cont. Ed. Pract. Vet. 2:243, 1980.

Fadok, V. A., and Janney, E.H: Thrombocytopenia and hemorrhage associated with gold salt therapy for bullous pemphigoid in a dog. J. Am. Vet. Med. Assoc. 181:261, 1982.

Griffin, C.E., and MacDonald, J.: A case of bullous pemphigoid in a dog. J. Am. Anim. Hosp. Assoc. 17:105, 1981.

Griffin, C.E., et al.: Canine discoid lupus erythematosus. Vet. Immunol. and Immunopathol. 1:79, 1979.

Halliwell, R.E.W.: Skin diseases associated with autoimmunity. Part II. The nonbullous autoimmune skin diseases. Compend. Cont. Ed. Pract. Vet. 2:156, 1981.

———: Skin diseases associated with autoimmunity. Part I. The bullous autoimmune skin diseases. Compend. Cont. Ed. Pract. Vet. 2:911, 1980.

Halliwell, R.E.W., and Goldschmidt, M.H.: Pemphigus foliaceus in the canine: A case report and discussion. J. Am. Anim. Hosp. Assoc. 13:431, 1977.

Halliwell, R.E.W., et al.: Dapsone for treatment of pruritic dermatitis (dermatitis herpetiformis and subcorneal pustular dermatosis) in dogs. J. Am. Vet. Med. Assoc. 170:697, 1977.

Hurvitz, A.I., and Feldman, E.: A disease in dogs resembling human pemphigus vulgaris: Case reports. J. Am. Vet. Med. Assoc. 166:585, 1975.

Kunkle, G., Goldschmidt, M.H., and Halliwell, R.E.W.: Bullous pemphigoid in a dog: A case report with immunofluorescent findings. J. Am. Anim. Hosp. Assoc. 14:52, 1978.

Manning, T.O., et al.: Three cases of canine pemphigus foliaceus and observations on chrysotherapy. J. Am. Anim. Hosp. Assoc. 16:189, 1980.

McKeever, P.J., and Dahl, M.V.: A disease in dogs resembling human subcorneal pustular dermatosis. J. Am. Vet. Med. Assoc. 170:704, 1977.

Schultz, K.T., and Goldschmidt, M.: Pemphigus vegetans in a dog. Cornell Vet. 67:374, 1977.

Scott, D.W.: Feline dermatology: A potpourri. *In* Proceedings of 48th Annual Meeting of the American Animal Hospital Association, 1981.

————: Immunologic disorders. J. Am. Anim. Hosp. Assoc. 16:384, 1980.

————: Immunologic skin disorders in the dog and cat. Vet. Clin. North Am. 8:641, 1978.

Scott, D.W., et al.: Observations on the immunopathology and therapy of canine pemphigus and pemphigoid. J. Am. Vet. Med. Assoc. 180:48, 1982.

————: The comparative pathology of non-viral bullous skin diseases in domestic animals. Vet. Pathol. 17:257, 1980.

————: Pemphigus erythematosus in the dog and cat. J. Am. Anim. Hosp Assoc. 16: 815, 1980.

————: Toxic epidermal necrolysis in two dogs and a cat. J. Am. Anim. Hosp. Assoc. 15:271, 1979.

————: A glucocorticoid-responsive dermatitis in cats resembling systemic lupus erythematosus in man. J. Am. Anim. Hosp. Assoc. 15:157, 1979.

Walton, D.K., et al.: Canine discoid lupus erythematosus. J. Am. Anim. Hosp. Assoc. 17:851, 1981.

11

Cutaneous Neoplastic and Cystic Diseases

Cutaneous neoplasms are the most frequently recognized neoplasms and represent more than 30% of all tumors in dogs and 20% of all tumors in cats. Mammary gland tumors, which are not always included in classifications of cutaneous tumors, especially in incidence surveys, are discussed in the section, "Neoplasms of Epithelial Origin."

ETIOLOGIC FACTORS

Specific etiologic factors of most cutaneous tumors are unknown. Both intrinsic and extrinsic factors have been implicated. Solar and ionizing radiation, as well as viral, chemical, hormonal, genetic, and immunologic factors all potentially play a role in the cause or origin of cutaneous tumors.

PATHOGENESIS

The pathogenesis of most cutaneous tumors is unknown. An irritant factor may act as an initiator, setting the stage for cell transformation. When the skin is exposed to another factor, called a promoter, overt clinical or histologic signs of cancer result.

HISTORY

The Canine Cutaneous Neoplastic and Cystic Disease Diagnostic Key (Appendix 1:11) outlines the pertinent historical and clinical findings and screening and definitive diagnostic tests that help to differentiate the most commonly encountered neoplasms and cysts. Similar data are presented in the Feline Cutaneous Neoplastic and Cystic Disease Diagnostic Key (Appendix 1:12).

Several breeds of dogs have a predilection for cutaneous tumors; these include the Boxer, Scottish Terrier, Kerry Blue Terrier, Norwegian Elkhound, Bassett Hound, and Weimaraner. No breed predilection has been reported in cats. It has been reported, however, that there is a lower incidence of skin tumors in Siamese cats than in other breeds.

CLASSIFICATION AND INCIDENCE

Cutaneous neoplasms are often classified according to their origin, i.e., as epithelial tumors, mesenchymal tumors, or tumors of melanin-producing cells. Multiple histologic types of skin tumors often occur simultaneously in the same animal.

Knowledge of the relative frequency and biologic behavior of skin tumors is important. Table 11–1 presents the origin, relative incidence, and biologic behavior of canine cutaneous neoplasms. Similar data for feline cutaneous tumors are found in Table 11–2. Relative incidence of cysts is not generally reported, although they are common in dogs and rare in cats.

TABLE 11–1.   THE ORIGIN, RELATIVE INCIDENCE, AND BIOLOGIC BEHAVIOR OF CANINE CUTANEOUS NEOPLASMS

Tumor or Cyst	Origin	Relative Incidence %*	Biologic Behavior		
			Always Benign	Occasionally Locally Invasive or Metastatic	Malignant
Lipoma	Mesenchymal	24.2	yes	no	no
Perianal gland adenoma	Epithelial	12.0	no	yes	no
Mast cell tumor	Mesenchymal	10.5	no	yes	yes
Squamous cell carcinoma	Epithelial	8.7	no	no	yes
Sebaceous gland adenoma	Epithelial	7.3	yes	no	no
Hemangiopericytoma	Mesenchymal	7.1	no	yes	no
Papilloma	Epithelial	4.4	yes	no	no
Melanoma	Melanin-producing cell	4.4	no	yes	yes
Basal cell tumor	Epithelial	4.1	no	yes	no
Histiocytoma	Mesenchymal	4.0	yes	no	no
Hemangioma	Mesenchymal	2.8	yes	no	no
Trichoepithelioma	Epithelial	2.1	no	yes	no
Sebaceous gland adenocarcinoma	Epithelial	1.9	no	no	yes
Fibroma	Mesenchymal	1.6	yes	no	no
Fibrosarcoma	Mesenchymal	1.3	no	no	yes
Cutaneous lymphosarcoma	Mesenchymal	1.2	no	yes	yes
Hemangiosarcoma	Mesenchymal	1.2	no	no	yes
Intracutaneous cornifying epithelioma	Epithelial	1.0	yes	no	no
Hair matrix tumor	Epithelial	0.9	yes	no	no
Neurofibroma	Mesenchymal	0.4	no	yes	no
Leiomyoma	Mesenchymal	0.3	yes	no	no
Myxosarcoma	Mesenchymal	0.3	no	no	yes
Sweat gland adenoma	Epithelial	0.25	yes	no	no
Sweat gland adenocarcinoma	Epithelial	0.2	no	no	yes
Liposarcoma	Mesenchymal	0.2	no	no	yes
Leiomyosarcoma	Mesenchymal	0.1	no	no	yes
Myxoma	Mesenchymal	0.1	yes	no	no
Mammary gland tumor	Epithelial	NR†	no	yes	yes

*Relative incidence is based on the averaging of data from Priester, W.A.: J. Natl. Cancer Inst. 50:457, 1973 and Theilen, G.H., and Madewell, B.R.: Veterinary Cancer Medicine, Lea & Febiger, 1979, p. 126.
†NR = not reported

TABLE 11–2.   THE ORIGIN, RELATIVE INCIDENCE, AND BIOLOGIC BEHAVIOR OF FELINE CUTANEOUS NEOPLASMS

Tumor	Origin	Relative Incidence %*	Biologic Behavior		
			Always Benign	Occasionally Locally Invasive or Metastatic	Malignant
Squamous cell carcinoma	Epithelial	26.2†	no	yes	yes
Fibrosarcoma	Mesenchymal	18.2	no	yes	yes
Basal cell tumor	Epithelial	15.7	yes	no	no
Mast cell tumor	Mesenchymal	10.4	no	yes	yes
Fibroma	Mesenchymal	4.1	yes	no	no
Trichoepithelioma	Epithelial	2.8	yes	no	no
Hemangioma	Mesenchymal	2.5	yes	no	no
Melanoma	Melanin-producing cell	2.1	no	yes	yes
Sebaceous gland adenoma	Epithelial	1.8	yes	no	no
Lipoma	Mesenchymal	1.8	yes	no	no
Sebaceous gland adenocarcinoma	Epithelial	1.0	no	yes	yes
Hemangiopericytoma	Mesenchymal	1.0	yes	no	no
Papilloma	Epithelial	1.0	yes	no	no
Leiomyoma	Mesenchymal	1.0	yes	no	no

*Relative incidence is based on the averaging of data from Priester, W.A.: J. Natl. Cancer Inst. 50:457, 1973 and Theilen, G.H., and Madewell, B.R.: Veterinary Cancer Medicine, Philadelphia, Lea & Febiger, 1979, p. 126.
†The incidence of feline squamous cell carcinoma is reported to be from 9 to 25% in other published reports.

Differentiating benign from malignant lesions is not always easy based on the gross appearance and history. Guidelines for differentiation of biologic activity are presented in Table 11–3. Cats have a higher proportion of malignant skin tumors than dogs. Only 3 of the 10 most common canine cutaneous tumors are considered to be malignant. The malignant tumors are mast cell tumor, squamous cell carcinoma, and melanoma. The more benign form of the mast cell tumor predominates in dogs. Squamous cell carcinoma is often highly invasive at the primary site, but is seldom metastatic. Only the oral and digital forms of melanoma are highly metastatic.

Of the 4 feline cutaneous tumors of highest incidence, 3 are usually malignant. These include fibrosarcoma, mast cell tumor, and squamous cell carcinoma.

Incidence of skin tumor types varies with geographic location. In some surveys, tumors of mesenchymal origin predominate, although those of epithelial origin have the highest incidence in others. Squamous cell carcinoma has a higher incidence in areas where animals are exposed to excessive amounts of sunlight. In both dogs and cats the incidence of skin cancer increases with age.

Neoplasms and Cysts of Epithelial Origin

EPIDERMOID, SEBACEOUS, AND EPIDERMAL INCLUSION CYSTS

Epidermoid, sebaceous, and epidermal inclusion cysts commonly occur in dogs and rarely in cats. They are observed most frequently in middle-aged and older dogs, but may be present when the dog is 1 to 2 years of age. The cysts are dermal or subcutaneous masses 0.2 to 3 cm in diameter (Plate 10:A). They may remain relatively static or may slowly increase in size. There is usually no discomfort or inflammation unless the cyst ruptures. The sebaceous cyst is filled with a doughy or semi-ifluid grey to brownish material (Plate 10:B) that is easily expressed with gentle pressure from most larger cysts. This procedure is not recommended, however, because a rupture of the cyst wall and release of the keratin can cause an inflammatory response in the adjacent dermis and subcutis.

PERIANAL GLAND ADENOMA

Perianal gland adenoma is a common tumor of older male and occasionally female dogs. The most common age of occurrence is 8 to 12 years. There is a predilection in the Dachshund, Cocker Spaniel, and German Shepherd.

Perianal gland tumors are located primarily around the anus. Occasionally they extend to the prepuce, the base of the tail, and along the sacral and lumbar regions of the back. They may be solitary or multiple nodules of variable size (Plate 10:C). Since pruritus is common, scooting and licking the tumor results in ulceration, hemorrhage, and sometimes secondary infection.

Although the majority of perianal gland tumors are benign, metastasis may occur to regional lymph nodes, especially in female dogs.

SQUAMOUS CELL CARCINOMA

Squamous cell carcinoma is one of the most common cutaneous tumors in dogs and cats. It is most prevalent in animals that are exposed excessively to sunlight. Dogs and cats of highest risk are at least 5-years-old and lack melanin pigment, e.g., white cats.

There may be a history of a previous solar dermatitis. In dogs, concurrent papillomas may also be observed in the same lesion. Often, there is a history of poor response to previous conservative treatment with antibiotics and steroids.

Squamous cell carcinoma has a predilection for mucocutaneous areas. In the dog, the oral cavity is the primary site with associated tumors of the lips and nose. The ventral abdomen of the dog is also a common site, and digital tumors rarely occur. The ears are the most common site for squamous cell carcinoma in cats (Plate 10:D) and nostril (Plate 10:E), and mammary glands are other sites of moderate to high incidence.

Clinical signs associated with squamous cell carcinoma vary depending on predisposing factors, and duration and degree of malignancy of the tumor. The early, precancerous lesion is erythematous and scaly; then, a thickened, infiltrative, fre-

TABLE 11–3. DIFFERENTIATION OF BENIGN AND MALIGNANT TUMORS ON THE BASIS OF HISTORY AND PHYSICAL EXAMINATION

Historical and Clinical Findings	
Benign	Malignant
Slow growth	Rapid growth
Well circumscribed	Poorly circumscribed
Nonulcerated	Often ulcerated
Not attached to surrounding structures	Fixation to overlying skin or underlying fascia
No local invasion	Local invasion
No regional lymphadenopathy	Regional lymphadenopathy
Long clinical course (weeks to years)	Rapid clinical course

quently ulcerated lesion develops. Pruritus may keep the lesion moist, thus causing a secondary infection. If the tumor becomes malignant, erosion and ulceration of the tissue and rapid local invasion as well as regional lymph node involvement may be seen. Squamous cell tumors of the digits are usually malignant with involvement of the foot pads and underlying bone.

SEBACEOUS GLAND TUMORS

Sebaceous gland tumors are divided into the following categories based on the level of maturation of the cells: nodular hyperplasia, sebaceous adenoma, sebaceous epithelioma, and sebaceous adenocarcinoma. These tumors are common in the Cocker Spaniel and Poodle. Sebaceous gland tumors are uncommon in cats.

Most of these tumors are observed incidentally by the owner and are asymptomatic. They often remain static in size and shape for years; adenocarcinoma, which is uncommon in dogs and rare in cats, is the exception with rapid growth observed.

Distribution is usually on the dorsal and lateral aspects of the trunk, legs, head, and neck. Sebaceous gland tumors may be solitary or multiple.

The most common type of sebaceous gland tumor is nodular hyperplasia, which is characterized as a discrete, lobulated, yellow mass, 2 to 5 mm in diameter (Plate 10:F). Sebaceous adenoma is wider in diameter (up to 2 cm), and less lobulated than a hyperplastic lesion (Plate 10:G). Sebaceous epithelioma is a firm, well-circumscribed, dermal mass that is frequently ulcerated and alopecic, and moves freely over underlying tissue. Sebaceous adenocarcinoma is characterized by rapid growth, ill-defined borders, and ulceration (Plate 10:H). Greasy sebaceous material may be forced from most sebaceous gland tumors. Histologic features assist in the characterization of the sebaceous gland tumor.

PAPILLOMA (WARTS)

Papillomas most commonly occur in the oral cavity and on the lips of dogs under 1 year of age. Such growths are occasionally seen on the medial aspect of the thighs. Papillomas are rare in cats. The growths may be observed by the owner before any other signs are noted. Hemorrhage from the lips and oral cavity may be noted as may a reluctance to eat.

Papillomas are initially smooth, white growths located around the lips that develop into roughened cauliflower-like surfaces (Plate 10:I). As the number of papillomas increases, more are observed on the tongue, hard palate, and medial cheek.

BASAL CELL TUMORS

Basal cell tumors are frequently seen in both dogs and cats over 6 years of age. They are slow-growing and often observed for years as asymptomatic, solitary tumors.

Basal cell tumors are most often found near the commissures of the mouth, eyes, pinnae, cheeks, and jaw; the trunk is less frequently affected. Tumors of this type are usually small, often less than 2.5 cm in diameter, circumscribed, encapsulated, and hairless with a pinkish-white glistening surface (Plate 10:J); they may also have a large central cyst. A large tumor may ulcerate. Feline basal tumors are often pigmented.

TRICHOEPITHELIOMA

Trichoepithelioma represents a small percentage of cutaneous skin tumors of dogs and cats. They range in diameter from 1 to 5 cm, and are found in the subcutaneous tissue, usually on the back. Ulceration may be observed.

INTRACUTANEOUS CORNIFYING EPITHELIOMA (KERATOACANTHOMA)

Intracutaneous cornifying epithelioma is most common in young male dogs, many under 5 years of age. There is a breed predilection in the Norwegian Elkhound and Keeshond for the multicentric form of the tumor. Athough many of these tumors are asymptomatic, there may be a history of biting at the site of the larger ones. Most tumors occur on the back, neck, thorax, and shoulders.

The gross appearance of intracutaneous cornifying epithelioma is variable. There is a dermal mass, usually from 1 to 4 cm in diameter, with a small central pore opening onto the skin surface from which a cheesy-like material can be expressed. At times a larger pore opening is observed, which contains a hard mass of keratin (Plate 10:K). A third type of epithelioma consists of multiple, small dermal masses within a large, protruding keratinized structure that emerges from the central pore.

MAMMARY GLAND TUMORS

Mammary gland tumors are the most common neoplasm in female dogs, and the third most frequently recognized tumors in cats. Unspayed females over 6 years of age have the highest incidences. Dogs and cats spayed prior to the first estrus have a low incidence. Spaying after $2\frac{1}{2}$ years of age does not have a marked effect on the incidence of mammary gland tumors.

The majority of mammary gland tumors in dogs are benign, however, most feline mammary tumors are malignant. Single or multiple glands may be involved.

In the dog, small nodules in the subcutaneous tissue near the nipples are usually benign (Plate 10:L). Larger tumors, and those which expand rapidly in size, tend to be more malignant and often ulcerate. The majority of feline mammary gland tumors are characterized by rapid growth, invasion, ulceration, and metastasis to regional lymph nodes, lungs, pleura, and liver.

Neoplasms of Mesenchymal Origin

LIPOMA

Lipoma is the most common cutaneous neoplasm in dogs; however, it is uncommon in cats. Incidence is highest in the older (7 or more years of age), overweight, female dog. Breeds reported to have the highest incidence include the Poodle, Dachshund, Weimaraner, Beagle, Cocker Spaniel, and Labrador Retriever.

Lipomas are slow-growing, usually asymptomatic, round to ovoid, well-circumscribed masses ranging in size from 0.5 to 20 cm in diameter (Plate 10:M). They are usually found in the subcutaneous tissue of the trunk and mammary gland areas. Occasionally, lipomas are found between intra-abdominal or intrathoracic muscle masses and can be soft or firm. A large ventral tumor can occasionally become traumatized and ulcerate.

MASTOCYTOMA (MAST CELL TUMOR)

Mastocytomas are frequently observed in both the dog and cat. The Boxer, Boston Terrier, English Bulldog, English Bull Terrier, and Fox Terrier have a predilection for mast cell tumors. The highest incidence is in dogs older than 6 years and the risk increases with age. Benign mast cell tumors may be slow-growing over a period of months to years. There may be a history of temporary, clinical response to steroids. In contrast, malignant mast cell tumors rapidly increase in size and usually show minimal if any response to steroids.

Cutaneous canine mastocytoma is usually benign. It is characterized by dermal or subcutaneous masses that have a predilection for the upper posterior limbs and perineal and preputial regions, but the tumors may be found on any part of the body. The tumors range in size from one to several centimeters in diameter and may be either solitary or multiple.

Benign tumors are firm, circumscribed, encapsulated, and are attached to the epidermis (Plate 10:N). In contrast, malignant tumors are nonencapsulated and extend deep into subcutaneous tissue. Ulceration, erythema, edema, and inflammation are common in the surrounding tissue. Metastasis to regional lymph nodes usually occurs. Systemic signs of duodenal and gastric ulceration, dysproteinemia, coagulopathies, and inflammatory glomerular disease have been associated with malignant canine mastocytoma.

Feline mastocytoma occurs at any age; no breed predilection has been reported; however, there is a higher incidence in males. There is usually a poor response to symptomatic therapy.

Feline mast cell tumors are usually malignant. Cutaneous tumors have variable clinical presentation. Most cats have multiple tumors in the region of the head and neck, which are usually firm, raised, dermal masses of 0.5 to 5 cm in diameter (Plates 10:O and 10:P). The borders are usually well demarcated although a few tumors are soft with nondiscrete borders. Color may be pink, yellow, or white. Lesions may be ulcerated, especially if they are large (Plate 10:Q). Splenomegaly and sometimes hepatomegaly are frequently associated with mast cell tumors, as are metastasis to regional lymph nodes and lungs.

CANINE HEMANGIOPERICYTOMA (SPINDLE CELL TUMOR, PERITHELIOMA)

Hemangiopericytoma occurs commonly in dogs over 5 years of age. There is a breed predilection for the Boxer, German Shepherd, Cocker Spaniel, and Beagle. Females are more commonly affected. Tumor growth is slow and progressive.

The majority of hemangiopericytomas are located on the extremities. They range in size from 0.5 to 25 cm in diameter. Small tumors are smooth or lobulated, well circumscribed, and move freely (Plate 10:R). Large tumors infiltrate the surrounding tissues, have indistinct borders, and frequently ulcerate. Secondary infection may follow.

CANINE CUTANEOUS HISTIOCYTOMA

Histiocytomas are common benign tumors that occur in young dogs. The average age is 2 years although immature dogs may be affected. The Boxer and Dachshund have the highest incidence. Tumors usually grow rapidly. Solitary tumors predominate although a multiple histiocytoma may occur.

Histiocytomas are usually located on the head, especially the ear pinna, neck, trunk, and legs. They are firm, well circumscribed, dome or button shaped and range in size from 0.3 to 2 cm in diameter (Plate 10:S). The surface is usually erythematous and may be ulcerated.

CUTANEOUS HEMANGIOMA

The incidence of hemangioma is low in both dogs and cats. It occurs most frequently in middle-aged or older dogs and cats, although occurrences have been noted in younger dogs.

Hemangiomas are characterized as soft or spongy, circumscribed, spherical to ovoid, dermal or subcutaneous masses, 0.5 to 2.0 cm in diameter. The overlying skin often has a dark red or bluish discoloration and may be alopecic (Plate 10:T). Some large tumors have an ulcerated surface and bleed easily.

CUTANEOUS HEMANGIOSARCOMA

Hemangiosarcoma occurs occasionally in dogs and rarely in cats. Male German Shepherd dogs are reported to have a higher incidence than other breeds.

Clinically, cutaneous hemangiosarcoma is usually a large, firm, poorly circumscribed, subcutaneous tumor. Marked inflammation and dark discoloration are observed in the surrounding tissue (Plate 10:U).

Systemic signs of metastasis are usually observed; the regional lymph nodes, liver, and lungs are the primary metastatic sites.

FIBROMA

Fibromas occur in both dogs and cats, although a higher incidence is reported in cats. There is no breed or sex predilection. Fibromas are more common in older animals. Solitary or multiple lesions are observed in the canine, although feline fibroma is usually solitary. Fibromas are usually asymptomatic unless traumatized. Canine fibroma has a predilection for areas lined by mucous membranes such as the gingiva, vagina, and rectum, and also for the limbs (Plate 10:V) and flank. There is no site predilection for feline fibroma.

Fibromas are characterized as firm or soft discrete masses of varying size located in the dermis and subcutis. The surface may be alopecic and the tumor may be pedunculated.

FIBROSARCOMA

Fibrosarcomas are the most frequently observed mesenchymal tumors and the second most com-

mon skin tumors in cats. They occur infrequently in dogs. Tumors may appear benign for a variable period of time before growing rapidly and metastasizing to regional lymph nodes and lungs. They respond poorly to symptomatic treatment.

Solitary nonviral-induced feline fibrosarcomas occur most commonly in older cats, with an average age of 11 years. Multicentric, viral-induced tumors occur in kittens under 4 months of age. These kittens are feline leukemia-test positive.

Fibrosarcomas are firm, poorly circumscribed masses of irregular size and shape (Plate 10:W). Ulceration, infection, and edema are common in advanced fibrosarcoma.

CUTANEOUS LYMPHOSARCOMA

Primary cutaneous lymphosarcoma is uncommon in dogs and rare in cats. The highest rate of occurrence is in older dogs; there is no breed or sex predilection. There is a history of poor response to systemic corticosteroids and antibiotics, The course of tumor growth may be weeks to years. Pruritus varies.

Cutaneous lymphosarcoma is characterized by variable clinical signs. Multiple nodules are present in the majority of dogs and cats (Plates 10:X and 10:Y) Alopecic, erythematous, scaly macules or patches may be observed (Plate 10:Z). Involvement of the mucocutaneous junctions and skin with diffuse infiltration of the tissue, erythema, ulceration, and crusting (Plates 10:AA and 10:BB) may be confused with signs of a bullous disease.

In advanced disease, peripheral lymphadenopathy may be noted.

Tumors of Melanin-Producing Cells

MELANOMA (JUNCTIONAL OR DERMAL MELANOCYTOMA, MALIGNANT MELANOMA)

Melanoma is commonly seen in dogs and infrequently in cats. Tumors occur in animals usually 7 years and older. The Scottish Terrier, Cocker Spaniel, Airedale, and Boston Terrier breeds have the highest incidence. Benign melanoma is usually solitary and may persist for years with minimal growth. Malignant melanoma usually grows rapidly and often metastasizes prior to the initial clinical examination. The majority of feline melanomas are malignant.

Melanoma may occur on any part of the body. The most common sites are the oral cavity, lips, eyelids, trunk and digits. Digital and oral melanomas are usually highly malignant.

Benign melanomas are usually brown to black growths, 0.5 to 4 cm in diameter. They may be round, ovoid, or pedunculated (Plate 10:CC). Malignant melanomas are discrete, dome-shaped, or sessile masses with infiltration into the surrounding tissue. They are usually pigmented, but may be amelanotic or nonpigmented. Necrosis, hemorrhage, and ulceration are common. Signs of metastasis to regional lymph nodes and lungs are frequently observed.

DIAGNOSIS

Definitive diagnosis of a specific tumor or type of cyst is often difficult to determine on the basis of history and clinical signs. Aspiration, incisional, and excisional biopsy are the diagnostic tests of choice.

Aspiration biopsy is of diagnostic value in the following types of tumor or cyst: epidermoid or sebaceous cyst, lipoma, mast cell tumor, and perianal gland adenoma. Results of aspiration biopsy are often suggestive but not definitive for a specific diagnosis. Figures 11–1 to 11–4 represent diagnostic characteristics of aspiration biopsies.

Tissue biopsy is the definitive diagnostic test

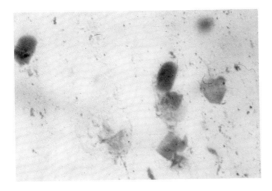

Fig. 11–1. Aspiration of sebaceous cyst. Note epithelial cells and absence of inflammatory cells.

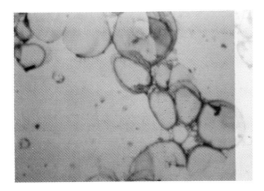

Fig. 11–2. Aspiration of lipoma. Note aggregates of lipocytes and absence of inflammatory cells.

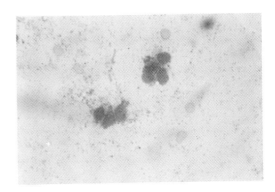

Fig. 11–3. Aspiration of mast cell. Note aggregates of mast cells and free mast cell granules.

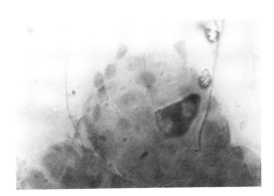

Fig. 11–4. Aspiration of perianal gland adenoma. Note sheets of hepatoid (epithelial) cells.

for all cutaneous neoplasms and cysts. Size, location, and suspected biologic behavior of the growth should be considered when selecting incisional as opposed to excisional biopsy.

The reader is referred to dermatopathology references for microscopic differentiation of the cutaneous cysts and tumors.

TREATMENT

Indications for specific therapeutic protocols and suggested therapy are given in the Cutaneous Neoplastic and Cystic Disease Therapeutic Key (Appendix 2:14).

The treatment of choice for most cutaneous tumors involves surgical excision. There are a few benign tumors and cysts that may not require any treatment, except for cosmetic reasons: these include the epidermoid cyst, lipoma, sebaceous gland nodular hyperplasia, adenoma, papilloma, and intracutaneous cornifying epithelioma. Adjunct therapy in the form of chemotherapy or immunotherapy is only indicated for the most malignant tumors, usually after metastasis has occurred. Neoplasms in this group include mast cell tumor, perianal gland tumor, mammary gland tumor, and sebaceous adenocarcinoma.

Squamous cell carcinoma, mast cell tumor, and perianal gland tumor are all partially responsive to radiotherapy.

SELECTED READINGS

Bevier, D.E., and Goldschmidt, M.H.: Skin tumors in the dog. Part I. Epithelial tumors and tumorlike lesions. Compend. Cont. Ed. Pract. Vet. 3:389, 1981.

————: Skin tumors in the dog. Part II. Tumors of the soft (mesenchymal) tissues. Compend. Cont. Ed. Pract. Vet. 3:506, 1981.

Gillete, E.L.: Radiotherapy. In Veterinary Cancer Medicine. Edited by G.H. Theilen and B.R. Madewell. Philadelphia, Lea & Febiger, 1979.

Hoover, E.A.: Pathologic features of canine cutaneous neoplasms. In Proceedings of Kal Kan Symposium for the treatment of dog and cat diseases. Vernon, California, Kal Kan Foods, 1980.

Macy, D.W., and Reynolds, H.A.: The incidence, characteristics and clinical management of skin tumors of cats. J. Am. Anim. Hosp. Assoc. 17:1026, 1981.

Madewell, B.R.: Therapy of cutaneous neoplasms in dogs and cats. In Proceedings of Kal Kan Symposium for the treatment of dog and cat diseases. Vernon, California, Kal Kan Foods, 1980.

Madewell, B.R., and Theilen, G.H. (eds.): Chemotherapy. In Veterinary Cancer Medicine. Philadelphia, Lea & Febiger, 1979.

Priester, W.A.: Epidemiology. In Veterinary Cancer Medicine. Edited by G.H. Theilen and B.R. Madewell. Philadelphia, Lea & Febiger, 1979.

————: Skin tumors in domestic animals: Data from 12 United States and Canadian Colleges of Veterinary Medicine. J. Natl. Cancer Inst. 50:457, 1973.

Robison, C.T.: Cryosurgery. In Veterinary Cancer Medicine. Edited by G.H. Theilen and B.R. Madewell. Philadelphia, Lea & Febiger, 1979.

Scott, D.W.: Neoplastic disorders. J. Am. Anim. Hosp. Assoc. 16:419, 1980.

Stannard, A.A., and Pulley, L.T.: Tumors of the skin and soft tissue. In Tumors of Domestic Animals. Edited by Jack Moulton. Berkeley, California, University of California Press, 1978.

————: Intracutaneous cornifying epithelioma (keratoacanthoma) in the dog: A retrospective study of 25 cases. J. Am. Vet. Med. Assoc. 167:385, 1975.

Theilen, G.H., and Madewell, B.R. (eds.): Tumors of skin and subcutaneous tissues. In Veterinary Cancer Medicine. Philadelphia, Lea & Febiger, 1979.

12

Miscellaneous Diseases

In the future, the etiologic factors of some of the canine and feline skin diseases discussed in this chapter will be further understood and the diseases will subsequently be classified more specifically. Pertinent historical and clinical findings and diagnostic tests are summarized in the Canine (Appendix 1:13) and Feline (Appendix 1:14) Miscellaneous Disease Diagnostic Keys. Suggested treatments are summarized in the Miscellaneous Disease Therapeutic Keys for Canine (Appendix 2:15) and Feline (Appendix 2:16).

PHYSICAL AND CHEMICAL DISORDERS

Irritant Contact Dermatitis

Irritant contact dermatitis is not immune mediated as is allergic contact dermatitis. Irritant contact dermatitis is the most common form of contact dermatitis in the dog and cat.

Etiologic Factors. Irritant contact dermatitis may be caused by either chemical or physical agents. The specific etiologic agents are similar for irritant and allergic contact dermatitis (Table 12–1). Some chemical and physical agents are primary irritants on the first exposure and act as allergens on subsequent exposures. It is often difficult to distinguish between an irritant and allergic reaction on the basis of history and clinical signs.

Pathogenesis. The pathogenesis of irritant

TABLE 12–1. ETIOLOGIC AGENTS OF IRRITANT CONTACT DERMATITIS IN DOGS AND CATS

Chemicals and ions	Materials and products
Chrome	Wool
Nickel	Synthetic fibers
Iodine	Rubber
Formaldehyde	Plastic
Dyes	Cleaning materials
Finishes (floor, fibers)	Polishes
Oleoresins	Leather
Sterols	Vehicles for drugs
Antioxidants	Flea collars
	Fertilizer

contact dermatitis is not as well understood as that of allergic contact dermatitis. Precise mechanisms by which chemicals cause irritation to skin are not known. These materials may not be toxic in themselves, but may be carried in a petroleum derivative which is toxic, or they may potentiate the toxicity of an otherwise mildly toxic material. Irritating qualities of petroleum distillate products are directly proportional to their fat solvent properties.

Substances that contact skin may cause varying degrees of damage to the epidermis. Heavy metals act as direct toxin to cells. Mildly irritant substances may dry the skin, which then becomes less resistant to further insults by the same or other materials. Severe or continued toxic damage by a contactant may result in the development of an acute edematous reaction which leads to epidermal necrosis and ulceration. Milder acting toxicants may result in thickened skin with minimal erythema. The most mild toxicants used over extended periods of time may cause only hyperpigmentation and slight fissuring of the epidermis.

History. Classical history for irritant contact dermatitis is a sudden onset at any age of pruritus and dermatitis associated with recent exposure to a potentially irritant chemical or physical agent. The lesions can be severe within a period of a few days or may gradually progress over a period of several weeks. It is common to observe lesions that persist for a variable period of time following removal from, or lack of contact with, the suspected irritant because of the initial damage to the skin.

Pruritus and self-trauma vary, but are often severe. Distribution of lesions is usually more variable with irritant than with allergic contact dermatitis. Many irritant contact problems are caused by liquids that may come in contact with any part of the body. Irritant reactions to the fibers of rugs or bedding result in a predominantly ventral and lateral distribution of lesions as is observed in the majority of allergic contact dermatitis reactions.

Clinical Signs. Physical examination reveals variable signs depending on many factors such as specific cause, severity of the pruritus, location of the lesions, and degree of secondary skin changes. Acute irritant contact dermatitis is usually characterized by erythema and a moist edematous lesion (Plate 11:A). The most common distribution is on the less haired areas of the body (ventral abdomen, medial thighs, axillae, footpads, and pinnae). A liquid irritant contactant may cause lesions on the haired areas also. With irritant reactions this often progresses rapidly to excoriation, ulceration, crusting, and alopecia (Plate 11:B). If there is a slower progression or less severe irritant reaction, excessive scaling and hyperpigmentation will be prominent. Lichenification may be observed and scarring may result from severe dermal inflammation.

Diagnosis. History of recent exposure to a potentially irritant chemical or physical agent supports a diagnosis of irritant contact dermatitis as does a history of improvement of clinical signs after isolation from the suspected irritant. Several screening diagnostic tests are indicated to rule out other primary and secondary causes. These include skin scraping, fungus culture, bacterial culture, and biopsy.

The most definitive diagnostic test for contact irritant dermatitis is isolation from the suspected irritant, followed by provocative exposure; however, such exposure is frequently avoided since many irritant reactions are severe. A presumptive diagnosis is justified on the basis of remission of clinical signs with the avoidance of the suspected irritant as long as other differential diagnoses have been ruled out.

Open or closed patch testing is seldom used for the purpose of identifying an irritant chemical or physical agent.

Treatment. Once a diagnosis of irritant contact dermatitis has been made, the best method of treatment is avoidance of exposure. Supportive therapy is often necessary until the lesions are in remission. If pruritus is a prominent clinical sign, oral or topical corticosteroids are indicated. Antibiotics, either oral or topical, should be used if there is concurrent pyoderma.

Care must be exercised when applying topical agents to lesions caused by irritants. When heavy crusting is present, warm water soaks without the application of topical medicaments are often helpful. If keratolytic agents are not irritating to the lesions, they may be indicated to help control scaling and crusting. See the Miscellaneous Disease Therapeutic Keys for specific drugs and dosages (Appendices 2:15 and 2:16).

Prevention of further self-trauma may be achieved with the use of an Elizabethan collar or similar device.

Prognosis. The prognosis for irritant contact dermatitis is usually favorable if the primary irritant agent is identified and avoided.

Solar Dermatitis (Actinic Dermatitis)

Solar dermatitis is defined as an actinic or photoaggravated reaction.

Etiologic Factors. Solar radiation (ultraviolet light waves of 3000 Angstrom unit band) and genetic predisposition are thought to play major roles in the cause of solar dermatitis. It has been suggested that several other factors, such as photodynamic agents or diseases may result in an indirect photosensitivity reaction that leads to the clinical signs of nasal solar dermatitis. Discoid lupus erythematosus is thought to be the major disease in most dogs (see Chap. 10).

Pathogenesis. The exact pathogenesis of solar dermatitis is unknown, although multiple factors are thought to be involved. Some evidence suggests that the ultraviolet rays alter deoxyribonucleic acid (DNA) synthesis and repair in the epidermis.

History. The usual history of a dog with nasal

solar dermatitis is exacerbation of irritation on the dorsum of the nose following extended exposure to greater than normal sun intensity. The tips and margins of the pinnae of white cats are usually involved. Subsequent improvement of lesions with decreased exposure to sunlight is commonly reported.

Incidence of solar dermatitis varies with geographic areas. It is most common in areas with long periods of intense sunlight, although reflection from snow can also result in severe reactions. The lesions tend to worsen each succeeding year unless treated. There is a tendency for the involved area to be easily traumatized.

The following breeds of dogs are predisposed to nasal solar dermatitis: white German Shepherd, Australian Shepherd, Welsh Corgi, and Weimaraner. There is no age or sex predilection. In cats, early lesions of solar dermatitis may be seen by 3 years of age, although the neoplastic process is usually observed over 7 years of age.

The drug history often includes a total or partial response to corticosteroids or sunscreens, especially if the lesions are less severe.

Clinical Signs. Initial lesions of canine nasal solar dermatitis are erythema and depigmentation at the junction of the haired and nonhaired areas of the dorsum of the nose (Plate 11:C), or on the planum nasale. Erosions and ulcerations are frequently present. Variable degrees of alopecia, crusting, excoriation, and secondary infection are observed. If the lesions are in a healing stage, they are often covered with a thin, dry, alopecic epithelium. A significant feature of nasal solar dermatitis is the localization of lesions to the nares and dorsum of the muzzle. If there are lesions on the pinnae or commissures of the mouth, other possibilities should be considered, such as immune-mediated disease.

In feline solar dermatitis there is an initial inflammatory reaction with erythema of the tips and margins of the pinnae. Alopecia, scaling, crusts, and pruritus follow as the lesions become more severe and chronic. The ear margins may begin to curl. Squamous cell carcinoma usually develops following several years of sunlight exposure. The neoplastic lesions are characterized by persistent ulcerative, locally invasive lesions of the pinnae.

Diagnosis. History and clinical findings are suggestive of solar dermatitis. Most of the diagnostic workup is for the purpose of ruling out other primary etiologic factors that may result in similar lesions. Diagnostic tests indicated for dogs include fungus and bacterial cultures, and cutaneous bi-opsy for histopathologic and immunofluorescent studies. Performing a biopsy of feline solar dermatitis lesions will differentiate between inflammatory and neoplastic lesions, although this procedure is seldom needed.

Treatment. Several different treatments have been suggested to control the lesions associated with solar dermatitis. These include confinement, topical sunscreens, topical and systemic corticosteroids, and tattooing in dogs. The specific drugs and dosages are summarized in the Miscellaneous Disease Therapeutic Keys (Appendices 2:15 and 2:16.)

Prognosis. Canine lesions that are not tattooed usually require continuous treatment during periods of exposure to sunlight. Tattooing usually controls the clinical signs; however, in time there is often gradual, partial depigmentation that requires retattooing of the area. Initial tattooing sometimes fails because of the presence of another disease, excessive inflammation, or poor technique. In some dogs with DLE, tattooing will exacerbate the clinical signs, causing increased inflammation and ulceration.

The long-term prognosis for untreated feline solar dermatitis is guarded, since most lesions develop into squamous cell carcinomas. However, early excision of the lesions results in a permanent remission in most cats. There is seldom metastasis.

CONGENITAL AND HEREDITARY DISEASES

Cutaneous Asthenia (Ehlers-Danlos Syndrome)

Cutaneous asthenia is an uncommon hereditary connective tissue disease characterized by hyperextensibility of the skin.

Etiologic Factor. Cutaneous asthenia is an autosomal dominant trait that results in dysplasia of the dermal connective tissue.

Pathogenesis. Activity of the enzyme procollagen peptidase is deficient, resulting in production of abnormal collagen molecules and weak connective tissue in the skin, thus causing the marked reduction of the tensile strength of the affected skin. There is probably some secondary hyperplasia of the elastic tissue since increased stretching of the collagen promotes elastofibrogenesis. This has not been demonstrated histopathologically. The loss of rigidity and tensile strength predisposes the affected skin to excessive tearing.

History. The owner may first observe multiple lacerations on the animal with no knowledge of trauma. The onset of hyperextensibility is gradual and may not be recognized by the owner in a young animal. It is not unusual to see a dog or cat with multiple alopecic, scarred areas on the back and legs.

There is breed predilection for the Springer Spaniel and Boxer. Other breeds reported to be affected include German Shepherd, Dachshund, and St. Bernard. No breed predilection is reported in cats.

Clinical Signs. Marked hyperextensibility of the skin is the most striking clinical sign (Plates 11:D, and 11:E). Excess skin hangs loosely on the dependent portions of the body. There are often multiple lacerations with large open wounds (Plate 11:F). There is minimal hemorrhage on the surface. Subcutaneous hematomas may develop at sites of trauma. Old lesions usually heal with scarring.

Diagnosis. History and clinical signs are usually sufficient to make a diagnosis. Histopathologic findings are variable. The collagenous fibers in the affected skin are small and sparse compared to control sections.

Treatment. There is no specific treatment for cutaneous asthenia. Lacerations must be sutured using tension patterns. The animal should be protected from any minor or major trauma.

Prognosis. The prognosis is unfavorable due to the hereditary, chronic course of the disease and the predisposition to injury.

Color Mutant Alopecia

Synonyms for color mutant alopecia include Blue Doberman Syndrome, Fawn Irish Setter Syndrome, and Blue Dog disease. The disease is a hereditary abnormality characterized by color mutation, alopecia, and papules.

Etiologic Factor. The specific genetic basis of the disease is unknown.

History. By the time the animal is 6 months of age, the owner notices a sparse hair coat, bluish-grey in color if the normal color is black, blonde in color if the normal color is fawn, and liver-colored if the normal color is red. There is a gradual development of scale and papules, especially dorsally, accompanied by thinning of the hair coat and partial alopecia. Usually by 2 years of age the lesions are fully manifested, although the age of onset is occasionally 1 to 2 years. There is often a history of poor response to a therapeutic trial of thyroid hormone. Minimal pruritus is reported unless it is associated with dry skin.

Clinical Signs. Generalized thin hair coat with patches of partial alopecia and multifocal papules on the dorsum are the most common signs of color mutant alopecia (Plate 11:G). Dry scale may also be present. Secondary superficial folliculitis is common.

Diagnosis. A diagnosis of color mutant alopecia is based on coat color, history, and clinical signs. Thyroid-function tests are recommended since a small number of color mutant alopecic dogs have concurrent hypothyroidism and show some response to thyroid replacement.

Treatment. All treatment is palliative. Antiseborrheic shampoos and oils are usually helpful. Antibiotics should be administered if bacterial folliculitis is observed.

Prognosis. The prognosis for a cure is unfavorable. Most dogs with color mutant alopecia require symptomatic treatment for life.

Ichthyosis (Fish Scale Disease)

Canine ichthyosis is a hereditary disease characterized by extreme hyperkeratosis and exaggerated thickening of the digital, carpal, and tarsal pads.

Etiologic Factors and Pathogenesis. Other than the fact that hereditary predisposition plays a role, the causes and pathogenesis of canine ichthyosis are unknown.

History and Clinical Signs. The incidence of canine ichthyosis is rare. A young dog (less than 6 months) is examined for excessive scaling, usually generalized, which progresses with age. There are tightly adhering tannish-gray scales and feathered keratinous projections. The digital pads are thickened with large accumulations of keratin at the margins of the pads; pain may also be associated with this disease.

Diagnosis. History and clinical appearance are diagnostic. Cutaneous biopsy rules out other etiologic factors and also results in the characteristic histopathologic findings of hyperkeratosis and hypergranulosis.

Treatment. Palliative treatment with warm water soaks and antiseborrheic and keratolytic shampoos are sometimes helpful. Emollient rinses may help prevent dryness of the skin (Miscellaneous Disease Therapeutic Key, Appendix 2:15).

Ectodermal Defect

Ectodermal defect is a hereditary congenital alopecia observed from birth. This defect has been reported to occur in the Miniature Poodle, Lhasa Apso, Whippet, and Cocker Spaniel breeds.

Pathogenesis. There is a total absence of hair follicles and associated adnexa in the alopecic skin. Abnormal dentition is reported in several of the alopecic dogs.

History and Clinical Signs. The regions of alopecia include the dorsum of the head, most of the lateral and ventral trunk, and the extremities except for the feet (Plate 11:*H*). The alopecic skin often becomes scaly and darker as the animal ages.

Diagnosis. The clinical signs of alopecia from birth are suggestive of an ectodermal defect. Biopsies are necessary to confirm the diagnosis.

Black Hair Follicular Dysplasia

Black hair follicular dysplasia is a tardive (not apparent at birth) hereditary alopecia in black and white spotted dogs. It has been observed in mongrel, Papillon, and Dachshund breeds.

Pathogenesis. Dysplasia of the follicle in the alopecic areas of black skin occurs with resulting abnormal hair development and shedding. The white skin is not affected.

History and Clinical Signs. The puppies are normal at birth. As the dog matures, hair on several of the black patches of skin fails to grow, while the hair on the adjacent white skin grows normally (Plate 11:*I*). There is sparse, fragile hair and scales on the alopecic areas.

Diagnosis. The clinical signs of alopecia limited to the black patches of skin on a spotted black and white dog are suggestive of follicular dysplasia.

NUTRITIONAL DISORDERS

Zinc-Responsive Dermatoses

Zinc-responsive dermatoses include the clinical skin conditions characterized by focal scaling and crusting lesions that respond to zinc supplementation.

Etiologic Factors. The specific cause of zinc-responsive syndrome is unknown. There may be relative zinc deficiency associated with mineral imbalance, defects in zinc absorption, or other causes.

CLINICAL SYNDROME I

History. The Siberian Husky is predisposed to the disease, although it has been reported in the Alaskan Malamute. The age of onset is approximately 1 year, although older dogs may be af-

fected. Stress-related factors such as pregnancy, lactation, or concurrent disease can precipitate clinical signs. No sex predilection has been noted. Pruritus is minimal unless a severe secondary infection is present.

Clinical Signs. Crusting, scaling, and secondary suppuration are observed around the mouth, chin, eyes, and ears (Plate 11:*J, K*). Thick crusts may be seen on the surface of various joints of the extremities, scrotum, prepuce, or vulva. Hyperpigmentation may be observed in chronic lesions.

Diagnosis. History and clinical signs suggest the possibility of zinc-responsive dermatosis. Screening diagnostic tests should be performed to rule out other primary etiologic factors. These tests include fungus culture and thyroid-function tests. Results of cutaneous biopsy with parakeratosis and hyperkeratosis support the diagnosis. The most definitive diagnostic test is a therapeutic trial with oral zinc supplementation.

Treatment. Zinc sulfate, zinc gluconate, or zinc methionine is given orally (Miscellaneous Disease Therapeutic Key, Appendix 2:15). It may be necessary to give the supplementation for life. Symptomatic treatment with antiseborrheic shampoos, emollient rinses, and antibiotics is usually indicated.

CLINICAL SYNDROME II

History. Puppies are examined for hyperkeratotic plaques resembling dry pyoderma over various parts of the body. Multiple animals in a litter may be affected. The severity of lesions in different litters and within litters varies. Most affected puppies appear normal, but some may be smaller, depressed, anorectic, or generally debilitated. The puppies may be on a high level of calcium supplementation. Infected lesions respond poorly to antibiotics.

Clinical Signs. The primary skin lesions are focal hyperkeratotic plaques and crusts over the head, trunk, and extremities. Thickening and fissuring of the footpads and planum nasale are common signs. Moderate lymphadenopathy may be observed.

Treatment. A balanced diet and oral zinc supplementation are recommended (Miscellaneous Disease Therapeutic Key, Appendix 2:15). The zinc supplementation can usually be discontinued at maturity.

DISEASES OF UNKNOWN OR MULTIPLE CAUSES

Nodular Panniculitis

Nodular panniculitis is an uncommon granulomatous inflammatory disease of the subcutaneous fat of dogs and cats.

Etiologic Factors. The specific causes are unknown but it has been suggested that the condition results from an autoimmune reaction against dermal fat tissues.

History. There is usually an acute onset of subcutaneous nodules, often accompanied or preceded by intermittent fever and anorexia. Some nodules are painful, and some may ulcerate and drain. The drug history is one of poor response to therapeutic trials with antibiotics; whereas corticosteroid therapeutic trials result in rapid improvement. Dogs often respond to anti-inflammatory dosages of glucocorticoids, although cats usually require immunosuppressive dosages.

The age of onset of nodular panniculitis in dogs is usually under 6 months of age. However, mature dogs do contract the disease. Adult cats of 5 to 9 years of age are most commonly affected.

The Dachshund and Collie breeds appear to be predisposed to nodular panniculitis. No breed predilection for cats or sex predilection for either species has been reported.

Clinical Signs. Multiple subcutaneous firm nodules, 0.5 to 5 cm in diameter, are found on the trunk and neck (Plate 11:L). Some nodules are fluctuant, and some rupture discharging an oily, brown or blood-tinged exudate (Plate 11:M). There may be evidence of scarring in the area of the ruptured nodules, and a secondary staphylococcal infection may occur following the rupture.

Diagnosis. History and clinical signs are suggestive of nodular panniculitis. Cutaneous biopsy reveals pyogranulomatous inflammation of the subcutaneous fat (Fig. 12–1). A therapeutic trial with anti-inflammatory dosages (dog) and immunosuppressive dosages (cat) of glucocorticoids is indicated. Bacterial culture of unruptured nodules is sterile, while Staphylococcus aureus may be cultured from draining nodules. Direct smear of the exudate reveals more fat droplets than expected with an abscess of primary bacterial origin.

Treatment. Administration of corticosteroids at 1 to 2 mg/kg/day for 7 to 14 days usually results in a rapid clinical response in the dog. In the cat, 4 mg/kg/day of prednisone is recommended. The steroids should be tapered on an alternate-day dosage schedule for an additional 7

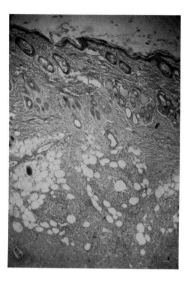

Fig. 12–1. Nodular panniculitis: Diffuse pyogranulomatous reaction in the subcutis. The dermis has a minimal involvement.

to 14 days. Antibiotics should be given concurrently. Long-haired animals should be shaved if there are many draining nodules causing matting of the hair. The use of an antibacterial shampoo is also indicated.

Prognosis. Prognosis for the immature dog is good with minimal chance of relapse. Adult-onset nodular panniculitis in the dog and cat has a less favorable prognosis for cure due to a higher recurrence rate following discontinuance of therapy.

Acanthosis Nigricans

Etiologic Factors. The cause of acanthosis nigricans is not clear. Frictional, endocrine, allergic, idiopathic, and malignant factors have all been suggested as being possibly related. It is probable that multiple factors are involved.

Pathogenesis. The pathogenesis of acanthotic and hyperpigmented lesions is unknown. Various endocrine-related pathways are possible, including TSH insufficiency (T_3 and T_4 levels are normal), either increased or decreased activity of the adrenal glands and gonads, and a relative excess of MSH, or a relative deficiency of melatonin.

Frictional acanthosis usually occurs when the conformation of the dog results in friction between the lower anterior chest and medial forearm. When the dog is obese, friction is exacerbated. Localized pruritus in the axilla and groin sometimes occurs in association with acanthotic nigrican-like lesions. Mechanical trauma apparently predisposes to the development of lesions similar to those caused by friction.

The idiopathic form of acanthosis nigricans is characterized by slowly developing symmetric lesions starting in the axilla. The marked breed predilection in the Dachshund suggests that hereditary factors may play a role in the pathogenesis of the disease.

History. Usually there is a history of a slowly progressing axillary hyperpigmentation that takes place over a period of months to years. A gradual thickening and increased scaling of skin in the axilla also occur. The primary complaint of the owner at initial examination may be onset of axillary pruritus, irritation, and odor. The Dachshund is the breed primarily affected, although the disease does occur in other breeds. Age of onset varies from 6 months to several years. Relapses are common.

Clinical Signs. The 3 clinical stages associated with acanthosis nigricans are: juvenile, axillary, and advanced.

The juvenile stage is characterized by a bilaterally symmetric oval brown patch in both axillae. There may be a transitory inflammatory reaction. The axillary stage is a progression to larger, grayish-black, thickened, and lichenified plaques (Plate 11:N). Seborrheic dermatitis with a greasy surface and rancid odor may be present. There may be excoriation following pruritus. The lesions may be secondarily infected. In the advanced stage, the lesions are extended to the forelegs (Plate 11:O), ventral thorax, and inguinal and perineal regions. Ear pinnae, commissures of the mouth, and the ventral neck may be involved. Bacterial infections and seborrheic dermatitis are prevalent.

Diagnosis. The diagnosis of acanthosis nigricans is based on the history, clinical signs, and ruling out of other primary causes such as those of allergic, endocrine, bacterial, and traumatic origin. Results of biopsy are nonspecific for acanthosis nigricans, but may rule out other specific primary causes (Fig. 12–2).

Treatment. The most specific therapy recommended is the administration of melatonin, an extract from the pineal gland that is not available commercially.[1] The most commonly used protocol for the axillary stage includes administration of alternate-day, low-dose corticosteroids and frequent use of antiseborrheic shampoos. The juvenile stage and mildly active axillary stage often respond to topical steroid creams. Antibiotics should be used when secondary infection is pres-

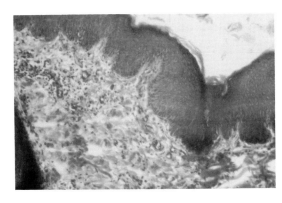

Fig. 12–2. Acanthosis nigricans: Note irregular acanthosis and focal hyperpigmentation (melanin deposition) in the basal cell layer. A mild inflammatory cell infiltration and edema are observed in the upper dermis.

ent. Specific drugs and dosages are listed in the Miscellaneous Disease Therapeutic Key, Appendix 2:15.

Prognosis. The prognosis for cure of acanthosis nigricans is unfavorable. Even with maintenance therapy, the disease tends to be slowly progressive, although there are usually periods of partial remission.

Canine Acral Lick Dermatitis

Acral lick dermatitis, lick granuloma, or acral pruritic nodule is a solitary lesion or multiple lesions on one or more extremities of a dog that result from excessive and persistent licking.

Etiologic Factors. Many factors have been suggested to predispose to or cause lick dermatitis. These include bacterial folliculitis, boredom, foreign bodies, local trauma, allergy, joint or bone disease, and psychogenic insults.

Pathogenesis. Specific pathogenesis is unknown. It is suggested that a primary folliculitis and release of mediators of pruritus are the major predisposing factors in acral lick dermatitis. Licking results in damage to the epidermis, leading to erosion and ulceration to a depth that elicits a chronic pruritic and/or pain sensation. Elimination of the epidermal protective barrier and continued trauma to the dermal tissue lead to deep folliculitis and dermal inflammation, involvement around apocrine sweat glands, and keratin plugging of the hair follicles. Epidermis on the periphery of the ulceration becomes hyperplastic, which leads to the development of a nodular plaque. Continued licking prevents normal re-epithelialization and perpetuates the dermal inflammatory response, thus persistence of the itch-lick cycle.

History. The owner's primary complaint is the

[1]Rickards' Research Foundation, 18235 Euclid Ave., Cleveland, OH 44112.

presence of lesions at sites of persistent licking. Large-breed dogs have a higher incidence of lick dermatitis. The most common site is the anterior carpal or metacarpal area. Onset of lesions can occur at any age, but it is more common in dogs over 5 years of age. Lesions tend to be recurrent, either at the same or different sites. There is often a history of poor or partial response to many therapeutic regimens.

Clinical Signs. Gross appearance of the lesions varies. Alopecia and some erosion or ulceration is usually present (Plate 11:*P*). In chronic conditions a nodular plaque is present, which may be mildly to markedly erythemic and moist or ulcerated. There is seldom any crust due to removal by licking.

Diagnosis. Diagnosis of acral lick dermatitis is based on the history, clinical signs, and elimination of other primary causes. Biopsy of the lesion is helpful in ruling out neoplasms and dermatomycosis. Fungus culture may also be indicated if a kerion is suspected. If joint or bone involvement is suspected, radiographs should be taken. If there is a history of generalized pruritus, either seasonal or nonseasonal, an allergy workup should be done.

Treatment. Many different therapies have been recommended for the treatment of acral lick granulomas. Almost all treatments have the primary goal of breaking the itch-lick cycle. The most commonly used treatment is intralesional corticosteroids. Topical triamcinolone and DMSO have given some favorable results. Intralesional orgotein has also been used. Recently, large dosages of lincomycin hydrochloride (Lincocin) have been reported to result in a good clinical response. Complete surgical excision can be accomplished in some dogs. Specific drugs and dosages are summarized in the Miscellaneous Disease Therapeutic Key, Appendix 2:15.

All local or systemic treatment should be accompanied by use of an Elizabethan collar, bucket, or other device to prevent the dog from reaching to lick the lesions(s).

Preventing boredom may be accomplished by more exercise, more animal or human companionship, or a new environment.

Acupuncture has been suggested as a method of treatment for acral lick granuloma.

Prognosis. The prognosis for curing lick dermatitis is unfavorable. The majority of dogs have recurrence either at the same site or a new site after treatment and removal of the restraint device.

Feline Eosinophilic Granuloma Complex

Eosinophilic granuloma complex refers to a group of feline lesions of different gross and microscopic appearances that respond to similar therapeutic agents. The lesions include eosinophilic ulcer (rodent ulcer), eosinophilic plaque, and linear granuloma.

Etiologic Factors and Pathogenesis. Etiologic factors of the clinical signs associated with eosinophilic granuloma complex are unknown. Because of the eosinophilic response in the blood and tissue of some lesions, a relationship to allergic disease and parasitic infection is possible. Evidence that eosinophilic granuloma complex is an immunologically mediated disease is based on the histologic appearance of the lesions and the possible relationship between immune complexes and eosinophils.

History. All three types of lesions are usually responsive to glucocorticoids or megestrol acetate.

Eosinophilic ulcers are usually nonpruritic, ulcerative lesions in cats ranging in age from 9 months to 9 years. There is a higher incidence in females than in males. Approximately 80% of the ulcerative lesions are found on the lips, although they may be observed on any part of the body and occasionally in the oral cavity. Eosinophilic ulcers may gradually resolve without therapy. In some cats there is a history of increasing severity leading to squamous cell carcinoma or fibrosarcoma. There may also be a history of concurrent feline leukemia.

Eosinophilic plaques are local, intensely pruritic lesions occurring most often in cats ranging in age from 2 to 6 years. Approximately 80% of the lesions occur on the abdomen and medial thighs, although they may be found on any part of the body or in the oral cavity.

Linear granuloma is seen most often in younger cats averaging about 1 year of age, and ranging in age from 6 months to 5 years. There is a higher incidence in females than in males. Most cats with linear granuloma are asymptomatic. Spontaneous remission may occur.

There may be multiple types of lesions occurring in the same animal. A history of relapse following the discontinuance of therapy is common with eosinophilic plaques and eosinophilic ulcer lesions. There are usually no systemic signs.

Clinical Signs. An eosinophilic ulcer is a well-circumscribed, ulcerated lesion of variable size most commonly found on the lips (Plates 11:*Q* and 11:*R*). The lesions usually have a necrotic center and ulcerated margins. If a squamous cell carcinoma or fibrosarcoma develops, there is local invasion of surrounding tissue with a loss of distinct borders.

Eosinophilic plaques are well-circumscribed, raised, erythematous lesions of variable size that occur most commonly on the abdomen and medial thighs (Plate 11:S). The surface is often moist, ulcerated, and exudative.

Linear granulomas are well-circumscribed, raised, firm, dermal masses arranged in a narrow linear pattern usually occurring on the posterior aspects of the hindlegs (Plate 11:T). They are usually 2- to 4-mm wide and 5- to 10-cm long. The surface is usually dry and yellow to pink in color. Occasionally there is ulceration.

Diagnosis. Diagnosis of eosinophilic granuloma complex is usually made on the basis of the history and clinical signs. Skin scrapings and fungus cultures may be performed. Specific tests for allergy including diet testing and intradermal tests are indicated. Microscopic examination of a biopsy specimen correlates with the gross appearance of the lesions, confirming a clinical diagnosis, but does not provide a definitive etiologic diagnosis. Tissue eosinophilia is a common finding in eosinophilic plaque lesions, but is relatively uncommon in the eosinophilic ulcer and linear granuloma lesions. A microscopic granulomatous reaction is only observed in the linear granuloma lesions.

Blood eosinophilia is often associated with eosinophilic plaques, but is not usually observed in the other types of lesions. There may be a moderate to marked nonspecific elevation of beta and gamma globulins in cats with multifocal lesions. A response to a therapeutic trial with glucocorticoids or megestrol acetate is supportive of a diagnosis of eosinophilic granuloma complex.

Treatment. Lesions associated with the eosinophilic granuloma complex are generally responsive to glucocorticoids and progestational compounds. Immunosuppressive doses of oral prednisolone or prednisone are frequently required initially, followed by alternate-day treatment in the evening. Injectable methylprednisolone acetate given subcutaneously every 2 weeks is usually effective. A minimum of 30 days of glucocorticoid therapy should be given.

The most widely used progestational compound for treating eosinophilic granuloma complex is megestrol acetate, although it is not approved for use in cats. Several dosage schedules are used, both for initial and maintenance therapy. High-induction doses are recommended to elicit a faster clinical response. Injectable progestational compounds are occasionally used. Refer to the Miscellaneous Disease Therapeutic Key (Appendix 2:16) for specific dosages and protocols.

Side effects of glucocorticoids are minimal in cats. Only prolonged, excessive doses of glucocorticoids have produced signs consistent with hyperadrenocorticism. Occasionally, increased water intake and appetite are observed.

More side effects are observed with the use of progestational compounds, especially megestrol acetate. An increase in appetite and weight gain are commonly reported, while polydipsia is uncommon. Redistribution of fat to the dorsal, caudal lumbar, and ventral abdominal regions is frequently seen. Mammary gland hyperplasia is common. Infrequently, mammary gland adenocarcinoma and diabetes mellitus follow chronic megestrol acetate therapy. Various personality changes are observed; some cats become more placid and friendly, while some seek seclusion.

Clinical response to glucocorticoids and progestational compounds is variable. Although the majority of cats respond to both types of medication, some cats respond to one and not to the other. Apparent refractiveness to a drug is occasionally observed following long-term use. A few cats with eosinophilic granuloma complex are refractive to both drugs. There tends to be more resistance to these medications following relapse of clinical signs.

Radiation therapy has been effectively used to treat solitary lesions of eosinophilic granuloma complex that were refractive to glucocorticoids and progestational compounds. The clinical response to radiation in multiple lesions is not generally satisfactory.

Levamisole hydrochloride and thiabendazole have been used as adjunct therapy in refractory cases.

Refer to the Miscellaneous Disease Therapeutic Key (Appendix 2:16) for specific drugs, dosages, and side effects.

Prognosis. Early lesions that are treated properly have up to a 25% chance of recurrence. Approximately 50% of all recurrent lesions, or those that are refractive to glucocorticoids or megestrol acetate, relapse following discontinuation of therapy.

Feline Miliary Eczema (Miliary Dermatitis)

Miliary eczema is a disease complex of multiple etiologic factors characterized clinically by small papules, crusts, and variable pruritus.

Etiologic Factors and Pathogenesis. There are diseases in most of the etiologic disease classifications that are associated with lesions consistent with miliary eczema. External parasites, especially fleas, are the most common cause of miliary eczema, although Cheyletiella mites and lice are occasionally associated with typical lesions. Dermatophytosis is the second most common cause of miliary eczema in many geographic areas. Other reported etiologic factors include bacterial dermatitis, intestinal parasitism, food allergy, drug eruption, fatty acid deficiency, biotin deficiency, and idiopathic factors.

Pathogenesis of miliary eczema is variable and depends on the primary cause. An increased number of mast cells and histamine in the skin has been reported.

History. History for miliary eczema varies depending on the etiologic factors involved. Pruritus is always present to some degree, manifested by licking, biting, or scratching. Hyperesthesia and personality changes may be observed. There is no age, sex, or breed predilection for idiopathic miliary eczema. Refer to the discussions under specific etiologic classifications in other chapters for further information.

Clinical Signs. Multifocal papules (Plate 11:U) or small crusts (Plate 11:V) are observed over the dorsum of the cat, although a generalized distribution is occasionally observed. External parasites or flea excrement may be seen. Acute inflammation and minimal alopecia are associated with the lesions.

Diagnosis. Diagnosis of miliary eczema is based on history, clinical signs, and screening and definitive diagnostic tests. Skin scrapings, fungal cultures, Wood's lamp examination, fecal examination, diet testing, and therapeutic trials with parasiticides are often indicated. Biopsy may be indicated as a screening diagnostic test, but will seldom confirm an etiologic diagnosis of miliary eczema. Idiopathic miliary eczema is considered when all of the above diagnostic tests fail to elicit a primary cause for the clinical signs.

Treatment. Treatment for miliary eczema should be specific for the primary cause if identified. Most idiopathic miliary eczema lesions are not responsive to glucocorticoids, although pruritus may decrease. Idiopathic miliary eczema usually responds to progestational compounds. Megestrol acetate, although not approved for cats, is used frequently. Intermittent life-time therapy is often required for miliary eczema, especially the idiopathic type.

Feline Neurodermatitis (Psychogenic Alopecia and Dermatitis)

Neurodermatitis is a syndrome associated with excessive licking or scratching of a local area.

Etiologic Factors and Pathogenesis. The most common suspected cause of neurodermatitis is anxiety neurosis or psychogenic insult, such as relocating the cat to a new environment or introducing new pets or people into the normal environment. Focal pruritic lesions have occasionally been associated with anal sac disease, tapeworm infestation, ectoparasites, urolithiasis, arthritis, psychomotor epilepsy, cauda equina syndrome, foreign bodies, and trauma.

The pathogenesis of neurodermatitis varies with the primary cause. Pathogenesis of lesions resulting from psychogenic factors is not completely understood. Once the cat starts licking or biting, the rough tongue surface causes superficial epidermal injury leading to inflammation, excoriation, and exposure of the sensory cutaneous nerve endings. Persistent irritation to the local area prevents healing of the surface.

History. There is a predilection for neurodermatitis in the Siamese, Burmese, Himalayan, and Abyssinian cat breeds; there is no age or sex predilection. A history of excessive licking, hair pulling, or scratching preceding or concurrent with the onset of the lesion is usually reported. The history usually reveals some change in the cat's life style immediately preceding the onset of clinical signs. Often there is a history of some displacement phenomena such as boarding, hospitalization, or a new pet or person in the household. There may be a drug history of poor clinical response to glucocorticoids.

Clinical Signs. Feline neurodermatitis is manifested by two rather distinct clinical signs. The first lesion, called the dermatitic form, is characterized by a solitary, discrete, excoriated, erosive, or ulcerated lesion (Plate 11:W), often with secondary infection. This lesion may be flat or raised, is usually moist, and varies in size. The dermatitic lesion is usually located on an extremity, the abdomen, or flank.

The second lesion, called the alopecic form, is characterized by solitary or multifocal areas of partial alopecia, broken hairs, and no inflammation of the skin (Plate 11:X). The distribution may be a strip on the dorsal back, or alopecic areas in the perineal, genital, medial posterior thigh, and abdominal areas. The stubs of hair remaining do not epilate easily.

Diagnosis. The history is the most important factor in the diagnosis of neurodermatitis, although clinical signs are suggestive. Screening diagnostic tests should be completed including skin scraping and fungus culture. A therapeutic trial with phenobarbital is often helpful. Direct examination of hairs should be done to determine if they are being broken off or are epilated. Results of biopsy are not diagnostic for neurodermatitis.

Treatment. Neurodermatitis is best treated by correcting the predisposing cause, if identified, and administering phenobarbital or progestational compounds (see Appendix 2:16) to break the itch-lick cycle.

Phenobarbital ($1/8$ g bid) usually stops the excessive licking within 2 to 4 days, which allows the dermatitic lesion to heal and stops the progression of the alopecic lesion. Diazepam has also been used as a centrally acting antianxiety medication.

The progestational drugs include progesterone (repositol form), medroxyprogesterone acetate, and megestrol acetate. The injectable drugs are given every 2 weeks. Megestrol acetate is initially given orally sid or q2d until clinical remission occurs. Maintenance protocol is then followed with a minimum treatment time of 1 month. The progestational drugs are not approved for cats. Some cats respond to one type of drug and not to another.

Prognosis. If a predisposing cause can be identified and eliminated, the prognosis is good. A relapse of clinical signs is common if there is recurrence of the predisposing factor. Some cats with neurodermatitis must be treated for life.

SELECTED READINGS

Anderson, R.K.: Canine acanthosis nigricans. Compend. Cont. Ed. Prac. Vet. 1:466, 1979.

Austin, V.: Blue dog disease. Mod. Vet. Pract. 56:31, 1975.

Baker, B.B., and Stannard, A.A.: Nodular panniculitis in the dog. J. Am. Vet. Med. Assoc. 167:752, 1975.

Collier, L.L, Leathers, C.W., and Counts, D.F.: A clinical description of dermatosparaxis in a Himalayan cat. Feline Pract. 10:25, 1980.

Halliwell, R.E.W.: Autoimmune skin diseases. In Current Veterinary Therapy VII: Small Animal Practice. Edited by R.W. Kirk. Philadelphia, W.B. Saunders, 1980.

Hargis, A.M.: A review of solar-induced lesions in domestic animals. Compend. Cont. Ed. Pract. Vet. 3:287, 1981.

Hegreberg, G.A., and Padgett, G.A.: Ehlers-Danlos syndrome in animals. Bull. Pathol. 8:247, 1967.

Hegreberg, G.A., et al.: A heritable connective tissue disease of dogs and mink resembling the Ehlers-Danlos syndrome of man. II: Mode of inheritance. J. Hered. 60:249, 1969.

Hegreberg, G.A., Padgett, G.A., and Ott, R.L.: Cutaneous asthenia in dogs. In Proceedings, 16th Gaines Veterinary Symposium. 1966.

Hess, P.W., and MacEwen, E.G.: Feline eosinophilic granuloma. In Current Veterinary Therapy VI: Small Animal Practice. Edited by R.W. Kirk. Philadelphia, W.B. Saunders, 1977.

Hutchinson, J.A.: Progestogen therapy for certain skin diseases of cats. Can. Vet. J. 19:324, 1978.

Ihrke, P.J.: Canine nasal solar dermatitis. In Current Veterinary Therapy VII: Small Animal Practice. Edited by R.W. Kirk. Philadelphia, W.B. Saunders, 1980.

Joshua, J.O.: The use of biotin in certain skin diseases of the cat. Vet. Rec. 71:102, 1959.

Kunkle, G.A.: Zinc-responsive dermatoses in dogs. In Current Veterinary Therapy VII: Small Animal Practice. Edited by R.W. Kirk. Philadelphia, W.B. Saunders, 1980.

Lane, J.G., and Graffeld-Jones, T.J.: Eosinophilic granuloma in cats. Vet. Rec. 100:251, 1977.

Muller, G.H.: Icthyosis in two dogs. J. Am. Vet. Med. Assoc. 169:1313, 1976.

Nesbitt, G.H.: Contact dermatitis. In Current Views in Veterinary Allergy and Dermatology. Gainesville, Fla., Division of Continuing Education, University of Florida, 1979.

O'Neill, C.S.: Hereditary skin disease in the dog and cat. Compend. Cont. Ed. Pract. Vet. 3:791, 1981.

Patterson, J.M.: Nasal solar dermatitis—A method of tattooing. J. Am. Anim. Hosp. Assoc. 14:370, 1978.

Pattison, P.F.: Eosinophilic granulomas in cats. Vet. Rec. 100:251, 1977.

Reid, J.S.: Acropruritic granuloma. In Current Veterinary Therapy V: Small Animal Practice. Edited by R.W. Kirk. Philadelphia, W.B. Saunders, 1974.

Scott, D.W.: Disorders of unknown or multiple origin. J. Am. Anim. Hosp. Assoc. 16:434, 1980.

————: Therapeutics. J. Am. Anim. Hosp. Assoc. 16:434, 1980

————: Miliary eczema in the cat: A review. In Proceedings of the 43rd Annual Meeting of the American Animal Hospital Association, 1976.

————: Observations on the eosinophilic granuloma complex in cats. J. Am. Anim. Hosp. Assoc. 11:261, 1975.

Stannard, A.A.: Actinic dermatoses. In Current Veterinary Therapy V: Small Animal Practice. Edited by R.W. Kirk. Philadelphia, W.B. Saunders, 1974.

Appendix 1

Diagnostic Keys

1:1 Dermatologic Disease

Etiologic classification	History	Clinical signs	Screening/Definitive tests
Allergic	Pruritus; responsive to corticosteroids; cats responsive to megestrol acetate	Variable excoriation, ulcers, plaques, crusts	Skin scrapings; therapeutic trials with parasiticides and megestrol acetate (cats); diet testing; skin testing
Parasitic (external including Demodex)	Parasites observed; responsive to parasiticides; variable pruritus; possible human contagion	Evidence of parasites (fleas, lice, Cheyletiella, Otodectes)	Skin scrapings; parasiticide therapeutic trial
Bacterial	Responsive to antibiotics; variable pruritus	Pustules, papules, crusts	Skin scrapings; bacterial culture; direct smear; biopsy; antibiotic therapeutic trial
Fungal	No response to antibiotics and corticosteroids; slowly progressive; pruritus—none to moderate	Scales, crusts, alopecia—focal or generalized	Skin scrapings; Wood's lamp; fungal culture; KOH preparation; biopsy
Endocrine	Pruritus—none to mild; slow regrowth of hair following clipping	Alopecia—partial to complete and focal to generalized; no inflammation scale	T_3/T_4, TSH stimulation; complete blood count; biochemical profile; ACTH stimulation
Bullous	No response to antibiotics or low-dose corticosteroids; variable pruritus	Bullae, vesicles, ulcers, crusts; distribution—often facial initially	Skin scrapings; biopsy (excisional); therapeutic trial with high-dose corticosteroids
Neoplastic	Poor response to antibiotics and corticosteroids; variable pruritus	Nodules, scales, crusts, excoriation	Skin scrapings; biopsy (excisional, incisional, needle, aspiration); direct smear
Seborrheic syndrome	Partial response to antibiotics, corticosteroids, and shampoos; progressive and/or persistent; often concurrent disease; variable pruritus	Scales (dandruff); oily or dry skin; variable inflammation; alopecia—partial, focal, regionalized or generalized	Skin scrapings; T_3/T_4, TSH stimulation; fungal culture; biopsy
Miscellaneous Physicochemical disorders Nutritional disorders Congenital-hereditary disorders Diseases of unknown or multiple cause	Variable; dependent upon specific disease entity	Variable	Skin scrapings; biopsy; therapeutic trials

1:2 Allergic Disease

Etiologic classification	History	Clinical signs	Screening/Definitive tests
Canine atopic dermatitis Feline inhalant dermatitis	Seasonal or nonseasonal pruritus; progressively worse with age; familial history (dogs); face-rubber, foot-licker, axillary pruritus (dogs); age of onset usually 1 to 4 years; cortisone-responsive; megestrol acetate responsive (cats)	Mild to severe erythema, excoriation, scales, crusts, papules, pustules, and alopecia; salivary stain (dogs); variable distribution of lesions	Intradermal skin testing
Allergic contact dermatitis	Nonseasonal pruritus; age of onset often > 2 yr; cortisone-responsive; megestrol acetate responsive (cats)	Ventral distribution most common; mild to severe excoriation, erythema, alopecia, crusts	Isolation and provocative exposure; patch test (open or closed)
Food allergy	Nonseasonal pruritus; age of onset often > 2 yr; cortisone-responsive; megestrol acetate responsive (cats)	Mild to severe erythema, excoriation, crusts, papules, alopecia; often head and neck distribution in the cat; variable distribution in the dog	Diet testing
Insect hypersensitivity	Pruritus associated with presence of external parasites; partial to total response to parasiticides; variable response to corticosteroids	Usually caudal, dorsal distribution, often dorsal neck (cats); fleas or flea excrement present; variable alopecia, excoriation, and crusts	Therapeutic trial with parasiticides; intradermal skin testing (dogs)

1:2 Allergic Disease *(continued)*

Etiologic classification	History	Clinical signs	Screening/Definitive tests
Drug eruptions	Onset of pruritus and/or dermatitis following administration of drug	Most common distribution on head and dorsal spine; variable erythema, scales, and excoriation	Withdrawal of drugs

1:3 Parasitic Disease

Etiologic classification	History	Clinical signs	Screening/Definitive tests
Fleas Ctenocephalides felis C. canis	Parasites observed; responsive to parasiticides; pruritus variable	Caudal and dorsal distribution of alopecia and scale, fleas or flea excrement	Parasiticide therapeutic trial
Mites Sarcoptes scabiei (dog)	Severe pruritus, nonresponsive to low-dose steroids; contagion to man or other animals	Excoriation, crusting of ear margins, elbows, and ventrum	Skin scrapings; parasiticide therapeutic trial
Notoedres cati (cat)	Intense pruritus; poor response to low-dose steroids and megestrol acetate; contagion to man or animals; often litters of young animals affected	Crusts, scales, excoriation of ears, face, and neck	Skin scrapings; parasiticide therapeutic trial
Cheyletiella yasguri (dog) C. blakei (cat)	Young animal; dorsal dandruff with minimal pruritus; contagion to man	Excessive dorsal dandruff; minimal to no inflammation; may be asymptomatic	Skin scrapings; parasiticide therapeutic trial
Demodex canis (dog) D. cati (cat)	Nonpruritic if no pyoderma; progressive focal or generalized alopecia; may resolve without treatment	Focal, alopecic hyperpigmented macules or patch on face, feet, or trunk; variable erythema; may be generalized alopecia with or without pyoderma	Skin scrapings; biopsy
Otodectes cynotis	Pruritus of ears; head shaking; waxy discharge from external ear canal	Mites, wax and debris in external ear canal; excoriation at base of ear; occasional focal alopecia, erythema and excoriation on head, neck, or back	Otoscopic examination of ear canal; skin scraping
Ticks Rhipicephalus sanguineus Dermacentor andersoni D. variabilis Amblyomma americanum	Observed parasites; history of exposure to endemic tick area; pruritus—none to minimal	Ticks present on head, neck, trunk, or feet; focal crusts and erythema at site of tick attachment	None required
Otobius megnini	Head shaking, pain, and pruritus of ear region	Mites and wax in ear canal; excoriation at base of ear	Otoscopic examination
Lice Trichodectes canis (dog) Heterodoxus spiniger (dog) Linognathus setosus (dog) Felicola subrostratus (cats)	Parasites of all stages observed; mild pruritus or asymptomatic	Lice present on haired areas of body; may be mild, focal alopecia and inflammation	None required
Pelodera strongyloides	Exposure to straw bedding; damp soil; intense ventral pruritus	Ventral erythema, papules, crusts, scales	Skin scrapings; larvae in washed bedding
Trombiculiasis Eutrombicula alfreddugesi	Pruritus; third stage orange-red larvae observed	Erythematous papules, scaling, alopecia on head, neck, axilla, and feet; parasites observed	Skin scrapings; parasiticide therapeutic trial
Myiasis Calliphorid flies Sarcophagid flies	Fly infested wound; foul odor from lesion; systemic signs common	Ulcerated lesion with fly larvae; tissue necrosis; may be signs of toxemia	None required

1:3 Parasitic Disease (continued)

Etiologic classification	History	Clinical signs	Screening/Definitive tests
Hookworm dermatitis (dog) Ancylostoma caninum Uncinaria stenocephala	Intense pruritus of all feet; history of hookworm exposure or infestation	Erythema, edema, and pain in all feet if acute; hyperkeratotic footpads if chronic; may have paronychia	Fecal; anthelmintic therapeutic trial
Cutaneous dirofilariasis Dirofilaria immitis (dogs)	Skin lesions concurrent with positive heartworm test or with heartworm disease	Erythema, alopecia, papules or ulcerating nodules of head, neck, trunk, and limbs	Microfilariae test; skin scraping; biopsy; therapeutic trial with dirofilaricide

1:4 Canine Bacterial Disease

Etiologic classification	Predisposing factors	History	Clinical signs	Screening/Definitive tests
Surface pyodermas Pyotraumatic dermatitis	Ectoparasites, trauma, poor grooming, otitis, anal sacculitis	More common in thick-coated dogs; often concurrent flea infestation; acute onset; rapid regression; pruritus, pain	Discrete, edematous erythematous, alopecic patch	Skin scraping; bacterial culture if refractory to symptomatic treatment; parasiticide therapeutic trial
Skin-fold pyoderma Lip fold	Anatomy	Cocker Spaniel, Setter breeds, Springer Spaniel predisposed; halitosis common	Ulcers; erythema; crusting in lip folds, often beneath tip of canine tooth	Same as above
Vulvar fold	Anatomy; obesity	Obesity; constant licking of vulvar region	Erosions, erythema, and crusting of vulvar margins and perivulvar	Same as above
Facial fold	Anatomy	Brachycephalic breeds predisposed; variable facial pruritus; foul odor	Moist surface; erosions; debris accumulation in facial folds	Same as above
Tail fold	Anatomy	Boston Terrier and English Bulldogs predisposed; minimal pruritus	Debris accumulation in tail folds; moist surface erosions	Same as above
Superficial pyodermas Impetigo	Unsanitary environment; crowding	Puppy 4–12 wk of age; distribution of lesions on nonhaired areas	Pustules and papules in groin and axilla	Scrapings; direct smear; antibiotic therapeutic trial
Superficial folliculitis	Various dermatologic problems (parasitic, allergic, endocrine)	Variable pruritus; often young dog; often secondary to another factor	Acute: pustules, papules, crusts, variable erythema Chronic: alopecia, hyperpigmented macule	Scrapings; direct smear; antibiotic therapeutic trial; bacterial culture if refractive to symptomatic treatment
Short-haired dog pyoderma	Hypothyroidism; seborrhea sicca	Smooth, short hair coats (Doberman, Great Dane, Dachshund, Dalmatian); "moth-eaten" appearance; pruritus variable	Occasional pustule and papule; multifocal alopecic lesions on dorsolateral trunk	Skin scraping; T_3/T_4; antibiotic therapeutic trial; direct smear; bacterial culture if poor initial response to therapy
Deep pyodermas Furunculosis	Demodicosis; immune deficiency	Often young dog < 1 yr of age; predisposition for muzzle, dorsum of nose, pressure points; German Shepherd—high incidence and usually recurrent	Fistulas with exudate, erythematous pustules and papules; scarring	Skin scrapings; bacterial culture from biopsy; biopsy
Cellulitis (Interdigital pyoderma, paronychia)	Demodicosis; immune deficiency	Often recurrent or chronic: poor or partial response to antibiotics	Warm, edematous, erythematous lesions; occasional suppuration with fistulous tracts	Skin scrapings; bacterial culture; biopsy

1:4 Canine Bacterial Disease *(continued)*

Etiologic classification	Predisposing factors	History	Clinical signs	Screening/Definitive tests
Hidradenitis suppurativa	Possibly immune mediated	Collies and Shetland Sheep Dogs predisposed; chronic course	Ulceration; well demarcated; groin or axillary lesions	Biopsy; bacterial culture
Perianal pyoderma	Possible anal sacculitis; hereditary	German Shepherd predisposed; pain; tenesmus	Perianal ulceration; fistulous tracts; excoriation; diarrhea or constipation may occur	None required
Miscellaneous pyodermas Juvenile pyoderma	Unknown	Puppies < 4 mo; predominantly facial; often several in a litter affected	Peripheral lymphadenopathy; edema; ulceration; fissures; abscess periorbital and perioral	Skin scrapings; antibiotic and corticosteroid therapeutic trials; bacterial culture if poor response to antibiotics
Dry pyoderma	Unknown	Puppies 4–9 mo; poor response to antibiotics; high incidence in Doberman Pinschers	Heavy, tightly adhered crusts and scales on face, extremities, pressure points	Skin scrapings; bacterial culture; zinc therapeutic trial

1:5 Feline Bacterial Disease

Etiologic classification	History	Clinical signs	Screening/Definitive tests
Surface pyodermas	Associated with "mouthing" by the queen; young kittens; no systemic signs	Alopecia, papules, pustules, and crusts on dorsal neck	Direct smear
Superficial pyodermas Folliculitis	Often associated with feline acne; variable pain, pruritus; antibiotic responsive	Alopecia, erosions, ulcers, and crusts	Culture; biopsy; direct smear
Deep pyodermas Folliculitis	Often associated with feline acne; variable pain, pruritus; variable response to antibiotics	Alopecia, erosions, ulcers, and crusts; fistulous tracts; may be peripheral lymphadenopathy	Culture; biopsy; direct smear
Subcutaneous abscess	Recent cat bites; acute onset of fluid-filled lesion; may notice after rupture; pyrexia; anorexia; pain	Fever; focal erythema; alopecia and crusts; abscess	Complete blood count; bacterial culture
Cellulitis	Recent cat bites; painful; heat; acute, diffuse, soft-tissue swelling on one limb; lameness; anorexia	Diffuse soft-tissue swelling; usually one extremity; erythema; fever; peripheral lymphadenopathy; alopecia or easy epilation of hair	Complete blood count; bacterial culture
Miscellaneous pyodermas Tuberculosis	Young adult cats; occurs in bovine tuberculous endemic areas; often no systemic signs	Single or multiple ulcers; abscesses; plaques; and nodules; thick yellow to green exudate; head, neck, and extremity distribution	Culture; biopsy with acid-fast stain
Feline leprosy (atypical mycobacterial granuloma)	No age predilection; subcutaneous nodules; poor response to antibiotics	Solitary or multiple nodules or abscess in subcutis; ulceration	Culture; biopsy with acid-fast stain

1:6 Fungal Disease

Etiologic classification	History	Clinical signs	Screening/Definitive tests
Dermatophytes Microsporum canis	Nonresponsive to antibiotics and steroids; variable pruritus; may be human or animal contagion	Focal or diffuse alopecia of head, neck, extremities, and trunk; variable scaling; cats frequently asymptomatic	Wood's lamp; KOH preparation; fungus culture; biopsy
M. gypseum	Nonresponsive to antibiotics and steroids; history of soil contact; variable pruritus	Heavy scales and crusts; focal alopecia; head and extremities most common distribution	KOH preparation; fungus culture; biopsy
Trichophyton mentagrophytes	Nonresponsive to antibiotics or steroids; often large areas of body involved; usually pruritic	Focal or diffuse alopecia, erythema, and hyperpigmentation; scaling	KOH preparation; fungus culture; biopsy
Subcutaneous mycoses Sporotrichosis Sporothrix schenckii	Often lymph node and cutaneous involvement; poor response to antibiotics and steroids; tender draining nodules	Subcutaneous nodules; often fistulous tracts with thick exudate	Direct smear of exudate; aspiration and culture; biopsy
Zygomycosis Mucor spp. Absidia Hyphomyces Entomophthora Basidiobolus Rhizopus	History of trauma and exposure to water and soil; breed predilection for German Shepherds; poor response to antibiotics and surgical excision of the lesion	Raised granulomas on extremities or near base of tail; fistulous tracts with thick exudate	Direct smear of exudate; fungus culture of exudate; biopsy
Mycetoma Actinomycoses Actinomyces Nocardia Actinomadura Streptomyces	Poor response to nonsulfa antibiotics and steroids; chronic draining lesions of feet and legs	Extremities mainly affected; subcutaneous swelling and fistulous tract; granules in exudate; may be ulceration	Direct smear of exudate; culture; biopsy
Eumycoses Allescheria boydii Curvularia geniculata Madurella spp.	Same as above	Same as above	Same as above
Aspergillosis Aspergillus fumigatus A. flavus	Respiratory signs (sneezing, nasal discharge); poor response to antibiotics and steroids	Subcutaneous nodules (granulomas) or deep cutaneous ulcers	Direct smear; fungal culture; biopsy
Systemic Mycoses Blastomycosis Blastomyces dermatitidis	Chronic debilitation; primary respiratory signs with later onset of skin lesions; poor response to antibiotics and steroids	Cutaneous and subcutaneous nodules, abscesses, ulcers, and fistulous tracts; marked lymphadenopathy; usually multiple lesions	Serologic tests (gel immunodiffusion); direct smears; biopsy
Histoplasmosis Histoplasma capsulatum	Chronic respiratory disease with late-onset skin lesions; poor response to antibiotics and steroids	Subcutaneous nodules, ulcers, and fistulous tracts	Serologic tests (complement fixation or gel immunodiffusion); direct smear; biopsy
Cryptococcosis	Cats more commonly affected; chronic multiple facial lesions following upper respiratory disease; unresponsive to antibiotics and steroids	Ulcers or nodules (granulomas); occasional abscesses with a mucoid exudate on the face	Direct smear of exudate; biopsy
Coccidioidomycosis Coccidioides immitis	Intermittent respiratory signs prior to onset of skin lesions; poor response to antibiotics and steroids	Granulomas, subcutaneous abscesses with fistulous tracts and occasional indolent ulcers in dogs; abscesses most common in cats	Serologic test (complement fixation); direct smear of exudate; biopsy

1:7 Endocrine Disease

Etiologic classification	History	Clinical signs	Screening/Definitive tests
Hypothyroidism	Nonpruritic to mildly pruritic; slowly progressive alopecia; lethargic; sensitive to cold; rare in cats	Symmetric alopecia of trunk or extremities; mild to marked scale; often dry, lusterless hair coat	Baseline T_3 and/or T_4; TSH-response test
Hyperadrenocorticism (Cushing's disease)	Polyuria and polydipsia (85%); polyphagia; progressive thinning of trunkal hair coat; rare in cats	Symmetric trunkal alopecia; mild to moderate hyperpigmentation; thin skin; pendulous abdomen; comedones on ventrum; may have calcinosis cutis; ecchymotic hemorrhages associated with venipuncture	Complete blood count; absolute eosinophil count; biochemical screen; ACTH-response test; dexamethasone-suppression tests
Pituitary dwarfism	50% normal size for breed or littermates; lack of normal coat development; predilection for German Shepherd dogs; adults often lethargic	Small size for age and breed; retention of secondary hairs; variable alopecia; seborrhea	Baseline T_3 and/or T_4; TSH-response test; ACTH-response test
Ovarian imbalance Type I (dog)	Intact middle to older female; abnormal estrus cycle; pruritus—none to moderate	Lichenification and hyperpigmentation with variable alopecia of posterior abdomen, perivulvar and perineal; gynecomastia; vulvar hyperplasia	Clinical response to ovariohysterectomy
Ovarian imbalance Type II (dog)	Middle-aged to older female; ovariohysterectomy at young age; progressive alopecia; responsive to estrogen replacement	Infantile hair coat on perineum, abdomen, ventral neck, and ears; alopecia; infantile vulva and nipples	Therapeutic trial with estrogens
Male feminizing syndrome (dog)	Middle to older intact male; chronic, progressive dermatoses; partial response to corticosteroids	Scaling and hyperpigmentation of flanks and perigenital regions; gynecomastia; normal palpating testicles	Therapeutic response to castration; testicular biopsy
Growth hormone responsive dermatosis—adult onset (dog)	Breed predilection for Keeshonds, Chow Chows, Pomeranians and Poodles; age of onset 1–2 years; poor response to thyroid hormone replacement and castration; nonpruritic; normal thyroid and adrenal function tests	Multifocal areas of alopecia with marked hyperpigmentation on neck, trunk, and perineum	Biopsy-elastin stains; therapeutic trial with growth hormone
Sertoli cell tumor (dog)	Breeds at risk (Chihuahua, Pomeranian, miniature Schnauzer, Poodles, Shetland Sheepdog, Siberian Husky, Boxers, Yorkshire Terrier); age of onset > 7 years; attraction of male dogs; often cryptorchid; pruritus with advanced clinical signs	Large cryptorchid testicle and small scrotal testicle; if both scrotal testicles—one large and one small; alopecia and hyperpigmentation of perineum, periscrotal, and posterolateral thigh; gynecomastia; prostatic hyperplasia	Abdominal radiographs; estrogen and testosterone serum levels; testicular biopsy
Seminoma (dog)	Cryptorchid > 7 yr old; mild alopecia; normal thyroid-function tests	Large cryptorchid testicle and small scrotal testicle; mild alopecia with minimal hyperpigmentation of perineum, ventral abdomen, and posterolateral trunk	Abdominal radiographs; testicular biopsy
Feline endocrine alopecia (cat)	Nonpruritic progressive alopecia; mostly neutered males and occasionally neutered females; middle-aged cats	Bilateral symmetric alopecia of perineum, ventral abdomen, and dorsum with sparing of the dorsal midline	Cutaneous biopsy; therapeutic trials with hormone replacement

1:8 Seborrheic Syndrome

Etiologic classification	History	Clinical signs	Screening/Definitive tests
Seborrhea Primary Secondary	Partial response to antibiotics, steroids, baths and rinses; usually concurrent specific dermatologic disease (90%); variable pruritus	Scale—mild to marked; dry or oily; variable erythema; may be superficial pyoderma; focal or generalized	T_3 and/or T_4; fungus culture; skin scrapings; therapeutic trial with parasiticide; diet testing; intradermal skin testing; dietary supplementation; biopsy
Schnauzer comedo syndrome	Miniature Schnauzer predisposition; recurrent or persistent dorsal eruptive dermatitis; pruritus—absent to minimal	Comedones or papules and crusts on dorsum of neck and back	T_3 and/or T_4; biopsy
Tail gland hyperplasia (dog)	Recurrent or persistent alopecia over tail gland area; possible biting in area with self-trauma	Alopecic, raised skin in area of tail gland; scale or crust; occasional pustule; inflammation variable	Skin scrapings; biopsy
Stud tail (cats)	Most common in intact male cats; predilection for Siamese, Persian, and Rex breeds; absence of pruritus; matting of hair over supracaudal organ	Comedones; waxy accumulation, scale and occasional crust on proximal dorsal tail	Scrapings; biopsy
Feline acne	Comedones on ventral chin; occasional pain and pruritus if infected; usually asymptomatic	Comedones on ventral chin and lower lips; occasional papules, pustules and edema	Scrapings; fungus culture; biopsy

1:9 Canine Bullous Disease

Etiologic classification	History	Clinical signs	Screening/Definitive tests
Autoimmune Pemphigus vulgaris	Poor response to antibiotics and low-dose steroids; may be systemic signs	Oral and mucocutaneous vesicles and ulcerations; nail bed involvement with sloughing of toe nail; focal or multifocal trunkal ulcerations and crusts	Biopsy; direct and indirect immunofluorescence
Pemphigus vegetans	Generalized proliferative dermatitis; poor response to antibiotics and low-dose steroids	Crusts, alopecia, and erythema; multifocal or diffuse, verrucose superficial lesions; some erosions and ulcerations; pustules common	Same as above
Pemphigus foliaceus	Facial and generalized proliferative dermatitis not involving mucocutaneous junctions; poor response to antibiotics and low-dose steroids; variable pruritus	Bullae, scales, crusts, erosions, erythema, alopecia, and pustules on face, ears, foot pads and trunk	Same as above
Pemphigus erythematosus	Lesions localized to face; poor response to antibiotics and steroids	Scale, crusts, and exudative lesions of nose, ears, and periorbitally; hypopigmentation	Same as above
Bullous pemphigoid	Usually mucocutaneous and oral lesions; poor response to antibiotics and steroids; variable pruritus	Vesicles, pustules, ulcers, crusts, and variable erythema; oral, periorbital, perioral, and occasionally trunkal distribution	Same as above
Systemic lupus erythematosus	Systemic disease concurrent with skin lesions; lesions exacerbated with sunlight; poor response to antibiotics; partial response to low-dose steroids	Papules, ulcerations, and crusts on face and ears, and occasionally on trunk; variable bacterial lesions	Biopsy; direct and indirect immunofluorescence; antinuclear antibody (ANA)

1:9 Canine Bullous Disease (continued)

Etiologic classification	History	Clinical signs	Screening/Definitive tests
Discoid lupus erythematosus	Facial dermatitis; poor response to antibiotics; partial response to low-dose steroids; lesions exacerbated with sunlight	Scales, crusts, erosions, and ulcerations on nasal planum and dorsal muzzle; hypopigmentation; variable erythema	Biopsy; direct immunofluorescence
Immune-mediated			
Dermatitis herpetiformis	Poor response to antibiotics and steroids; usually pruritic; generalized distribution of lesions	Vesicles, papules, and pustules; irregular scaling; erythema	Biopsy; therapeutic trial with dapsone (Avlosulfon, Ayerst)
Toxic epidermal necrolysis	Painful ulcerative lesions; slow healing; concurrent systemic disease	Diffuse, deep focal or multifocal ulceration	Biopsy
Drug eruption	Skin lesions following administration of drug; remission upon withdrawal of drug	Variable lesions including vesicles, erosions, ulcers, crusts, papules, and pustules	Provocative exposure to drug (usually done inadvertently)
Hereditary			
Epidermolysis bullosa simplex	Age of onset in young dog < 6 mo; Collies and Shetland Sheepdogs predisposed; lesions worse in warm weather	Lesions on face and bony prominences of extremities; alopecia on dorsum of nose and periorbitally; variable erosions, vesicles, ulcers, erythema, plaques, scales, and crusts	Biopsy following induced focal trauma
Idiopathic			
Subcorneal pustular dermatosis	Poor response to antibiotics and steroids; sterile bacterial cultures; varaiable pruritus	Trunkal and facial distribution of erythematous macules, papules, pustules, and crusts	Biopsy; therapeutic trial with dapsone (Avlosulfon, Ayerst)

1:10 Feline Bullous Disease

Etiologic classification	History	Clinical signs	Screening/Definitive tests
Autoimmune			
Pemphigus vulgaris	Poor response to antibiotics and low-dose steroids; anorexia and depression	Erythema, ulcers, and crusts of oral cavity and mucocutaneous junctions; occasional vesicle	Direct impression smear; direct and indirect immunofluorescence; biopsy
Pemphigus foliaceus	Facial lesions initially; poor response to antibiotics, low-dose steroids, and megestrol acetate; variable pruritus	Vesicles, pustules, erosions, erythema, crust, scales, and alopecia on head, trunk, and extremities	Same as above
Pemphigus erythematosus	Same as above	Vesicles, pustules, erosions, erythema, crusts, scale, and alopecia localized to head region	Direct impression smear; direct immunofluorescence; biopsy, antinuclear antibody (ANA)
Systemic lupus erythematosus	Poor response to antibiotics, steroids, and megestrol acetate; generalized chronic dermatitis, depression, and anorexia	Erythema, vesicles, and ulcerations with generalized distribution; fever; lymphadenopathy	Biopsy; direct immunofluorescence; antinuclear antibody (ANA)
Immune-mediated			
Toxic epidermal necrolysis	Concurrent systemic disease; fever, anorexia, and depression; painful lesion	Severe ulcers and vesicles of large focal or multifocal areas	Biopsy

1:11 Canine Cutaneous Neoplastic and Cystic Disease

Histologic classification	History	Clinical signs	Screening/Definitive tests
Cysts of epithelial origin Epidermoid, sebaceous, and epidermal inclusion cysts	No discomfort or inflammation unless ruptured; slow enlargement or static size	Fluctuant or firm nodule of varying size in dermis or subcutis; grey to brownish cheesy contents in lumen (sebaceous); hair in lumen (inclusion)	Aspiration biopsy; excision biopsy
Tumors of epithelial origin Perianal gland adenoma	Breeds at risk: Dachshund, Cocker Spaniel, German Shepherd; male dogs 8–12 yr; rare in females; often pruritic	Solitary or multiple erythematous nodules located perianally and occasionally on prepuce; may be ulcerated	Aspiration biopsy; excision biopsy
Squamous cell carcinoma	Predisposed or exacerbated by sunlight on white skin; starts as local irritation and depigmentation; progressive erosion of lip and nose; poor response to antibiotics and steroids	Erosion and ulceration of lips and nose; local invasion; may be diffuse ulceration of digit, pad, ventral abdomen, and eyelids	Incision biopsy; excision biopsy; radiographs of bone under lesion
Sebaceous gland tumor Nodular hyperplasia Adenoma Epithelioma	Breeds at risk: Cocker Spaniel, Poodle, Boston Terrier; slow growing, often static for years; usually no discomfort or inflammation	Firm, solitary or multiple 0.2 to 2 cm discrete dome or pedunculated nodules that are hairless and multilobulated	Excision biopsy
Papilloma (wart)	Common in mouth of young dogs; usually multiple; occasionally dysphagic; spontaneous remission in 6–8 wk	Initially small, whitish-raised mass on oral mucosa and lips; later rough, cauliflower-like surface; occasional small solitary or multiple nodule on medial thigh, face, or eyelid	Excision biopsy
Basal cell tumor	Cocker Spaniel at risk; slow growth; age of onset > 6 yr; solitary	Firm, circumscribed, hairless discrete tumor; usually pink, glistening surface on lips, eyelids, pinna, trunk, or legs	Excision biopsy
Trichoepithelioma	Locally invasive subcutaneous dorsal nodule	1–5 cm firm subcutaneous tumor on trunk; may be ulcerated	Excision biopsy
Sebaceous gland adenocarcinoma	Rapidly growing; locally invasive and metastatic, often local inflammation	Large, raised ulcerated mass lacking discrete borders	Excision biopsy
Intracutaneous cornifying epithelioma (keratoacanthoma)	Norwegian Elkhound male at risk for generalized form; both solitary and multiple growths; age of onset 2–5 yr	Dermal or subcutaneous nodules 0.5–4 cm with a pore opening to surface; keratin plug in pore; back, neck, thorax, and shoulder most common distribution	Excision biopsy
Mammary gland tumor	Females > 6 yr old highest incidence; single or multiple glands; 50% of lesions benign; variable growth rates	Subcutaneous tumor mass of varying size in one or multiple mammary glands; large tumors may ulcerate	Aspiration biopsy; incision biopsy (large mass); excision biopsy
Tumors of mesenchymal origin Lipoma	Dachshunds and Poodles at risk; middle-aged to older dog; slowly growing asymptomatic subcutaneous mass	Well-circumscribed oval or round subcutaneous mass of varying size; consistency may be soft to firm	Aspiration biopsy; excision biopsy
Mast cell tumor	Breeds at risk: Boston Terrier, English Bulldog, English Bull Terrier; age of onset > 6 yr; single or multiple	Firm, solitary, or multiple dermal or subcutaneous tumors of varying size; may be ulcerated; may have systemic signs with peripheral lymphadenopathy	Aspiration biopsy; excision biopsy; hemogram; buffy-coat smear
Hemangiopericytoma (spindle cell tumor)	Breeds at risk: Boxer, German Shepherd, and Cocker Spaniel; onset > 5 yr of age; slow growing	Firm, raised, smooth or lobulated mass on extremities, often with indistinct borders; ulceration and infection common	Incision biopsy; excision biopsy

1:11 Canine Cutaneous Neoplastic and Cystic Disease *(continued)*

Histologic classification	History	Clinical signs	Screening/Definitive tests
Histiocytoma	Breeds at risk: Boxers, Great Dane, Dachshund; age of onset < 3 yr of age; rapid growing; may spontaneously regress in 2–3 mo	Solitary 0.3 to 5 cm dome or "button" shaped, firm, well-circumscribed erythematous mass; occasionally ulcerated; rarely multiple	Excision biopsy
Hemangioma	Most common in middle-aged dogs with range of 6 mo to 15 yr; ulcerated lesion that bleeds easily; solitary or multiple	0.5–2.0 cm ovoid, soft, spongy discrete, dark red tumor of dermis or subcutis; often ulcerated	Aspiration biopsy; excision biopsy
Fibroma	Aged dog; solitary or multiple dermal masses; slow growing	Firm or soft discrete raised tumors of variable size and shape; occasionally pedunculated; may have alopecia of surface	Excision biopsy
Fibrosarcoma	Rapid course; locally invasive and metastatic	Firm, irregular-shaped, poorly circumscribed tumor; often ulcerated; edema and secondary infection common	Hemogram; biochemical profile; radiographs; excision biopsy
Cutaneous lymphosarcoma	Older dog of any sex or breed; poor response to antibiotics and steroids; usually generalized; course of weeks to years; pruritus variable	Variable clinical signs and distribution; nodules, crusts, erythema, ulceration, and alopecia	Punch biopsy; incision biopsy; excision biopsy
Hemangiosarcoma	Rapid growth; appears as subcutaneous hemorrhage; metastatic	Large, firm, poorly circumscribed tumor; inflammation in surrounding tissue	Hemogram; biochemical profile; radiographs; excision biopsy
Tumors of melanin-producing cells Melanoma	Breeds at risk: Scottish Terrier, Cocker Spaniel; tumors in mouth or on feet usually malignant and fast growing; solitary tumors on skin usually benign and slow growing; age of onset > 7 yr	Benign tumors are discrete, hairless, pedunculated dark masses of 1–4 cm diameter on lips, eyelids, and occasionally trunk; Malignant tumors are poorly demarcated, variably pigmented, flattened or rounded tumors in the mouth or on the feet	Excision biopsy

1:12 Feline Cutaneous Neoplastic and Cystic Disease

Histologic classification	History	Clinical signs	Screening/Definitive tests
Tumors of epithelial origin Squamous cell carcinoma	High incidence in areas of intensive sunlight; white cats predisposed; middle to older age cats; poor response to steroids and megestrol acetate	Usually solitary; firm, locally invasive ulcerative lesions with irregular borders on the pinnas, lips, nose, or eyelids	Excision biopsy; incision biopsy
Basal cell tumor	Slow growing; > 9 yr average age of onset; usually small and solitary	Firm, well-circumscribed, round or dome-shaped; often pigmented and ulcerated; occasionally has large central cyst	Excision biopsy
Trichoepithelioma	Slow growing; small and solitary	Small, firm, elevated growth; may be ulcerated	Excision biopsy
Sebaceous gland tumor (nodular hyperplasia, adenoma)	Older cat; usually asymptomatic	Solitary; < 0.5-cm diameter, smooth or rough surface	Excision biopsy
Papilloma (wart)	Older cat; predilection for face and limbs; usually solitary	Solitary; firm, discrete border; pedunculated; < 0.5-cm diameter; cauliflower-like surface	Excision biopsy
Sebaceous gland adenocarcinoma	Rare; older cat; locally invasive and metastatic; rapid growth	Solitary; firm, ulcerated mass lacking discrete borders; lymphadenopathy; lung lesions	Excision biopsy

1:12 Feline Cutaneous Neoplastic and Cystic Disease (continued)

Histologic classification	History	Clinical signs	Screening/Definitive tests
Tumors of mesenchymal origin			
Fibrosarcoma	Solitary tumors of aged cats; multiple tumors in kittens < 4 mo of age; locally invasive and metastatic	Aged cat: solitary, irregular or nodular growth of variable size; frequent ulceration; Kitten: multiple tumors on trunk; often evidence of metastasis to lymph nodes and lung	Excision biopsy
Mast cell tumor	No age or breed predilection; higher incidence in males; majority are malignant; single or multiple; partial response to steroids or megestrol acetate	Firm, raised, dermal masses; 0.5- to 5-cm diameter; most have discrete borders; color variable—pink, white, or yellow	Aspiration biopsy; excision biopsy
Fibroma	Aged cat; usually solitary	Firm or soft; elevated; discrete border; variable size	Excision biopsy
Hemangioma	Adult to aged cat; usually solitary	Discrete, 0.5- to 2-cm diameter, round, bluish-red dermal or subcutaneous mass; friable	Excision biopsy
Lipoma	Adult to aged cat; slow growing	Well-circumscribed, subcutaneous mass of variable size and shape	Aspiration biopsy; excision biopsy
Tumors of melanin-producing cells			
Melanoma	Uncommon; usually solitary; majority are malignant with metastasis at time of initial examination	Discrete, brown-to-black dome-shaped or pedunculated growth; variable size	Excision biopsy

1:13 Canine Miscellaneous Disease

Etiologic Classification	History	Clinical Signs	Screening/Definitive tests
Physical and Chemical Disorders			
Irritant contact dermatitis	Sudden onset of pruritus at any age; clinical signs associated with recent exposure to potentially irritant physical or chemical agent	Acute inflammation with erythema and edema; severe or chronic lesions with crusting, ulcerations, excoriation, and alopecia; may be scaling, hyperpigmentation or scarring	Isolation and provocative exposure; skin scraping; fungus culture; biopsy
Nasal solar dermatitis	Progressive lesions on muzzle and other lightly pigmented skin; aggravated by sunlight; partial to complete response to steroids; may complete all criteria for diagnosis of discoid lupus erythematosus	Erythema, ulceration, crust, and scale at junction of haired and non-haired skin of muzzle; dorsal muzzle and pinnae may be involved with similar lesions	Biopsy, direct immunofluorescence
Congenital and Hereditary Diseases			
Cutaneous asthenia (Ehlers-Danlos syndrome)	Multiple lacerations noted without trauma; breed predilection for Springer Spaniels and Boxers; skin tears easily, sags and stretches excessively	Marked hyperextensibility of the skin; multiple lacerations with large open wounds; subcutaneous hematomas at sites of trauma	Biopsy
Ichthyosis	Rare; progressive scaling; pads may be painful	Tightly adhered grey scales with generalized distribution; digital pads hyperkeratotic	Biopsy
Color mutant alopecia	Breed predilection for blue Doberman Pinscher, Dachshund, and Whippet, and fawn Irish Setter; sparse hair coat and slowly progressing alopecia at < 1 yr of age; poor response to symptomatic therapy	Generalized thin hair coat with patches of alopecia; papules and scale; often superficial folliculitis	T_3 and/or T_4

1:13 Canine Miscellaneous Disease *(continued)*

Etiologic classification	History	Clinical signs	Screening/Definitive tests
Nutritional Disorder Zinc-responsive dermatoses Clinical syndrome I	Siberian Husky predisposed; age of onset about 1 yr of age; clinical signs may be precipitated by stress	Crusting and scaling around mouth, chin, eyes, and ears; thick crusts on surface of joints of extremities, scrotum, prepuce, or vulva; variable hyperpigmentation	Fungus culture; T_3 and/or T_4; biopsy, therapeutic trial with zinc replacement
Clinical syndrome II	Puppies; often several in litter; may be depressed and anorexic	Multiple hyperkeratotic plaques; fissures of foot pads common; may be infected	Biopsy; therapeutic trial with zinc
Diseases of Unknown or Multiple Cause Nodular panniculitis	Acute onset; intermittent fever and anorexia; poor response to antibiotics; good response to steroids; age of onset usually < 6 mo; occurs in older dogs	1.0 to 5 cm multiple firm subcutaneous nodules on trunk and neck; often ruptured with oily, brown discharge; possible secondary infection	Direct smear of discharge; deep biopsy; therapeutic corticosteroid trial
Acanthosis nigricans	Slowly progressive hyperpigmentation of axillae; variable pruritus; foul odor; Dachshunds predisposed	Bilateral symmetric brown patch in axillae; large grey to black acanthotic and lichenified patches; often seborrheic dermatitis; advanced lesions may involve forelegs, ventral thorax, and posterior abdomen	Biopsy
Acral lick granuloma	Constant licking of localized area(s) of extremities; tendency for recurrence at same or new site following treatment; higher incidence in large breeds	Alopecic eroded or ulcerated plaques on extremities; variable size	Biopsy; radiographs

1:14 Feline Miscellaneous Disease

Etiologic classification	History	Clinical signs	Screening/Definitive tests
Physical and Chemical Disorders Irritant contact dermatitis	Sudden onset of pruritus at any age; clinical signs associated with recent exposure to potentially irritant physical or chemical agent	Acute inflammation with erythema and edema; severe or chronic lesions with crusting, ulcerations, excoriation, and alopecia; may be scaling, hyperpigmentation or scarring	Isolation and provocative exposure; skin scraping; fungus culture; biopsy
Feline solar dermatitis	White cats with intensified or prolonged exposure to sunlight; clinical improvement with decreased sunlight exposure; chronic and progressive over years; variable pruritus	Initial: erythema of tips and margins of pinnae; alopecia, scaling, and crusts with chronicity; ear margins may curl Neoplastic stage: persistent ulceration; local invasion	Fungus culture; biopsy
Congenital and Hereditary Diseases Cutaneous asthenia (Ehlers-Danlos syndrome)	Markedly loose skin; stretches excessively; tears easily; multiple lacerations without history of trauma and scarring	Hyperextensibility of skin; multiple lacerations; alopecic scars; subcutaneous hemorrhage at sites of trauma	Biopsy
Diseases of Unknown or Multiple Cause Nodular panniculitis	Age of onset 5–9 yr; usually systemic signs (anorexia, depression, fever) preceding cutaneous signs; cutaneous nodules may be painful; poor response to antibiotics and megestrol acetate	Multiple dermal nodules; well-demarcated, firm, 0.5- to 2-cm diameter; nodules become fluctuant and rupture; ulcerations and fistulous tracts; thick, bloody, oily exudate	Complete blood count; aspiration biopsy; excision biopsy

1:14 Feline Miscellaneous Disease *(continued)*

Etiologic classification	History	Clinical signs	Screening/Definitive tests
Eosinophilic granuloma complex			
Eosinophilic ulcer (rodent ulcer)	Nonpruritic; all ages; higher incidence in females; lesions may resolve without therapy; may have feline leukemia; responsive to steroids and megestrol acetate	Well-circumscribed with ulcerated, necrotic center; variable size; 80% of lesions on lips; if neoplastic, local invasion with indistinct borders	Feline leukemia test; complete blood count; biopsy; diet testing; intradermal skin tests; therapeutic trial with megestrol acetate or steroids
Eosinophilic plaque	Intense focal pruritus; age of onset 2–6 yr; megestrol acetate and steroid responsive; eosinophilia common	Well-circumscribed, raised, and erythematous; variable size; surface moist, ulcerated, and often exudative; most lesions on abdomen and thighs	Same as above
Linear granuloma	Young cat with average age of onset 1 yr; higher incidence in females; often asymptomatic; spontaneous remission may occur; megestrol acetate and steroid responsive	Well-circumscribed, raised firm dermal masses in narrow linear pattern; dry surface; most common on posterior of hind legs	Same as above
Miliary eczema (miliary dermatitis)	Pruritus; may have hyperasthesia; personality changes; always associated with some primary cause (fleas and dermatophytes most often)	Multifocal papules or small crusts on dorsum; external parasites or flea excrement may be seen; minimal alopecia	Skin scrapings; Wood's lamp; fungus culture; fecal examination; complete blood counts; diet testing; intradermal skin testing; therapeutic trials with parasiticides
Neurodermatitis (psychogenic alopecia)	Predilection for Burmese, Siamese, Himalayan, and Abyssinian breeds; usually some change in life style preceding clinical signs; poor response to steroids	Dermatitic form: solitary discrete, excoriated, erosive, or ulcerated lesion; variable size; usually on an extremity, abdomen, or flank Alopecic form: solitary or multifocal; partial alopecia with broken hairs; no inflammation	Skin scrapings; fungus culture; therapeutic trial with phenobarbital

Appendix 2

Therapeutic Keys

2:1 Topical Dermatologic Agents—Shampoos

Drug: generic name (commercial name, manufacturer)	Action	Indications	Dosage/Administration	Comments
Sulfur, 2–10%; salicylic acid, 5–50%; coal tar, 1–10%: (Mycodex Tar and Sulfur, Beecham) (Thiomar, EVSCO) (Lytar, DVM) (Sebutone, Westwood)	Keratolytic; keratoplastic; antipruritic; antibacterial; antifungal	Seborrheic syndrome; pruritus; crusts and scale; pyoderma	Bathe q3d–q14d prn; leave in contact for 10 min and rinse well	Coal tar may be irritating or toxic for cats; not approved for cats; may stain light-coated dogs
Coal tar 0.5–8% (Pragmatar, Norden) (Pentrax, Texas Pharmacal)	Keratolytic; keratoplastic	Seborrheic syndrome; pruritus; crusts and scale	Same as above	Same as above
Sulfur 2–5%; sodium salicylate 0.5%, hexachlorophene 3%: (Sebbafon, Winthrop)	Keratolytic; keratoplastic; antipruritic; antifungal; antibacterial	Seborrheic syndrome; pruritus; crusts and scale; pyoderma	Same as above	Safe and approved for cats
Benzoyl peroxide 2.5–5% (OxyDex, DVM)	Keratolytic; keratoplastic; antibacterial; follicular flushing	Seborrheic syndrome; pruritus; crusts and scale; pyoderma; acne	Same as above	5% concentration may be irritating
Chlorhexidine (Nolvosan 2% solution; 0.5% shampoo; Ft. Dodge)	Antibacterial; antifungal	Dermatophytosis; pyoderma, pododermatitis	Bathe q3d–q14d prn; leave in contact for 10 min and rinse well	Safe and nonirritating for cats
Selenium disulfide 0.9% (Seleen Suspension, Diamond)	Keratolytic	Seborrheic syndrome	Same as above	Poor antibacterial action
Salicylic acid, 2%; captan 2%; sulfur 1% (Casteen, Burns-Biotec)	Keratolytic; keratoplastic; antibacterial; antifungal	Seborrheic syndrome; pyoderma; dermatophytosis	Same as above	Safe for cats
Polyalkyleneglycoliodine complex (Welladol, Pitman-Moore)	Antibacterial; antifungal	Pyoderma; dermatophytosis	Same as above	May be irritating

2:2 Topical Dermatologic Agents—Parasiticides

Drug: generic name (commercial name, manufacturer)	Action	Indications	Dosage/Administration	Comment
Parasiticidal dips Organophosphate-organochlorines (Dermaton II, Wellcome Animal Health) (Kil-A-Mite, Wellcome Animal Health) (Paramite, Vet-Kem)	Cholinesterase inhibitor; contact poison	Flea, tick and lice prophylaxis and treatment; fly and mosquito prophylaxis; Cheyletiella mange; sarcoptic mange	Use as dip q7d–q14d; do not rinse off	Dermaton not for sarcoptic mange; Paramite approved for cats; organophosphate toxicity
Lindane (Gamma Rx, Carson)	Contact and ingestant poison	Same as above	Same as above	Not approved for cats
Organophosphate (Ectoral, Pitman-Moore)	Cholinesterase inhibitor	Same as above	Same as above	Not approved for cats
Carbamate (VIP Flea and Tick Dip, Florida Vet)	Cholinesterase inhibitor	Flea, tick, and Cheyletiella mange prophylaxis and treatment	Same as above	Resistance develops frequently when used continuously; approved for cats

2:2 Topical Dermatologic Agents—Parasiticides (*continued*)

Drug: generic name (commercial name, manufacturer)	Action	Indications	Dosage/Administration	Comment
Carbamate-lindane (Para Dip, Haver-Lockhart)	Cholinesterase inhibitor; contact and ingestant poison	Flea, tick, Cheyletiella mange, and lice prophylaxis and treatment	Same as above	Not approved for cats or nursing puppies
(Mycodex Dip, Beecham)	Same as above	Flea, tick, lice, and Cheyletiella mange prophylaxis and treatment	Same as above	Not approved for cats
Sulfurated lime (Vlem Dome, Dome) (Orthorix, Chevron Chemical Co.) (Lym-Dyp, DVM)	Unknown	Sarcoptic mange; Cheyletiella, lice, and chiggers	Same as above	Safe for neonates, cats, and exotic species; will discolor light hair
Parasiticidal sprays Carbaryl-pyrethrins (Pet Spray, Vet-Kem) (Norsect, Norden) (Sect-a-Spray, EVSCO)	Cholinesterase inhibitor; contact poison	Flea, lice, tick, and Cheyletiella mange treatment and prophylaxis	q7d	Spray must penetrate hair to reach skin; poor residual action; approved for dogs and cats
Parasiticidal shampoo Carbamate (Mycodex Pet Shampoo with Carbaryl, Beecham)	Cholinesterase inhibitor	Flea, Cheyletiella, tick, and chigger treatment	As needed	Poor residual action; not approved for cats
Resmethrin (DuraKyl, DVM)	Ingestant poison	Flea and Cheyletiella mange treatment and prophylaxis	Bathe q5d	Five day residual effect; approved for cats; can use concurrently with organophosphates
Lindane (Mycodex Pet Shampoo with Lindane, Beecham)	Contact and ingestant poison	Flea, tick, lice, and Cheyletiella mange treatment	Bathe as needed	Poor residual action; not approved for cats
Pyrethrins (Fleavol, Norden) (K.F.J. Insecticide Shampoo, Pitman-Moore) (Mycodex Pet Shampoo, Beecham)	Contact poison	Flea and Cheyletiella mange treatment	Bathe as needed	Poor residual action; approved for cats
Parasiticidal powders Carbamate (Mycodex Powder, Beecham) (Sevin, Thuron) (Diryl, Pitman-Moore) (Vet-Kem Flea and Tick Powder, Vet-Kem)	Cholinesterase inhibitor	Flea, tick, lice, and Cheyletiella mange treatment and prophylaxis	q3d-q7d	Approved for cats; short residual effect; must work through hair to skin
Organophosphate (Phosmet) (Paramite Insecticidal Dust, Vet-Kem)	Cholinesterase inhibitor	Flea, tick, Cheyletiella mange, and lice prophylaxis and treatment	q7d-q21d	Residual flea control up to 21 days; tick control up to 14 days
Parasiticidal collars Carbamate (Tick and Flea Collars, Vet-Kem) (Mycodex Flea Collar, Beecham) Dichlorvos, DDVP, Vapona	Cholinesterase inhibitor	Flea and tick control	Change q4m	Select specific collars indicated for dogs or cats; lack of efficacy on long-haired or large animals; do not use other organic phosphate drugs concurrently
(Flea Collars, E.R. Squibb & Sons)	Cholinesterase inhibitor	Flea and tick control	Change q4mo	Same as above

2:2 Topical Dermatologic Agents—Parasiticides *(continued)*

Drug: generic name (commercial name, manufacturer)	Action	Indications	Dosage/Administration	Comment
Organophosphate (Phosmet)	Cholinesterase inhibitor	Same as above	Change q7mo	Residual flea and tick control up to 7 mo
(Paramite Insecticidal Collar, Vet-Kem) Premise Parasiticides Resmethrin (DuraKyl Pet, Yard, and Kennel Spray, DVM)	Ingestant poison	Premise treatment for fleas	Spray areas q2wk-q4wk	
Malathion	Cholinesterase inhibitor	Premise treatment for fleas, ticks, and flies	Same as above	
Delnav, DDVP, pyrethrin (Vet-Kem Yard and Kennel Spray, Vet-Kem)	Cholinesterase inhibitor, contact poison	Same as above	Same as above	

2:3 Topical Dermatologic Agents–Glucocorticosteroids

Drug: generic name (commercial name, manufacturer)	Action	Indications	Dosage/Administration	Comment
Hydrocortisone 1–2% cream, ointment	Antipruritic; anti-inflammatory; superficial effect	Focal excoriation; erythema	Tid–qid initially; then sid–bid	Not practical for large areas
Prednisolone 0.5% cream (Meti-Derm, Schering)	Same as above	Same as above	Same as above	Same as above
Triamcinolone acetonide 0.5%, cream (Vetalog, E.R. Squibb & Sons)	Same as above	Same as above	Bid–tid initially; then sid–bid	Same as above
Desoximetasone 0.25% cream (Topicort, Hoechst)	Antipruritic; anti-inflammatory; marked penetration	Same as above	Same as above	Marked anti-inflammatory effect; not practical for large areas
Betamethasone 17-valerate 0.1% cream, ointment (Valisone, Schering)	Same as above	Same as above	Same as above	Same as above
Fluocinonide 0.05% cream (Lidex, Syntex)	Same as above	Same as above	Same as above	Same as above

2:4 Topical Dermatologic Agents–Combined Glucocorticosteroids and Antibiotics

Drug: generic name commercial name, manufacturer)	Action	Indications	Dosage/Administration	Comment
Nystatin, Neomycin sulfate, thiostrepton, triamcinolone acetonide: cream, ointment (Panalog, E. R. Squibb & Sons)	Antipruritic; anti-inflammatory; antibacterial; anticandidal	Focal excoriation; erythema; otitis externa	Bid–tid	There is no efficacy for dermatophytes
Neomycin sulfate, fluocinolone acetonide; cream (Neo-synalar, Diamond)	Antipruritic; anti-inflammatory; antibacterial	Focal excoriation; erythema	Bid–tid	
Thiabendazole, dexamethasone, neomycin sulfate: solution (Tresaderm, Merck)	Antipruritic; anti-inflammatory; antibacterial; antifungal	Focal excoriation; erythema; otitis externa	Bid–tid	

2:5 Systemic Dermatologic Agents–Glucocorticosteroids

Drug: generic name (commercial name, manufacturer)	Action	Indications	Dosage/Administration	Comment
Short-acting Prednisone Prednisolone Methylprednisolone (Medrol, Upjohn)	Antipruritic; anti-inflammatory	Pruritus (acute or chronic)	Loading dose: 0.5–1 mg/kg sid–bid for 2–5 day PO Maintenance dose: 0.5–1 mg/kg q2d or as needed PO	Polyuria, polydipsia, polyphagia; iatrogenic hyperadrenocorticism may result from chronic daily administration
Long-acting Dexamethasone (Azium, Schering)	Antipruritic; anti-inflammatory	Acute pruritus of expected short duration	0.25–2 mg sid PO or IM	Polyuria, polydipsia, polyphagia; do not use in chronic pruritus requiring long-term steroids; potential for iatrogenic hyperadrenocorticism
Residual Triamcinolone acetonide (Vetalog, E.R. Squibb & Sons)	Same as above	Acute pruritus of expected short duration	0.25–2 mg sid PO or IM	Same as above
Methylprednisolone acetate (Depo-Medrol, Upjohn)	Same as above	Dogs: Acute pruritus of expected short duration Cats: Eosinophilic granuloma complex and nonspecific pruritus	Dogs: 1 mg/kg IM Cats: 20 mg q6wk SC	Do not repeat more than once in dogs; no side effects reported with repeated injections in cats

2:6 Systemic Dermatologic Agents–Antibiotics

Drug: generic name (commercial name, manufacturer)	Action	Indications	Dosage/Administration	Comment
Cephalexin (Keflex, Lilly & Co.)	Bactericidal	Deep pyoderma; recurrent superficial pyoderma; nonresponsive pyoderma	20–30 mg/kg bid PO	High efficacy
Cephradine (Velosef, E.R. Squibb & Sons)	Bactericidal	Same as above	20–30 mg/kg bid PO	Same as above
Trimethoprim-sulfadiazine (Tribrissen, Wellcome Animal Health)	Bactericidal	Same as above	30 mg/kg sid or divided bid PO	Decreased tear production with long-term use
Gentamicin sulfate (Gentocin, Schering Corp.)	Bactericidal	Deep pyodermas resistant to all other antibiotics; Pseudomonas spp. and Proteus spp infections	4 mg/kg bid (day 1): then sid SC	Potentially nephrotoxic; no oral form; high efficacy
Kanamycin sulfate (Kantrim, Bristol Lab)	Bactericidal	Recurrent superficial pyoderma; deep pyoderma; nonresponsive pyoderma	6–8 mg/kg bid SC	Not absorbed through intestinal tract
Nafcillin (Unipen, Wyeth)	Bactericidal	First occurrence superficial pyoderma	20 mg/kg tid PO	Penicillinase resistant antibiotic
Oxacillin sodium (Prostaphilin, Bristol Lab)	Bactericidal	Same as above	12 mg/kg tid PO	Penicillinase resistant antibiotic
Cloxacillin sodium (Tegopen, Bristol Lab)	Bactericidal	Same as above	12 mg/kg tid PO	Susceptible to penicillinase; rapid development of bacterial resistance
Ampicillin	Bactericidal	Same as above	22 mg/kg tid PO	Susceptible to penicillinase; low efficacy
Penicillin G	Bactericidal	Same as above	20,000 U/kg qid PO	Same as above
Lincomycin (Lincocin, Upjohn)	Bacteriostatic	All first occurrence superficial pyoderma; may be used for first occurrence deep pyoderma if no apparent immunosuppression	20 mg/kg bid PO	
Erythromycin	Bacteriostatic	Same as above	10–15 mg/kg tid PO	Vomiting common
Chloramphenicol	Bacteriostatic	All first occurrence superficial pyodermas	20–50 mg/kg tid PO	
Troleandomycin (TAO), Roerig)	Bacteriostatic	Same as above	20 mg/kg tid PO	

2:7 Allergic Disease

Drug: generic name (commercial name, manufacturer)	Action	Indications	Dosage/Administration	Comments
Shampoos: refer to Appendix 2:1 Topical glucocorticosteroids: refer to Appendix 2:3 and 2:4 Systemic glucocorticosteroids: refer to Appendix 2:5 Systemic antibiotics: refer to Appendix 2:6 Antihistamines:				
Promethazine hydrochloride (Phenergan-D, Wyeth)	Antihistamine; antipruritic	Pruritus; adjunct therapy for atopic dog, urticaria	0.2–1 mg/kg tid–qid PO, SC	
Trimeprazine tartrate (Temaril, SmithKline)	Antihistamine; antipruritic; sedative	Same as above	1–2 mg/kg bid PO, SC	Marked sedative effect
Diphenhydramine (Benadryl Hydrochloride, Parke-Davis)	Antihistamine; antipruritic; anticholinergic	Same as above	1–2 mg/kg bid–tid PO	
Chlorpheniramine (Chlor-Trimeton, Schering)	Antihistamine; antipruritic; weakly sedative	Same as above	0.5–2 mg/kg bid–tid PO	Excitation at high doses
Allergen extracts: Aqueous allergenic extracts (Barry Lab) (Center Lab) (Iatric) (Hollister-Stier Lab)	Hyposensitization	Atopic dermatitis	Series SC (see Table 4–5 for suggested protocol)	Least expensive; frequent interval for injections; large selection of allergens
Alum-precipitated allergenic extracts (Center-al, Center Lab) (Allpyral, Miles Lab)	Hyposensitization	Atopic dermatitis	Series SC (see Table 4–6 for suggested protocol)	Expensive; residual effect; longer interval and fewer injections than aqueous extracts; limited selection of allergens

2:8 Parasitic Disease

Drug: generic name (commercial name, manufacturer)	Action	Indications	Dosage/Administration	Comments
Topical parasiticidal drugs (dips, shampoos, powders, sprays, and collars): refer to Appendix 2:2.				
Systemic parasiticide				
Proban cythioate (Proban, American Cyanamid)	Cholinesterase inhibitor	Flea prophylaxis	3.3 mg/kg q3d	Do not use other organophosphate drugs concurrently; not approved for cats
Demodex therapeutic agents				
Rotenone (Goodwinol, Goodwinol Products Corp.)	Unknown	Localized demodicosis	sid	Efficacy not proven
Ronnel 4% in propylene glycol (60 ml Ectoral emulsifiable concentrate, Pitman-Moore: 330 ml propylene glycol)	Unknown	Generalized demodectic mange	Apply solution to one third of body daily for 8 wk or longer	Mild weight loss; excessive scale; hepatotoxicity; relapses may occur
Amitraz (Mitaban Liquid 19.9% concentrate, Upjohn)	Unknown	Local or generalized demodicosis: sarcoptic mange	5.3 ml/1 gal water, wash on entire body and airdry, do not rinse off; repeat q2wk for minimum of 3 to maximum of 18 treatments for Demodex; can repeat series of 3–6 applications q2wk prn	Clip medium- and long-haired dogs; post-treatment lethargy for 24 hr; no eye irritation; usually 1 or 2 treatments required for sarcoptic mange; safety not proved for dogs < 4 mo of age; do not use for cats; do not save unused portion of diluted material

2:9 Bacterial Disease

Drug: generic name (commercial name, manufacturer)	Action	Indications	Dosage/Administration	Comments
Systemic antibiotics: refer to Appendix 2:6				
Topical antibiotics (creams, ointments, gels, solutions)				
Cuprimyxin (Unitop cream, Hoffmann-LaRoche)	Antibacterial; keratolytic; fungicidal	Surface and superficial pyoderma	bid	Local contact dermatitis is possible
Bacitracin-polymixin B	Antibacterial	Same as above	bid	Same as above
Furacin	Antibacterial	Same as above	bid	Same as above
Benzoyl peroxide hydrous (OxyDex Gel, DVM)	Antibacterial; follicular flushing; keratolytic; keratoplastic	Surface and superficial pyoderma; acne	sid–bid	Same as above
Povidone-iodine (Betadine solution, Purdue Frederick Co.)	Antibacterial; antifungal	All pyodermas	sid on local lesions as soak or in whirlpool	May have severe irritation; not recommended for cats

2.9 Bacterial Disease *(continued)*

Drug: generic name (commercial name, manufacturer)	Action	Indications	Dosage/Administration	Comments
Immunotherapy Bacteriophage (Staphage lystate, Delmont Lab)	Nonspecific immune stimulation	Chronic, recurrent superficial or deep pyoderma; staphylococcal hypersensitivity	Day 1: 0.2 ml SC Day 2: 0.4 ml SC Day 3: 0.6 ml SC Day 4: 0.8 ml SC Day 5: 1.0 ml SC Day 12: 1.5 ml SC Boosters: 1.5 ml SC weekly, then q2wk, then q4wk based on clinical response	Use concurrently with antibiotics until lesions are resolved; then discontinue antibiotics
Staphylococcus bacterin (Staphoid A–B, Jen-Sal) (Lysigin, Bioceutic Lab)	Nonspecific immune stimulation	Same as above	Day 1: 0.1 ml ID; 0.15 ml SC Day 2: 0.1 ml ID; 0.40 ml SC Day 3: 0.1 ml ID; 0.65 ml SC Day 4: 0.1 ml ID; 0.90 ml SC Day 5: 0.1 ml ID; 1.15 ml SC Day 12: 0.1 ml ID; 1.40 ml SC Day 19: 0.1 ml ID; 1.65 ml SC Day 26: 0.1 ml ID; 1.90 ml SC Boosters: 0.1 ml ID; 1.90 ml SC every 1–3 mo as needed	
Autogenous bacterin	Nonspecific immune stimulation	Same as above	No set protocol	Suggest using one of the protocols above

2:10 Fungal Disease

Drug: generic name (commercial name, manufacturer)	Action	Indications	Dosage/Administration	Comments
Topical				
Shampoos, solutions, rinses				
Povidone-iodine (Betadine solution, Purdue Frederick)	Antifungal; antibacterial	All dermatophytes	Shampoo q3d–q7d; or apply to focal lesion sid; dilute with water one part Betadine to 4–6 parts water	May be irritating to skin, especially for cats
Polyalkyleneglycoliodine (Welladol, Pitman-Moore)	Antifungal; antibacterial	All dermatophytes	Same as above	Same as above
Chlorhexidine (Nolvasan 2% solution; 0.5% shampoo; Ft. Dodge)	Antifungal; antibacterial	All dermatophytes	Same as above	Safe and usually nonirritating for cats
Sulfurated Lime (Vlem Dome, Dome) (Orthorix spray, Chevron Chemical Co.)	Fungicidal; antibacterial; keratolytic	All dermatophytes	Saturate skin after bath; do not rinse dip off; dilute to 1:40 solution for whole body; 1:20 solution for local treatment q3d–q7d	Safe for cats; odiferous; will discolor light hair
Captan (Orthocide spray, Chevron Chemical Co.)	Antifungal	All dermatophytes	Shampoo animal q3d–q7d with 2–3% solution	Safe for cats; inexpensive
Captan 2%, sulfur 1%, salicyclic acid 2% (Casteen, Burns-Biotec)	Antifungal; antibacterial; keratolytic	All dermatophytes	Shampoo q3d–q7d	Safe for cats
Creams and lotions				
Miconazole (Conofite, Pitman-Moore)	Fungicidal	All dermatophytes	Apply to local lesions bid	Occasional contact dermatitis
Cuprimyxin (Unitop, Hoffmann LaRoche)	Bactericidal; fungicidal; keratolytic	All dermatophytes; Candida albicans	Same as above	
Tolnaftate (Tinavet Cream, Schering) (Tinactin, Schering)	Fungistatic	Microsporum gypseum	Same as above	Minimal efficacy for most dermatophytosis
Clotrimazole (Veltrim, Haver-Lockhart) (Lotrimin, Schering)	Fungicidal	All dermatophytes; Candida albicans	Same as above	
Environmental disinfectants: Hypochlorite solution	Antifungal; sporocidal	Disinfection of the environment	Wash all surfaces well sid–q3d	Helps to prevent animal reinfection
Systemic: Griseofulvin (Fulvicin-U/F, Schering)	Fungistatic	All dermatophytes	Treatment: 70–130 mg/kg divided bid PO Prophylaxis: 200–220 mg/kg in 1 bolus PO Add vegetable oil or animal fat to diet sid	Therapy should be continued for 2 weeks after animal is asymptomatic; teratogenic; occasional bone marrow suppression in cats; oil or fat aids the intestinal absorption

2:10 Fungal Disease *(continued)*

Drug: generic name (commercial name, manufacturer)	Action	Indications	Dosage/Administration	Comments
Griseofulvin (Cont'd) (Gris-PEG, Dorsey)	Fungistatic	All dermatophytes	35–65 mg/kg sid PO	No fat or oil supplementation needed for adequate absorption
Sodium iodide 20%	Sporocidal	Cutaneolymphatic and cutaneous sporotrichosis	0.22 ml/kg tid PO	May cause vomiting, depression, cardiac collapse
Amphotericin B (Fungizone, E.R. Squibb & Sons)	Fungistatic or fungicidal	Sporotrichosis (disseminated); zygomycosis; blastomycosis; cryptococcosis; coccidioidomycosis	0.5 mg/kg IV diluted in 250 ml dextrose 5% and water first day; then 1.0 mg/kg diluted in dextrose 5% and water q2d IV	May cause vomiting; nephrotoxic; phlebitis if extravascular
Penicillin	Bactericidal	Actinomycosis	80,000–100,000 U/kg IM sid	
Trimethoprim-sulfadiazine (Tribrissen, Wellcome Animal Health)	Bactericidal	Mycetomas	30 mg/kg sid or divided bid	Decreased tearing with chronic use
Ketoconazole (Nizoral, Janssen Pharmaceutica)	Fungistatic	Cryptococcosis, blastomycoses, dermatophytosis	10–30 mg/kg sid-tid PO	Not approved for dogs or cats; observe for possible hepatotoxicity

2:11 Endocrine Disease

Drug: generic name (commercial name, manufacturer)	Action	Indications	Dosage/Administration	Comments
Thyroid:				
Thyroxine (Synthroid, Flint) (Soloxine, Daniels Pharm.)	T_4 replacement	Canine hypothyroidism as initial therapy	0.02 mg/kg q12h-q24h PO	Polydipsia and nervousness if excessive dosage
Triiodothyronine (Cytobin, Norden) (Cytomel, SmithKline)	T_3 replacement	Canine hypothyroidism if poor response to thyroxine	4.4 µg/kg q8h PO	Depresses serum T_4 values
Combination thyroxine and triiodothyronine (Euthroid, Parke-Davis) (Thyrolar, Armour)	T_3 and T_4 replacement	Canine hypothyroidism if poor response to thyroxine	Calculate dosage on basis of thyroxine content (0.02 mg/kg q8h-q12h) PO	
Desiccated thyroid	T_3 and T_4 replacement	Same as above	0.02 gr/kg q8h-q12h PO	Short shelf life
Androgens:				
Methyltestosterone Fluoxymesterone (Halotestin, Upjohn)	Testosterone replacement; increases sebum production	Sertoli cell tumor—postsurgery; hypoandrogenism; seborrhea sicca	0.5 mg/kg daily PO	
Testosterone propionate (Repotest, Burns-Biotec)	Testosterone replacement	Hypoandrogenism; Sertoli cell tumor—postsurgery; feline endocrine alopecia	2.2 mg/kg IM; repeat q2wk for dogs and q4-6wk for cats	
Progestins:				
Progesterone (Repository) (Repogest, Burns-Biotec Lab) (Progesterone injection, Med-Tech, Inc.)	Progesterone replacement	Feline endocrine alopecia	2.2-20 mg/kg IM; repeat in 6 wk if poor regrowth of hair	

2:11 Endocrine Disease *(continued)*

Drug: generic name (commercial name, manufacturer)	Action	Indications	Dosage/Administration	Comments
Megestrol acetate (Ovaban, Schering) (Megace, Mead Johnson)	Progesterone replacement	Feline endocrine alopecia	2.5–5 mg/cat q2d until regrowth of hair; then maintenance dose 2.5–5 mg q3d to q7d; PO	Not approved for cats in the United States: adverse reactions may include polyuria, polyphagia, mammary hyperplasia; personality change; diabetes mellitus
Estrogen: Diethylstilbestrol	Estrogen replacement; decrease sebum production	Ovarian imbalance Type II; seborrhea oleosa in spayed female	0.02 mg/kg daily × 2 wks PO; then q2d as needed	Monitor bone marrow if long-term usage; drug is not available in U.S.
o,p'-DDD (Lysodren, Bristol Lab)	Adrenocorticolytic	Pituitary dependent hyperadrenocorticism in dogs	Loading: 50 mg/kg daily × 10 days PO or until decrease in water intake Maintenance: 50 mg/kg weekly or divided biweekly	Give 0.2–0.4 mg/kg of prednisone daily until 3–4 days after stopping loading dose; vomiting; diarrhea; weakness, lethargy; depression
Growth Hormone (Bovine and Porcine growth hormone, Sigma)	Growth hormone replacement	Growth hormone responsive dermatosis	5 units q2d SC × 10 doses	Difficult to obtain commercially

2:12 Seborrheic Syndrome

Drug: generic name (commercial name, manufacturer)	Action	Indications	Dosage/Administration	Comments
Antiseborrheic shampoos: Refer to Appendix 2:1				
Parasiticidal agents: Refer to Appendix 2:2				
Systemic glucocorticosteroids: Refer to Appendix 2:5				
Systemic antibiotics: Refer to Appendix 2:6				
Hormones: Refer to Appendix 2:11				
Miscellaneous antiseborrheic drugs:				
Water	Keratolytic; antipruritic	Seborrhea sicca; pruritus	15-min warm water soaks daily or as needed	
Zinc Zinc methionine 15 mg elemental zinc (Zinpro Corp)	Normalization of keratinization	Zinc-responsive dermatoses	1.7–2 mg/kg of elemental zinc PO daily or divided q12h	Occasionally causes vomiting
Zinc sulfate 220 mg (50 mg elemental zinc)				
Oil rinses (Alpha-Keri therapeutic bath oil, Westwood) (HyLyt EFA, DVM) (Veterinary Formula Rinse, Med-Tech)	Surfactant; protection of surface of skin	Seborrhea sicca; pruritus	Dilute 1–2 ml/qt of water; apply after bathing or between baths; do not rinse off	

2:13 Bullous Disease

Drug: generic name (commercial name, manufacturer)	Action	Indications	Dosage/Administration	Comments
Topical glucocorticosteroids: Refer to Appendix 2:3				
Systemic glucocorticosteroids:				
Prednisone Prednisolone	Anti-inflammatory; immunosuppressive; antipruritic	All bullous diseases except subcorneal pustular dermatosis	Loading dose: 2–4 mg/kg PO: Maintenance: gradual taper to lowest q2d dosage to control signs	Marked polydipsia, polyuria, and polyphagia; often some abdominal bloating; prolonged high dosage may lead to iatrogenic Cushing's disease
Chemotherapeutic agents:				
Cyclophosphamide (Cytoxan, Mead Johnson)	Alkylating agent; immunosuppression	Pemphigus vulgaris; pemphigus foliaceus; pemphigus vegetans; pemphigus erythematosus; bullous pemphigoid	1.5 mg/kg or 50 mg/m^2 daily 4 consecutive days/wk	Leukopenia; hemorrhagic cystitis
Azathioprine (Imuran, Burroughs Wellcome)	Antimetabolite; immunosuppression	Same as above	1.0–1.5 mg/kg daily or q2d	Leukopenia
Chlorambucil (Leukeran, Burroughs Wellcome)	Alkylating agent; immunosuppression	Same as above	0.2 mg/kg daily	Usually no adverse effects noted; occasional bone marrow suppression
Miscellaneous drugs:				
Avlosulfon (Dapsone, Ayerst)	Unknown	Subcorneal pustular dermatosis; dermatitis herpetiformis	Initial: 1.1–1.5 mg/kg q6h-q12h; Maintenance: 0.3–0.6 mg/kg q12hr	Anemia; leukopenia; thrombocytopenia; elevated liver enzymes
Aurothioglucose (Solganal, Schering)	Anticomplementary; inhibit T-cell function; inhibit macrophage and neutrophil chemotaxis; depress immunoglobulin synthesis	Pemphigus vulgaris; pemphigus foliaceus; pemphigus vegetans; pemphigus erythematosus; bullous pemphigoid	Test dose: first week 1–5 mg IM; second week 2–10 mg IM; Treatment: 1 mg/kg q7d × 2–3 mo; then q30d	Contraindicated in systemic lupus erythematosus; thrombocytopenia and hemorrhage are reported
Vitamin E	Unknown	Discoid lupus erythematosus; systemic lupus erythematosus	200 IU q12h PO	
Topical sunscreens p-amino benzoic acid (PABA) (Presun Lotion, Westwood)	Sunscreen	Discoid lupus erythematosus; systemic lupus erythematosus	Apply 30 min prior to exposure to direct sunlight	

2:14 Cutaneous Neoplastic and Cystic Disease

Tumor or cyst	Surgical indication	Surgical procedure	Adjunct therapy		Prognosis
			Indication	Treatment	
Epidermoid cyst Dermoid cyst	Fast growing with potential to rupture; ruptured cyst; discomfort; cosmetic	Total excision	None		Good with excision; potential for new cysts at another site
Basal cell tumor	Diagnosis; therapy	Excision	None		Good
Fibroma	Diagnosis; therapy	Excision	None		Good
Fibrosarcoma	Diagnosis; therapy	Wide excision	Metastasis	Chemotherapy	Poor to guarded; often metastasis and local invasion
Hemangioma	Diagnosis; therapy	Wide excision; cryosurgery	None		Good with wide excision
Hemangiopericytoma	Diagnosis; therapy	Excision	None		Guarded; frequent recurrence
Hemangiosarcoma	Diagnosis; therapy	Wide excision	None		Poor due to metastasis
Histiocytoma	Diagnosis; therapy	Excision	Multiple tumors	Immunotherapy	Good for solitary tumor; guarded for multiple tumor
Intracutaneous cornifying epithelioma	Diagnosis; therapy	Excision	None		Good for solitary lesion; guarded for multiple lesions due to new tumors at other sites
Lipoma	Fast growing; traumatized mass; interference with function; cosmetic	Excision	None		Good; potential for new tumors at other sites
Cutaneous lymphosarcoma	Solitary lesion	Excision	Multiple tumors	Prednisone 2–4 mg/kg daily PO	Good for solitary lesion; poor for multiple lesions
Mast cell tumor	Solitary tumor; easily resectable mass	Wide excision	Nonresectable lesion	Radiotherapy	Variable survival time; if over 30 week survival postsurgery—good prognosis
	Cosmetic effect	Cryosurgery	Progressive disease; metastatic disease; recurring tumor	Vinblastine sulfate 0.7 mg/m² IV q7d; cyclophosphamide 1.5 mg/kg or 50 mg/m² daily 4 consecutive days each week; prednisone 2 mg/kg q2d	Favorable for welldifferentiated; poor for poorly differentiated cell types
Mammary gland tumor	Diagnosis; therapy	Excision	Malignant tumor	Chemotherapy; immunotherapy; (experimental protocols)	Favorable if well-differentiated; guarded to poor if malignant
Melanoma	Diagnosis; therapy	Excision	None		Good for benign; poor for malignant
Papilloma	Traumatized mass; interference with function; cosmetic	Excision	Endemic environment; cosmetic	Autogenous vaccine	Good

2:14 Cutaneous Neoplastic and Cystic Disease *(continued)*

Tumor or cyst	Surgical indication	Surgical procedure	Adjunct therapy		Prognosis
			Indication	Treatment	
Perianal gland tumor	Ulcerated, necrotic; solitary tumor Intact male Advanced stages with multiple tumors	Wide excision Castration Cryosurgery	Adenocarcinoma with metastasis	Cyclophosphamide 1.5 mg/kg or 50 mg/m² PO daily for 4 consecutive days each week; Vincristine sulfate 0.5 mg/m² q4d-q7d	Favorable for perianal adenoma; unfavorable for adenocarcinoma
			Intact male without castration	Estradiol cypionate 1–2 mg IM q4wk-q6wk	
			Multiple tumors; extensive inflammation and edema	Radiation therapy	Long-term therapy may result in thrombocytopenia and anemia
Squamous cell carcinoma	Carcinoma of lip, nose, ears, abdomen Carcinoma of digit	Wide excision; cryosurgery Amputation	Postsurgery	Radiation therapy	Chance for local recurrence; seldom metastatic
Sebaceous gland tumors Nodular hyperplasia Adenoma Epithelioma	Cosmetic; rapidly growing; traumatized	Excision	None		Good; chance for new tumor at other site
Adenocarcinoma	Diagnosis; therapy	Wide excision	Metastasis	Cyclophosphamide 1.5 mg/kg or 50 mg/m² PO daily for 4 days each week	Poor due to frequent metastasis

2:15 Canine Miscellaneous Disease

Disease	Drug: generic name (commercial name, manufacturer)	Dosage/Administration	Comments
Irritant contact dermatitis	Water	Warm water soaks 10–15 min q12h	Nonirritating; inexpensive; effective for removing crusts
	Topical corticosteroids	q12h	(See Appendix 2:3.)
	Prednisone; prednisolone	1–2 mg/kg daily PO	Often not needed. (See Appendix 2:5.)
	Systemic antibiotics		Use if lesion is secondarily infected. (See Appendix 2:6.)
Nasal solar dermatitis	Topical sunscreens		
	p-amino benzoic acid (PABA) (Presun Lotion, Westwood)	Apply 30 min prior to exposure to direct sunlight	
	Topical corticosteroids	q8h-q12h	(See Appendix 2:3.)
	Prednisone; prednisolone	1–2 mg/kg daily PO; taper to q2d; may need loading dose of 2–4 mg/kg daily PO if bullous disease (see Appendix 2:13)	If poor response to anti-inflammatory dosage, suspect another primary cause. (See Appendix 2:5.)
	Tattoo ink (Peliken ink, Gunther Wagner)	Infiltrate intralesionally to effect; may need to repeat focal areas in 3–4 wks; often need to reinject focal areas annually	If area is inflamed, expect less retention of ink; may be increased erosion or ulceration
	Hyaluronidase (Wydase, Wyeth)	Mix 1.0 ml hyaluronidase with 0.5 ml tattoo ink and 50,000 U crystalline penicillin	Improves dispersion of the ink through the tissue
Cutaneous asthenia (Ehlers-Danlos syndrome)	None		There is no specific treatment. Lesions are treated symptomatically

2:15 Canine Miscellaneous Disease (continued)

Disease	Drug: generic name (commercial name, manufacturer)	Dosage/Administration	Comments
Color mutant alopecia	Antiseborrheic shampoos	Bathe as needed to control scale	(See Appendix 2:1.)
	Systemic antibiotics		Use if bacterial dermatitis. (See Appendix 2:6.)
	Emollient rinses (Alpha-Keri therapeutic bath oil, Westwood) (HyLyt EFA, DVM) (Veterinary Formula Rinse, Med-Tech)	Dilute 2–4 ml/qt of water; apply after bathing or between baths; do not rinse off	
	Thyroxine	0.02 mg/kg q12h or daily PO	If serum thyroxine is low, use for a therapeutic trial. (See Appendix 2:11.)
Ichthyosis	Water	Warm water soaks for 10–15 min daily or as needed	
	Keratolytic shampoos	Bathe q3d-q7d or as needed	(See Appendix 2:1.)
	Emollient rinse (Alpha-Keri therapeutic bath oil, Westwood) (HyLyt EFA, DVM) (Veterinary Formula Rinse, Med-Tech)	Dilute 2–4 ml/qt of water; apply after bathing or between baths; do not rinse	
Zinc-responsive dermatosis	Zinc Zinc methionine 15 mg elemental zinc (Zinpro Corp) Zinc sulfate 220 mg (50 mg elemental zinc)	1.7–2.0 mg/kg of elemental zinc PO daily or divided q12h	Occasionally causes vomiting
	Keratolytic shampoos	Bathe q3d-q7d or as needed	(See Appendix 2:1.)
	Emollient rinse	Dilute 2–4 ml/qt of water; apply after bathing or between baths; do not rinse	(See Appendix 2:1.)
	Systemic antibiotics		Use if secondary bacterial infection.(See Appendix 2:6.)
Nodular panniculitis	Prednisone; prednisolone	1–2 mg/kg daily PO	(See Appendix 2:5.)
	Tar-sulfur shampoos	Bathe q3d-q7d or as needed	(See Appendix 2:1.)
	Systemic antibiotics		Use if secondary bacterial infection. (See Appendix 2:6.)
Acanthosis nigricans	Topical corticosteroids Fluocinonide (Lidex 0.25% cream, Syntex) Desoximetasone (Topicort, Hoechst) Hydrocortisone 1% cream	Apply q8h-q24h as needed	Use fluocinonide or desoximetasone if moderately severe to severe; if mild use hydrocortisone cream; in general, use the steroid cream with the least anti-inflammatory effect which will control clinical signs
	Prednisone, prednisolone	1–2 mg/kg daily; taper to q2d	(See Appendix 2:5.)
	Melatonin (Rickards Research Foundation)	2 mg q2d SC × 4 injections; then q2wk	
	Systemic antibiotics		Use if secondary bacterial infection. (See Appendix 2:6.)
Acral lick dermatitis (Acral pruritic nodule)	Systemic antibiotics		Use therapeutic dosages for prolonged time (6–8 wks minimum). (See Appendix 2:6.)
	Topical corticosteroids with DMSO	10 ml triamcinolone acetonide in 30 ml DMSO; apply daily	
	Triamcinolone acetonide 2 mg/ml (Vetalog, E.R. Squibb & Sons)	0.5–3.0 ml intralesional	
	DMSO (Domoso, Diamond)	Apply daily as needed	

2:15 Canine Miscellaneous Disease *(continued)*

Disease	Drug: generic name (commercial name, manufacturer)	Dosage/Administration	Comments
	Systemic corticosteroids		Do not use residual steroids on repeated basis; if necessary to use systemic steroids for an extended period use short-acting drugs. (See Appendix 2:5.)
	Orgotein (Palosein, Diagnostic Data)	5 mg intralesional; repeat in 7 days	

2:16 Feline Miscellaneous Disease

Disease	Drug: generic name (commercial name, manufacturer)	Dosage/Administration	Comments
Irritant contact dermatitis	Water	Warm water soaks 10–15 min q12h	Nonirritating; inexpensive; effective for removing crusts
	Topical corticosteroids	q12h	(See Appendix 2:3.)
	Prednisone; prednisolone	1–2 mg/kg daily	Often not needed. (See Appendix 2:5.)
	Systemic antibiotic		Use if lesion is secondarily infected. (See Appendix 2:6.)
Feline solar dermatitis	Topical corticosteroids	q12h as needed	(See Appendix 2:3.)
	Prednisone; prednisolone	1–2 mg/kg daily	(See Appendix 2:5.)
Cutaneous asthenia (Ehlers-Danlos syndrome)	None		There is no specific treatment; lesions are treated symptomatically
Nodular panniculitis	Prednisone; prednisolone	2–4 mg/kg daily; taper to 2qd	(See Appendix 2:5.)
	Systemic antibiotic		Use if secondarily infected. (See Appendix 2:6.)
	Shampoo	Bathe q3d-q7d or as needed	(See Appendix 2:1.)
Eosinophilic granuloma complex	Prednisone; prednisolone	2–4 mg/kg daily: PO; then taper to q2d	(See Appendix 2:5.)
(Eosinophilic ulcer) (Eosinophilic plaque) (Eosinophilic granuloma)	Megestrol acetate (Ovaban, Schering) (Megace, Mead-Johnson)	5 mg PO daily × 5–7 d; then 2.5–5 mg q2d and taper to q7d-q14d	Megestrol acetate is not an approved drug for use in cats in the United States; adverse reactions may include polyuria, polyphagia, mammary hyperplasia, occasionally diabetes mellitus and mammary adenocarcinoma; personality change
	Methylprednisolone acetate (Depo-Medrol, Upjohn)	20 mg SC q4wk-q6wk	There are minimal adverse side effects reported on long-term use at the recommended dosage and frequency
	Progesterone (Repository) (Repogest, Burns-Biotec) (Progesterone injection, Med-Tech, Inc.)	2.2–22 mg/kg SC or IM q2wk	
	Beta-radiation	Based on individual lesion	
Miliary eczema (Miliary dermatitis)	Megestrol acetate (Ovaban, Schering) (Megace, Mead-Johnson)	5 mg PO daily × 5–7 d: then 2.5–5 mg q2d and taper to q7d-q14d	Use for idiopathic miliary eczema; drug is not approved for cats in the United States; adverse reactions, see above
	Antifungal agents		(See Appendix 2:10.)
	Shampoos	Bathe as needed	(See Appendix 2:1.)
	Topical parasiticides		(See Appendix 2:2.)
	Systemic antibiotics		(See Appendix 2:6.)

2:16 Feline Miscellaneous Disease *(continued)*

Disease	Drug: generic name (commercial name, manufacturer)	Dosage/Administration	Comments
Neurodermatitis (Psychogenic alopecia)	Phenobarbital	1/8 gr q12h PO; 2.2–6.6 mg/kg q12h PO	If the predisposing factor is eliminated, long-term therapy is not required
	Diazepam (Valium, Roche)	1.25–2.5 mg q12h PO	
	Megestrol acetate (Ovaban, Schering) (Megace, Mead-Johnson)	5 mg daily × 7 d PO; then 2.5–5 mg q2d	Same as above; adverse reactions; see above

Appendix 3

Color Plates

Plate 1. Gross Morphologic Lesions—Primary

A, Macule (arrow) and patch (double arrow): Hyperpigmented alopecic areas without elevation or depression on the surface. B, Papule: Small erythematous solid elevated superficial lesion. C, Nodule: Palpable, solid mass with its base in the deep dermal or subcutaneous layers. D, Hyperkeratotic plaque: Large, elevated area with a flattened, hyperkeratotic surface. E, Erythematous plaque: Large, elevated area with flattened erythematous surface. F, Tumor (papilloma): Firm nodules containing neoplastic cells. G, Pustule: Circumscribed superficial elevated lesion containing purulent exudate. H, Wheal: Superficial elevation with smooth, rounded surface containing edema fluid. I, Bulla: Circumscribed elevated lesion on tongue containing clear fluid.

Plate 1

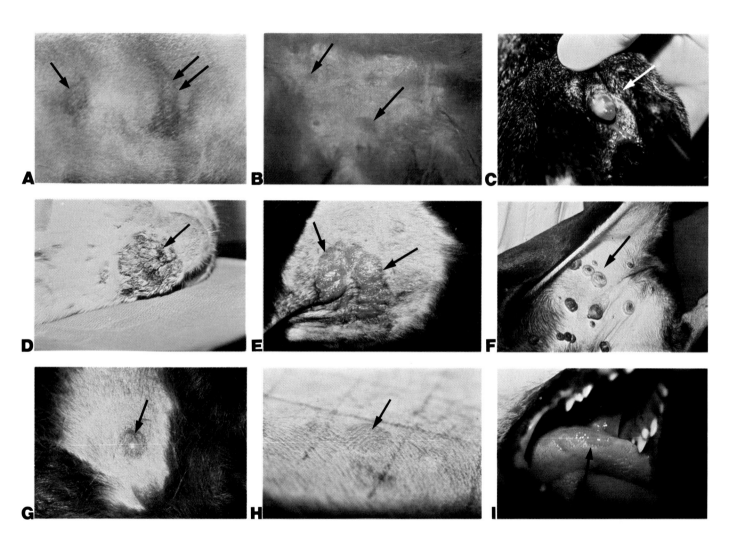

Plate 2. Gross Morphologic Lesions—Secondary and Miscellaneous

A, Excoriation: Superficial excavations of epidermis (arrows). B, Scale: Accumulation of loose fragments of the stratum corneum. C, Crust: Dried exudate, debris, and necrotic cells on the surface of the skin (arrows). D, Scar: Alopecic lesion on the dorsum of muzzle consisting of fibrous tissue. E, Ulcer: Destruction of all layers of the epidermis and superficial dermis. F, Lichenification and hyperpigmentation: Thickened firm skin with exaggerated superficial skin markings and excessive dark coloration. G, Hyperkeratosis: Increased thickness of stratum corneum of the footpads resulting in scale formation. H, Erosion: Multifocal areas of loss of superficial epidermis of the dorsal trunk (arrows). I, Furuncle: Multifocal areas of deep necrotic, exudative lesions associated with hair follicles. J, Abscess and sinus: Solitary slightly elevated lesion with an exudate-filled cavity in the subcutaneous layer and a tract (arrow) leading to the surface. K, Cyst: Fluid-filled apocrine glands (arrow) containing a clear liquid. L, Cyst: Ruptured sebaceous cyst with semisolid, doughy material on the surface (arrow).

Plate 2

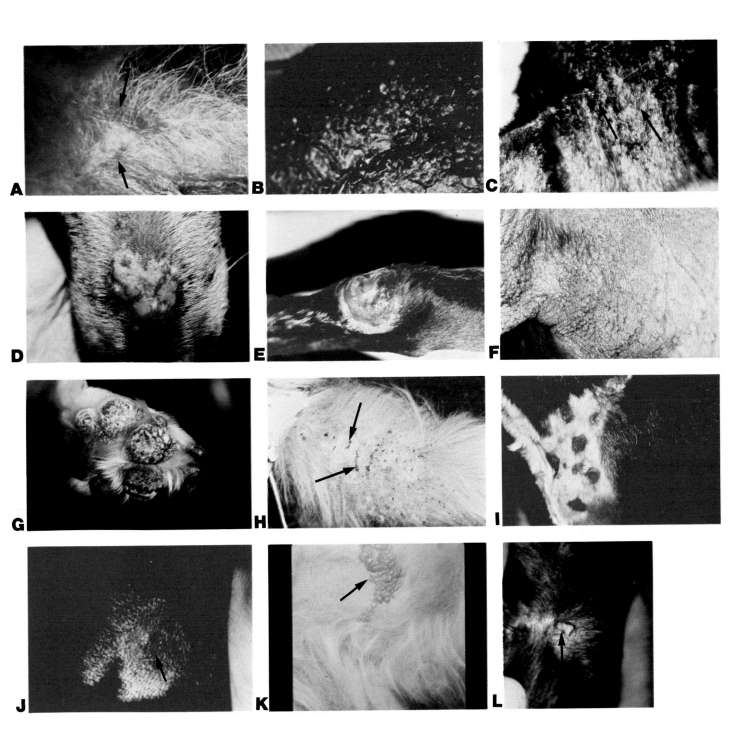

Plate 3. Allergic Diseases

A, Acute atopic dermatitis: Diffuse erythema of ventral abdomen and medial thighs. B, Acute atopic dermatitis: Alopecia and generalized erythema and excoriation of axillae and ventral thorax. C, Allergic otitis: Erythema of distal portion of medial pinna associated with atopic dermatitis. D, Chronic atopic dermatitis: Generalized alopecia, lichenification, erythema, excoriation, and hyperpigmentation. E, Chronic atopic dermatitis: Brownish discoloration (saliva stain) on the foot resulting from licking. F, Feline allergic dermatitis associated with airborne allergens: Facial alopecia, erythema, and mild excoriation. G, Acute allergic contact dermatitis: Diffuse erythema of the ventral abdomen. H, Chronic allergic contact dermatitis: Diffuse hyperpigmentation of ventral abdomen. I, Canine food allergy: Erythematous papules and focal crusts on the ventral abdomen. J, Feline food allergy: Diffuse partial alopecia, erythema, and excoriation on head, ears, and neck. K, Feline food allergy: Erythematous plaques on the ventral abdomen. L, Acute fleabite allergic dermatitis (canine): Multifocal erythemic partially alopecic patches on dorsal caudal back and dorsal cranial tail region. M, Chronic fleabite allergic dermatitis (canine): Diffuse alopecia, hyperpigmentation, and scale over dorsal caudal back. N, Fleabite allergic dermatitis (feline): Multifocal alopecic lesions and miliary crust on dorsal trunk.

Plate 3

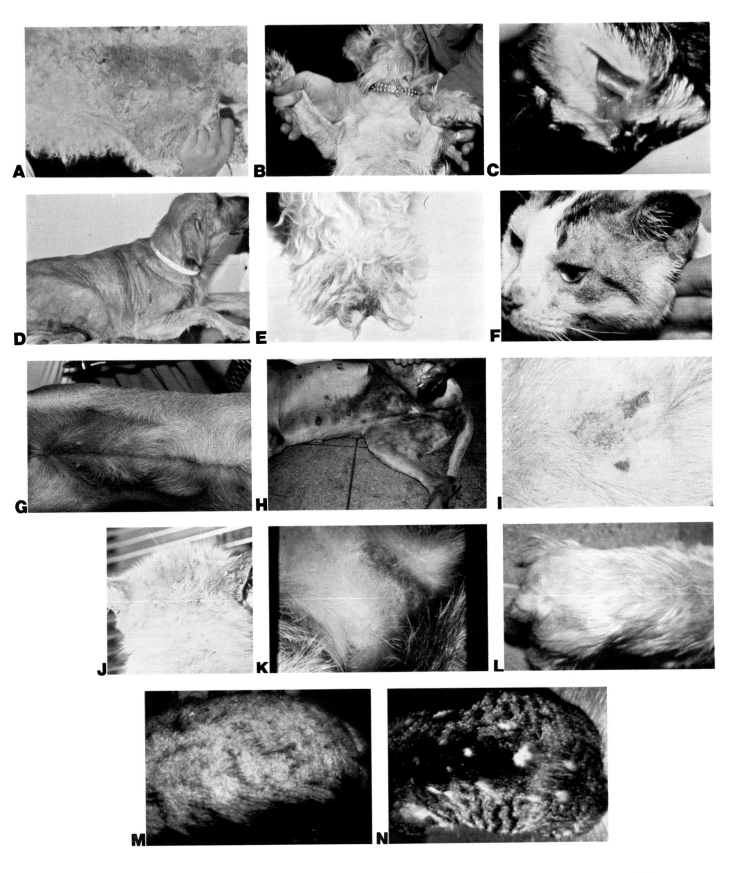

Plate 4

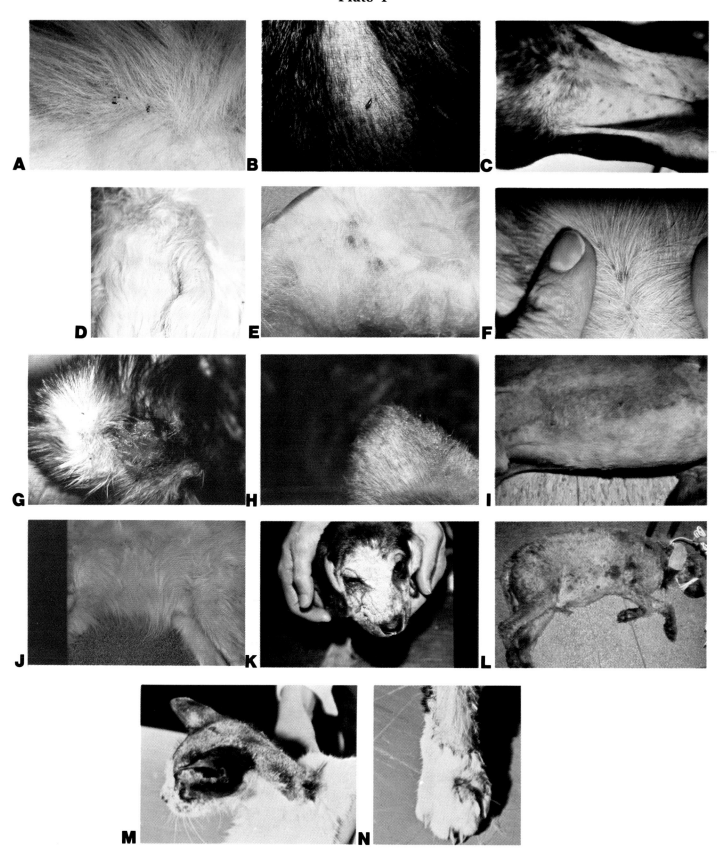

Plate 4. Parasitic Diseases

A, Flea dermatitis: Brown flea excrement on dorsal caudal back. B, Flea dermatitis: Adult flea on diffuse, alopecic area of dorsal caudal back. C, Flea dermatitis: Multifocal erythematous papules on ventral abdomen. D, Acute canine flea dermatitis: Patchy alopecia and erythema of dorsal and lateral proximal tail. E, Acute canine flea dermatitis: Excoriation and diffuse erythema of medial thigh. F, Feline flea dermatitis: Erythematous, miliary crusts and focal alopecia on dorsal caudal back. G, Feline flea dermatitis: Focal excoriation on dorsal neck. H, Sarcoptic mange: Alopecia and crusting of pinna margin. I, Sarcoptic mange: Multiple erythematous, pruritic papules and excoriations on the ventrum. J, Sarcoptic mange: Diffuse erythema and excoriation of elbow, axilla, ventral and lateral trunk, and extremities. K, Sarcoptic mange: Severe diffuse crusting of the face of 3-month-old dog. L, Sarcoptic mange: Generalized alopecia and multifocal excoriations on unshaven dog. M, Notoedric mange: Diffuse alopecia, crusting, and scaling on face and dorsal neck. N, Notoedric mange: Alopecia and mild ulceration on metacarpus and foot.

Plate 4 continued

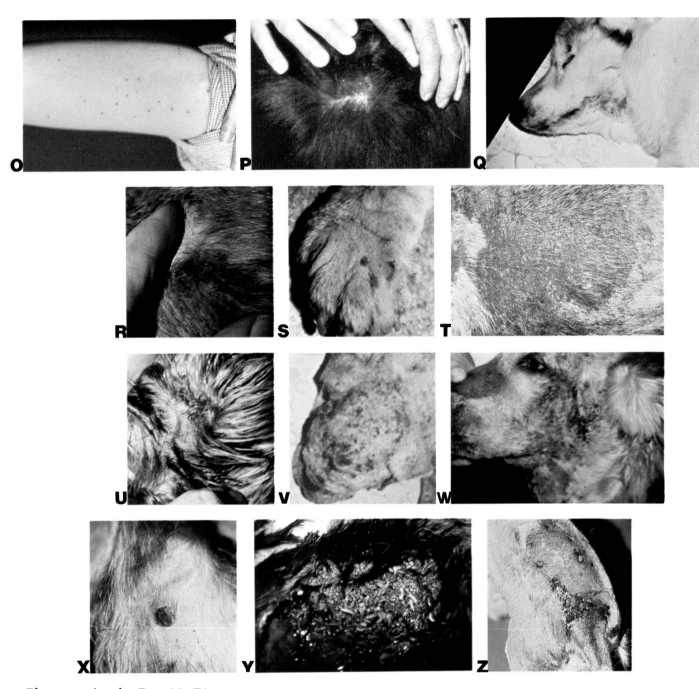

Plate 4 continued.   Parasitic Diseases

O, Cheyletiella mange: Multiple erythematous papules on arm of person infected with feline cheyletiellosis. *P,* Cheyletiella mange: Mild dandruff on dorsum of a cat. *Q,* Localized demodicosis: Patches of alopecia and mild erythema on lateral muzzle, lip, and mandible of 1-year-old dog. *R,* Localized demodicosis: Alopecic hyperpigmented patch. *S,* Generalized demodicosis: Diffuse alopecia and erythema of foot and metacarpus of 6-month-old dog. *T,* Generalized demodicosis: Diffuse alopecia, hyperpigmentation, and scaling of skin of 2-year-old dog. *U,* Generalized demodicosis: Erythema, pyoderma, and crusting of periauricular region in adult dog. *V,* Generalized demodicosis: Alopecia, erythema, crusting, and severe deep pyoderma of head of 4-month-old dog. *W,* Generalized demodicosis: Patchy alopecia, hyperpigmentation, and focal excoriation with crusts of a 4-year-old dog. *X,* Tick attached to skin of a dog. Note erythema associated with the attachment site. *Y,* Myiasis: Large ulcerated lesion filled with larvae on the back of a cat. *Z,* Myiasis: Multifocal ulcerative lesions on dorsal caudal back of a dog following removal of larvae from the lesions.

Plate 5. Bacterial Diseases

A, Surface pyoderma (acute moist dermatitis): Diffuse erythema and erosions on ventral neck. *B,* Lip fold pyoderma: Focal erythema and erosion on lower lip. *C,* Facial fold pyoderma: Erythematous patch in facial fold of English Bulldog. *D,* Vulvar fold pyoderma: Brownish discoloration of vulvar fold associated with chronic irritation secondary to obesity. There is a concurrent erythematous papular eruption on ventral abdomen. *E,* Superficial folliculitis: Erythematous papules and pustules on ventral abdomen. *F,* Superficial folliculitis: Focal crust with erythematous margin (arrow). *G,* Superficial folliculitis: Multiple focal hyperpigmented macules with an epidermal collarette and erythema at the periphery. Also note erythematous papules and focal crusts. *H,* Superficial folliculitis: Multifocal alopecic macules with epidermal collarette at margins. Note absence of acute inflammation. *I,* Superficial folliculitis: Multifocal hyperpigmented macules with new hair growth.

Plate 5

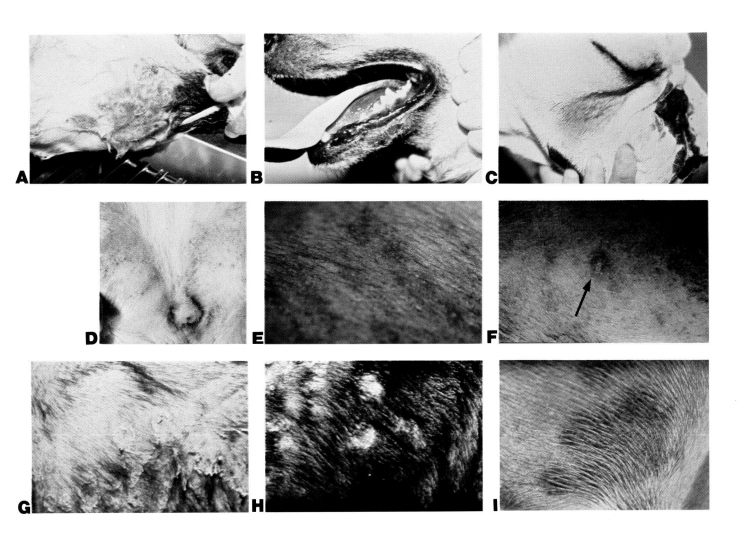

Plate 5 continued. Bacterial Diseases

J, Canine acne and pyoderma: Alopecia and comedones on ventral chin accompanied by focal erythematous ulceration and furunculosis. *K,* Deep pyoderma: Solitary furunculosis lesion with an ulcerative center and erythematous, raised margin. *L,* Deep pyoderma: Generalized multifocal ulceration on the trunk associated with furunculosis. *M,* Deep pyoderma: Partial alopecia, focal scarring, and hyperpigmentation of foot and metacarpus associated with chronic furunculosis. *N,* Callous pyoderma: Heavy crusting, erosions, and hyperpigmentation on the callous and erythematous papules on the adjacent skin. *O,* Interdigital pyoderma: Deep ulcerations and erythema in the interdigital space. *P,* Deep pyoderma: Multiple pustules on the ventral foot located between the footpads. *Q,* Perianal pyoderma: Multiple fistulous tracts lateral to the anus. *R,* Feline acne and pyoderma: Swelling of ventral chin with multiple ulcerative areas associated with furunculosis. *S,* Abscess: Ruptured abscess on face of a cat secondary to a cat bite. *T,* Feline leprosy: Microscopic section with macrophages filled with acid-fast bacilli (Ziehl-Neelsen stain) (high power).

Plate 5 continued

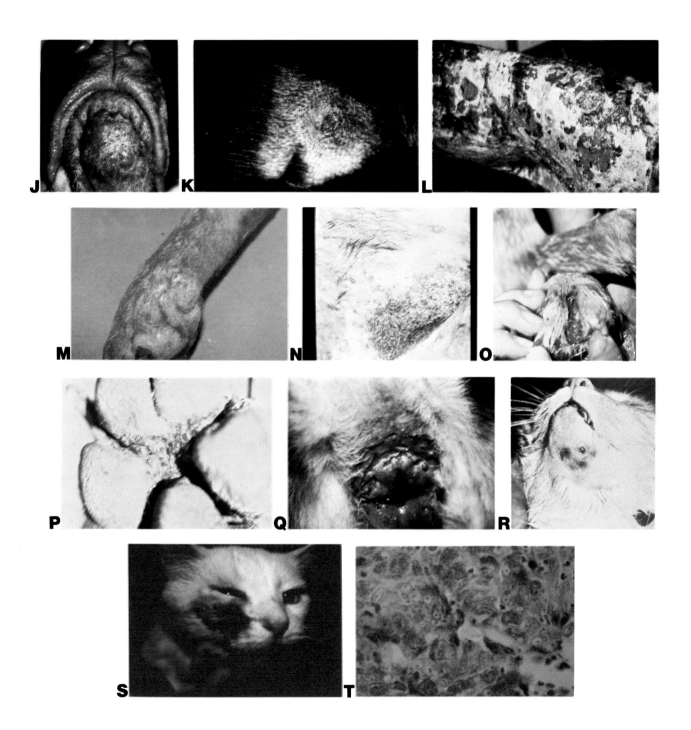

Plate 6. Fungal Diseases

A, Trichophyton mentagrophytes: Diffuse alopecia, erythema, and scale on the ventral abdomen and medial thigh of a dog. *B*, Microsporum gypseum: Alopecic, hyperpigmented, scaly patch cranial to the ear of a dog. *C*, M. canis: Diffuse alopecia and mild erythema of dorsal head, neck, and shoulders of an adult dog. *D*, M. canis: Focal patch of broken hair shafts and scale on the dorsum of the head of a kitten. *E*, M. canis: Diffuse alopecia and scale on the dorsum of the head and lateral pinna of an adult cat. *F*, M. canis: Linear alopecic area with mild scale on the dorsal midline of an adult cat. *G*, Kerion: Solitary ulcerated nodule caused by M. gypseum on the distal limb of a dog. (Courtesy of Carol O'Neill.) *H*, Dermatophyte test medium: M. canis culture five-days-old. Note all of medium is red with a small amount of white colony growth. *I*, Dermatophyte test medium: Contaminant growth of 21 days of Penicillium spp. Note that the medium turned red after the dark colony growth occurred. *J*, Sporotrichosis: Multiple ulcerated subcutaneous nodules on the head and pinna of a cat. (Courtesy of Nita Gulbas.) *K*, Sporotrichosis: Multiple subcutaneous ulcerated nodules and some crusts on the front feet and legs of a cat. (Courtesy of Nita Gulbas.) *L*, Blastomycosis: Granulomatous nodule on the lateral aspect of the foot of a dog. (Courtesy of Al Legendre.) *M*, Blastomycosis: Ulcerated granulomatous nodule on the anterior aspect of the upper lip of a dog. (Courtesy of Al Legendre.) *N*, Cryptococcosis: Multiple ulcerated granulomatous nodules on the face of a cat. (Courtesy of Nita Gulbas.)

Plate 6

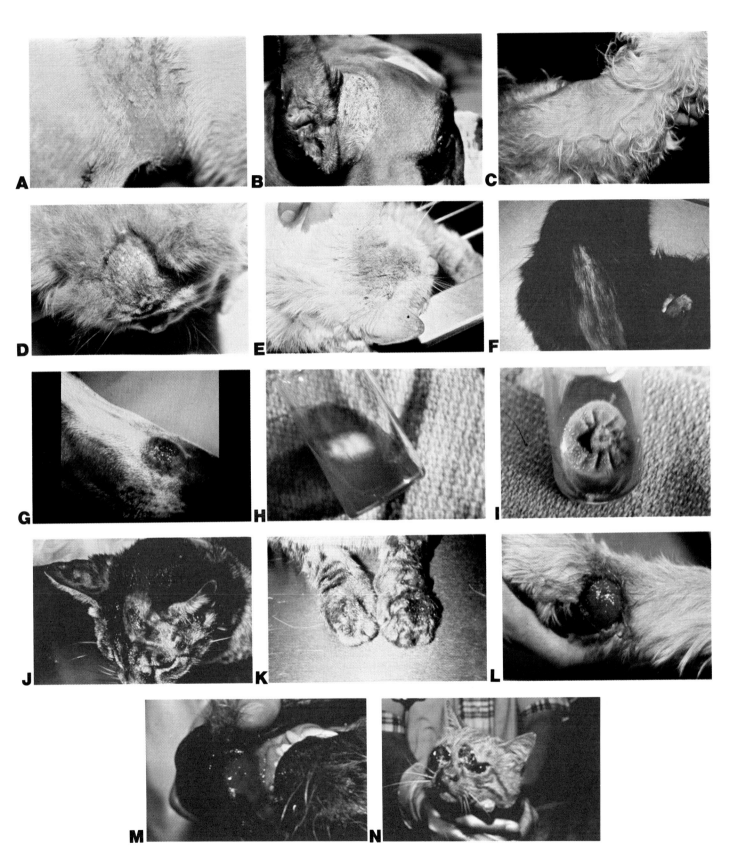

Plate 7. Endocrine Diseases

A, Hypothyroidism: Diffuse alopecia and hyperpigmentation on dorsal neck and shoulder associated with friction from a collar. *B,* Hypothyroidism: Diffuse alopecia of perineum and posterior thighs. *C,* Hypothyroidism: Multifocal alopecic areas on lateral aspect of the trunk of a dog. *D,* Hypothyroidism: Total trunkal alopecia and focal excoriation of a dog. *E,* Hyperadrenocorticism: Total trunkal alopecia and mild hyperpigmentation. The head and forelegs are not affected with alopecia. *F,* Hyperadrenocorticism: Diffuse alopecia of the dorsal trunk. Excoriation associated with calcinosis cutis is observed. *G,* Hyperadrenocorticism: Prominent ventral abdominal veins and comedones. *H,* Hyperadrenocorticism: Ecchymotic hemorrhage on ventral neck following jugular venipuncture. *I,* Hyperadrenocorticism: Hyperkeratotic plaque and excoriation associated with calcinosis cutis. *J,* Hyperadrenocorticism: Plaque associated with calcinosis cutis on the dorsal neck. Note the absence of inflammation. *K,* Ovarian imbalance Type I: Alopecia and mild hyperpigmentation of ventral caudal abdomen and medial thighs of intact female dog. Note mild gynecomastia. *L,* Ovarian imbalance Type I: Partial alopecia, hyperpigmentation, and scale on posterolateral thigh and lateral flank in an intact female dog.

Plate 7

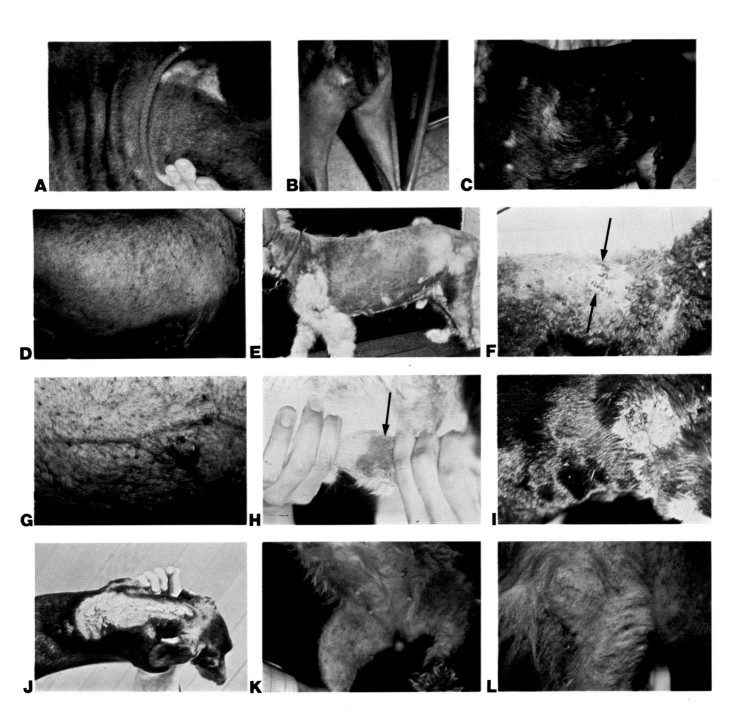

Plate 7 continued. Endocrine Diseases

M, Ovarian imbalance Type II: Diffuse alopecia of ventrum and abnormally soft, smooth skin in a spayed Weimaraner. Note the small vulva. N, Ovarian imbalance Type II: Patchy alopecia on dorsum of head. O, Sertoli cell tumor: Symmetric alopecia and hyperpigmentation on posterolateral thighs associated with a large scrotal testis. P, Sertoli cell tumor: Marked hyperpigmentation and lichenification of ventral caudal abdomen and scrotum associated with large scrotal testis. Q, Sertoli cell tumor: Focal alopecia and hyperpigmentation of lateral stifle and pendulous hyperpigmented prepuce associated with large scrotal testicle. R, Seminoma: Partial diffuse alopecia and mild hyperpigmentation of the lateral trunk associated with an inguinal testis. S, Feline endocrine alopecia: Diffuse alopecia with soft noninflamed skin on ventrum of trunk and medial thighs. T, Feline endocrine alopecia: Bilateral symmetric alopecia of lateral trunk. U, Feline endocrine alopecia: Bilateral alopecia of posterior aspect of forelegs and partial alopecia of ventral caudal abdomen. V, Pituitary dwarfism: Four-year-old German Shepherd cross that had a progressive thinning of hair and lethargy. Note size of dog (8 kg). W, Growth hormone responsive dermatosis: Multifocal patchy alopecia and hyperpigmentation of shoulder, lateral trunk, and perineum in intact male Pomeranian. X, Growth hormone responsive dermatosis: Diffuse alopecia of ventrum of neck and trunk in intact male Pomeranian. Y, Growth hormone responsive dermatosis: Total alopecia and marked hyperpigmentation of neck and thinning of hair of the thigh in intact male Chow Chow.

Plate 7 continued

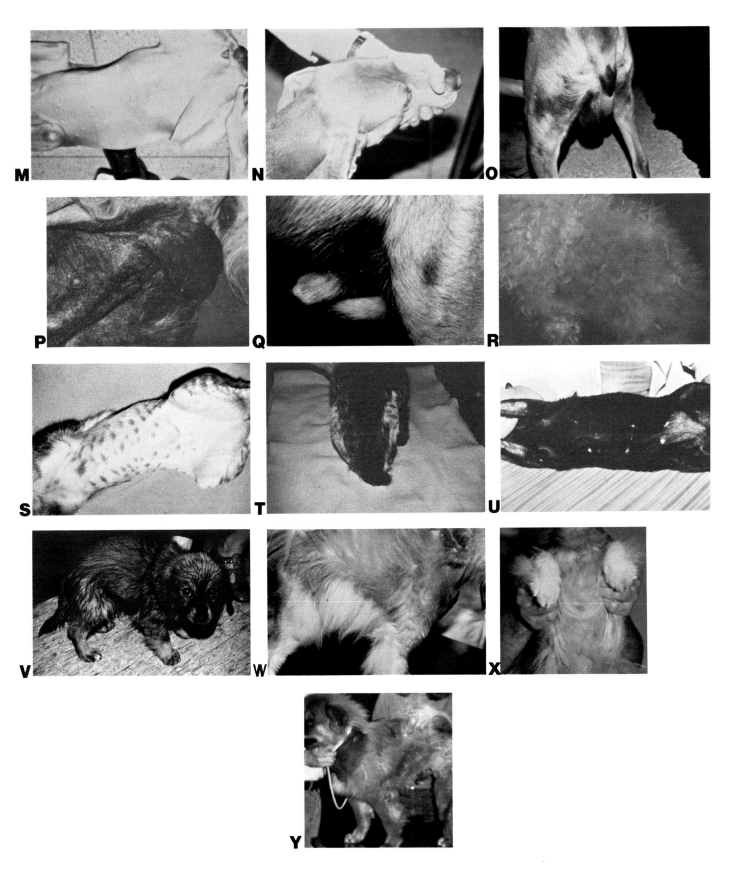

Plate 8. Seborrheic Syndrome

A, Seborrhea sicca: Generalized scaling (dandruff) on the dorsum of a dog. B, Seborrhea oleosa: Greasy, matted hair coat and scales on the hair of a dog. C, Seborrheic dermatitis: Large alopecic, erythematous patch with scales and crusts on the flank of a dog. D, Seborrhea sicca: Diffuse, partial alopecia and scale on the leg of a cat associated with Microsporum canis infection. E, Seborrhea oleosa: Generalized alopecia and greasy scale on a cat with pleural effusion and cardiomyopathy. F, Tail gland hyperplasia: Raised alopecic patch on the dorsal tail of a dog about five cm from the tail base. G, Feline acne: Comedone formation on ventral chin. A few crusts are present at the posterior margin of the lesion.

Plate 8

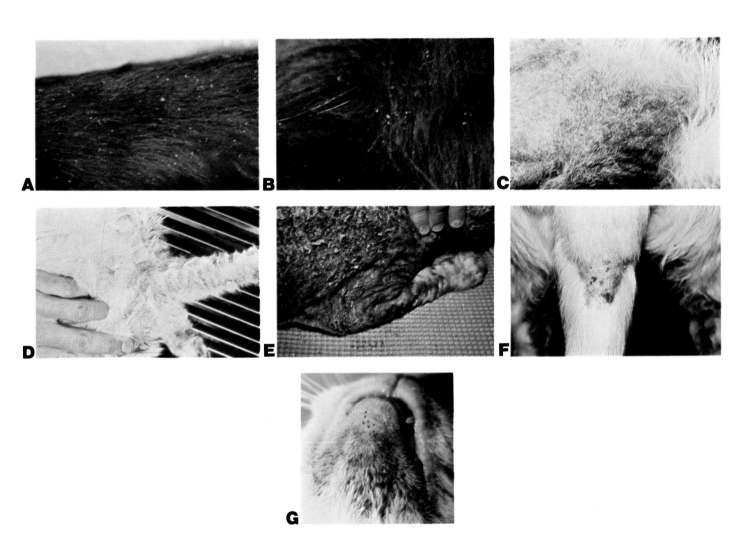

Plate 9. Bullous Diseases

A, Pemphigus vulgaris: Crusting at the mucocutaneous junctions of the upper lip on a dog. *B,* Pemphigus vulgaris: Ulceration and crusting of the anal mucosa and mucocutaneous junction of a dog. *C,* Pemphigus vulgaris: Ulceration and crusting of the ear pinna of a cat. (Courtesy of Nancy Brown.) *D,* Pemphigus foliaceus: Diffuse alopecia and crusting of dorsal muzzle, anterior face, and medial pinnae in a dog. *E,* Pemphigus foliaceus: Hyperkeratotic footpads in a dog. *F,* Bullous pemphigoid: Ulcerations of the oral mucosa (posterior hard palate) of a dog. *G,* Bullous pemphigoid: Ulceration and crusting of medial ear pinna of a dog. *H,* Discoid lupus erythematosus: Hypopigmentation and ulceration of the planum nasale and dorsal anterior muzzle of a dog. *I,* Acantholytic cells: A direct impression smear of an erosive lesion associated with pemphigus foliaceus. (Courtesy of Tom Manning.) *J,* Immunofluorescence testing of a skin lesion from a dog with pemphigus foliaceus or pemphigus vulgaris. Note the intercellular deposition of immunoglobulin in the epidermis. (Courtesy of R.M. Lewis and Teena Smith.) *K,* Immunofluorescence testing of a skin lesion from a dog with bullous pemphigoid. Note the deposition of immunoglobulin at the basement membrane zone. (Courtesy of R.M. Lewis and Teena Smith.) *L,* Toxic epidermal necrolysis: Multifocal ulcerative lesions on the neck of a cat. (Courtesy of William Miller.) *M,* Epidermolysis bullosa simplex: Mild focal scarring of the dorsal periorbital region and mild erythema and scaling ventral to the eye of a Collie. *N,* Subcorneal pustular dermatosis: Multifocal pustules and crust on the dorsal neck region of a dog. *O,* Subcorneal pustular dermatosis: Diffuse crusting of medial pinna.

Plate 9

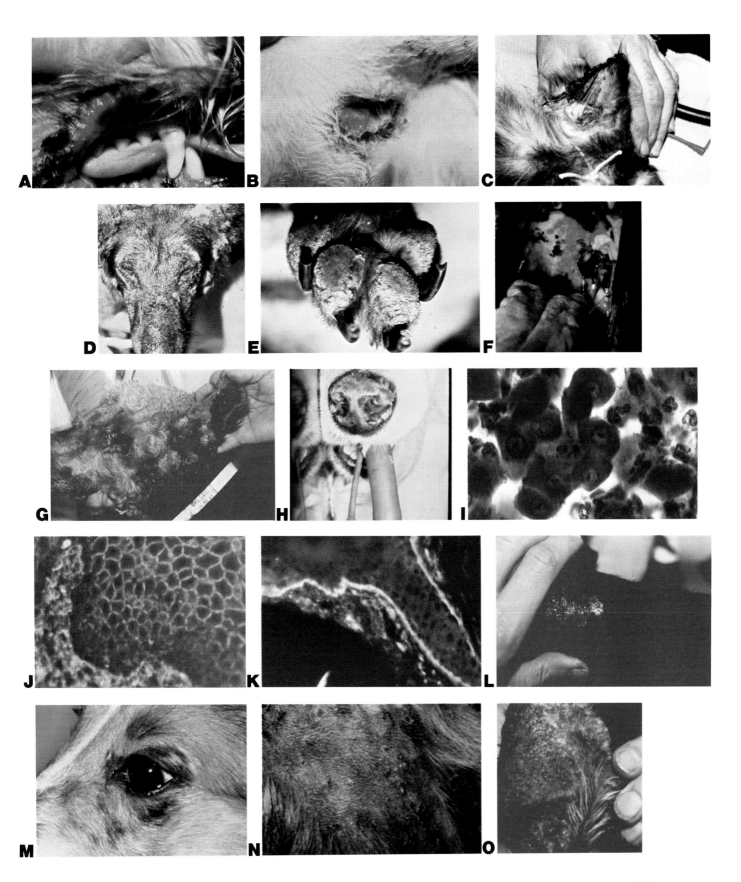

Plate 10. Neoplastic and Cystic Diseases

A, Epidermal inclusion cyst: A cyst opened surgically. Small dark structures within the cyst were filled with hair implanted into the dermis and subcutis by a dog bite. B, Sebaceous cyst: Ruptured cyst with semisolid doughy contents on the surface of the skin. C, Perianal adenoma: Solitary tumor in the perianal region. (Courtesy of E. Gregory MacEwen.) D, Squamous cell carcinoma: Erosion and crusting of tip of ear of white cat. (Courtesy of Daryl Biery.) E, Squamous cell carcinoma: Ulceration and destruction of tissue of rostral nares of white cat. (Courtesy of Daryl Biery.) F, Sebaceous gland tumor (nodular hyperplasia): Discrete lobulated tumor approximately 5 mm in diameter. G, Sebaceous gland tumor (adenoma): Solitary tumor of 1.5 cm in diameter with smooth, alopecic surface. H, Sebaceous gland adenocarcinoma: Large firm, irregularly shaped mass removed from the dorsum of a dog. The mass has been divided into halves. I, Oral papilloma: Multiple, whitish growths with irregular rough surfaces on the lips of a young dog. J, Basal cell tumor: Solitary, circumscribed tumor with a smooth, glistening surface on the leg of a dog. K, Intracutaneous cornifying epithelioma: Solitary tumor on back of dog with a keratinized plug. (Courtesy of Peter Ihrke and William Brewer.) L, Canine mammary gland tumor: Firm, subcutaneous nodules located near the nipples. M, Lipoma: Smooth, moderately firm, well-circumscribed, subcutaneous nodules on the ventral abdomen of a dog. N, Canine mastocytoma: Solitary, circumscribed tumor with a smooth surface on the stifle.

Plate 10

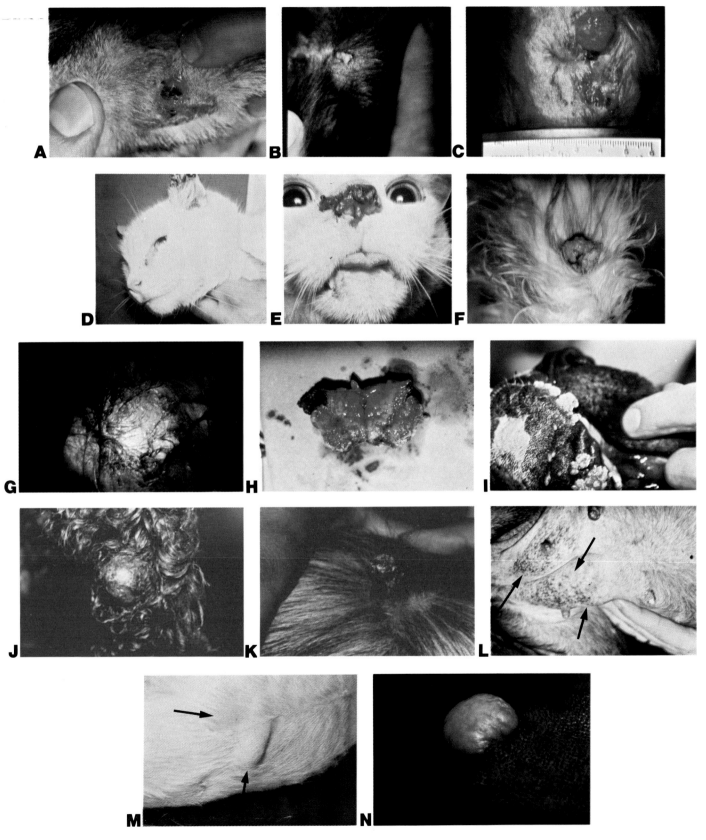

Plate 10 continued. Neoplastic and Cystic Diseases

O, Feline mastocytoma: Multiple, irregular erythematous plaques on the ventral abdomen. P, Feline mastocytoma: Rapidly growing ulcerated tumor on the face. Q, Feline mastocytoma: Diffuse, chronic ulceration of the anterior aspect of the forelimb. R, Canine hemangiopericytoma: Solitary, smooth, erythematous, dermal tumor located near the anus. (Courtesy of E. Gregory MacEwen.) S, Canine cutaneous histiocytoma: Small, circumscribed smooth, dermal tumor with mildly erythemic surface. T, Cutaneous hemangioma: Large, alopecic, soft, smooth, circumscribed, solitary tumor of dark blue color on a dog. U, Cutaneous hemangiosarcoma: Large alopecic tumor with poorly defined borders and bluish coloration on the metatarsus of a dog. V, Fibroma: Multiple circumscribed, rounded dermal nodules on extremity of a dog. W, Fibrosarcoma: Large circumscribed mass with invasion into surrounding tissue on dorsum of aged cat. (Courtesy of Richard L. Bradley.) X, Cutaneous lymphosarcoma: Dog with multiple, discrete, raised, dermal masses over trunk and extremities. Y, Cutaneous lymphosarcoma: Cat with ulcerated, circumscribed tumor on head. (Courtesy of Paul Caciolo.) Z, Cutaneous lymphosarcoma (Mycosis fungoides-like): Multifocal alopecic, scaly macules with excoriation on a dog. AA, Cutaneous lymphosarcoma: Diffuse infiltration and erythema and mild crusting of lips and buccal mucosa of a dog. BB, Cutaneous lymphosarcoma: Irregular erythematous, ulcerated plaque posterior to the elbow in a cat. (Courtesy of Paul Caciolo.) CC, Melanoma: Pedunculated, firm, discrete, hyperpigmented tumor on the dorsal toe of a dog.

Plate 10 continued

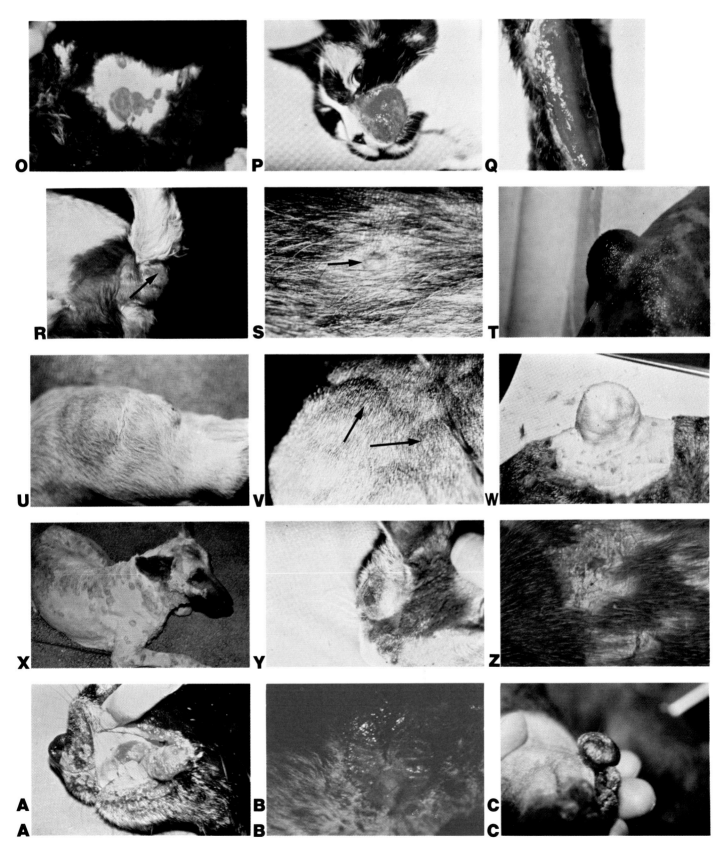

Plate 11. Miscellaneous Diseases

A, Irritant contact dermatitis: Diffuse erythema and erosion on ventral abdomen of a dog caused by an ammoniated floor cleaner. *B*, Irritant contact dermatitis: Diffuse alopecia and excoriation on dorsal head and neck of a cat following repeated applications of an iodine solution. *C*, Nasal solar dermatitis: Erythema and erosion on the anterior dorsal muzzle. *D*, Cutaneous asthenia: A 1-year-old Siamese cat with marked hyperextensibility of the skin. *E*, Cutaneous asthenia: Boxer with marked hyperextensibility of the skin. (Courtesy of Anthony Stannard.) *F*, Cutaneous asthenia: A 3-year-old cat with a new laceration on the shoulder and an alopecic, healing lesion on the dorsal thorax. *G*, Color mutant alopecia: An 8-month-old Doberman Pinscher with a bluish-grey coat color and large, irregular patches of alopecia on head, neck, extremities, and trunk. *H*, Ectodermal defect: Note the total alopecia of the dorsolateral neck and trunk of a Miniature Poodle. *I*, Black hair follicular dysplasia: Short, sparse hair coat on the black patches of skin with normal hair coat on the white skin. *J*, Zinc responsive dermatoses: Partially alopecic, scaly patches on lateral muzzle and ventral chin of a Siberian Husky. *K*, Zinc responsive dermatoses: Alopecia, scaly, hyperpigmented patches on the periorbital and lateral face region of a Siberian Husky. *L*, Nodular panniculitis: Multiple deep draining nodules on the trunk of a 3-month-old dog. *M*, Nodular panniculitis: Oily, blood-tinged discharge from subcutaneous nodule of 3-month-old dog.

Plate 11

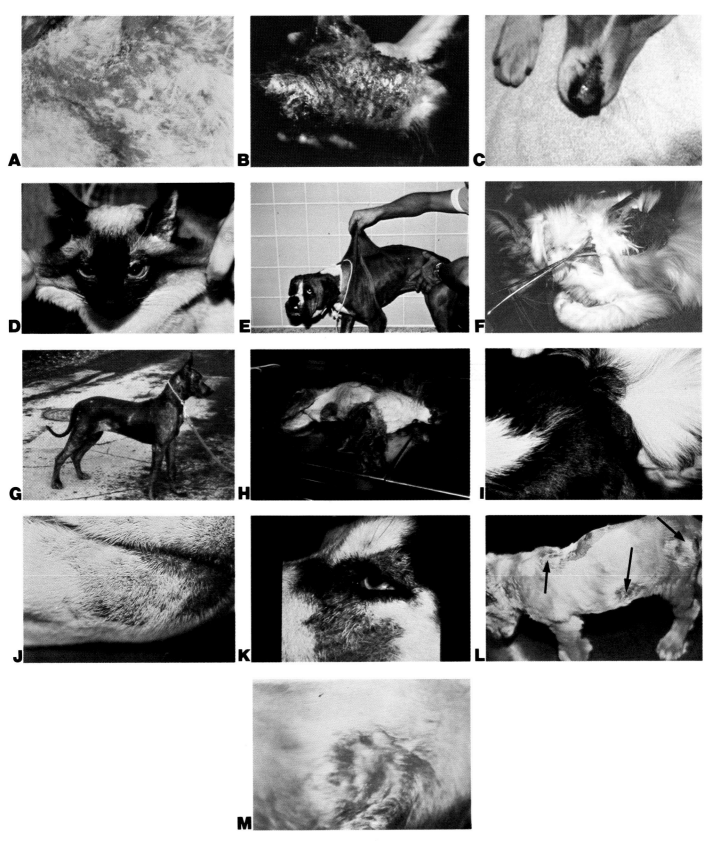

Plate 11 continued. Miscellaneous Diseases

N, Acanthosis nigricans: Axillary stage with moderate axillary hyperpigmentation and lichenification in an Irish Setter. O, Acanthosis nigricans: Advanced stage with marked axillary and medial forelimb hyperpigmentation and lichenification. P, Acral lick dermatitis: Large, alopecic plaque with erosion and focal exudate on the forelimb of a dog. Q, Eosinophilic ulcer: Diffuse ulceration and thickening of upper anterior lip of a cat with crusting on the surface. Note eosinophilic granuloma on hard palate (arrow). R, Eosinophilic ulcer: Focal ulcerative lesion on abdomen of a cat. S, Eosinophilic plaque: Focal plaque with a moist, erythematous, ulcerative surface on the abdomen of a cat. T, Linear granuloma: Linear pattern of multiple, raised, dry, plaques on posterior thigh of a cat. (Courtesy of Paul Caciolo.) U, Miliary dermatitis: Multiple erythematous papules on the lateral thorax of a cat. (Courtesy of Gail Kunkle.) V, Miliary dermatitis: Multiple small crusts on the dorsum of a cat. W, Neurodermatitis (dermatitic form): Focal area of alopecia on lateral forelimb with erythema and multifocal erosions. X, Neurodermatitis (alopecic form): Alopecic noninflamed patch on the lateral abdomen of a cat.

206

Plate 11 continued

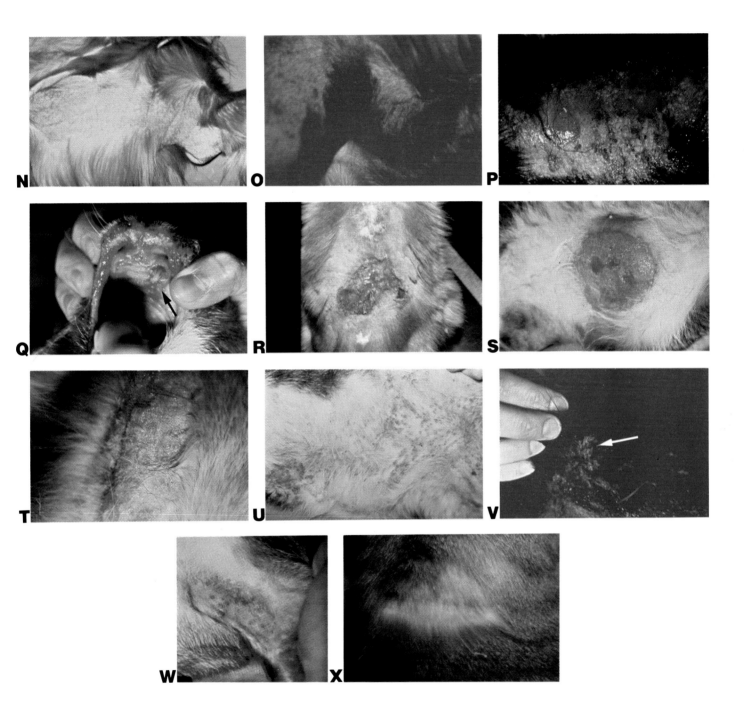

Appendix 4

Client Information Series

4:1 CANINE ATOPIC DERMATITIS—
ALLERGIC INHALANT DERMATITIS (AID), CANINE ATOPY

General Facts

1. Canine atopic dermatitis is an inherited predisposition to allergic symptoms following repeated exposure to inhalant allergens.
2. Age of onset is usually between 6 months and 3 years.
3. Due to the hereditary nature of the disease several breeds such as Golden Retrievers, most Terriers, and Irish Setters have a higher incidence. Many mixed breed dogs are also affected.
4. Symptoms may be seasonal or year-round and tend to worsen for longer periods of time as the dog ages.
5. Common causes of canine atopic dermatitis include pollens (trees, weeds, grasses), molds, dust, wool, cat dander, and feathers.
6. Allergic signs are aggravated by concurrent flea infestation. Therefore, continuous flea control should be maintained.

Clinical Signs

1. The primary clinical sign is scratching, most often in one or more of the following areas: under front legs (armpit area), between back legs, lower abdomen, face (rubbing), and feet (licking). Other types of allergies may affect the same areas.
2. Secondary lesions that result from scratching are common and include hair loss, redness, seborrhea (scaly skin with bad odor), and hyperpigmentation (dark skin).

Diagnosis

The only way to identify specific allergens is to skin test the dog. The dog *must not* be under the influence of cortisone (steroids). Waiting time following the oral administration of cortisone may vary from 2 to 4 weeks. There may be up to 2 months waiting time afer a long-acting cortisone injection. Type of cortisone, frequency of use, and dosage are factors to consider.

Treatment

1. Hyposensitization
   A. The preferred method of treatment is hyposensitization using allergy vaccine.
   B. An initial series of injections, usually every 3 days for 6 weeks, is injected under the skin.
   C. Periodic boosters, often every 1 to 4 weeks, may be required for life. If scratching is seasonal, the vaccine may not have to be given year-round.
   D. A common mistake is to discontinue the vaccine when improvement is noted, rather than continuing with boosters.
   E. A period of several months may be required to see significant improvement. Approximately 70 to 75% of the dogs improve with hyposensitization. In about 25% of these dogs some cortisone will still be required in doses and frequency less than that required before hyposensitization.
   F. Cortisone in minimal dosages may be given while hyposensitizing.
2. Cortisone
   A. Cortisone is the only drug that is consistently effective in masking the allergic symptoms.
   B. Administer the cortisone orally in the morning on alternate days to minimize side effects.
   C. Known common side effects of most cortisone therapy include increased water intake and frequency of urination as well as an increased appetite.
   D. Long-term treatment may cause increased susceptibility to infection, hair loss, thin skin, liver damage, gastrointestinal problems, and muscle weakness.

4:2 AQUEOUS HYPOSENSITIZATION SCHEDULE

Date: _____

ID number: _____   Referral veterinarian: _____

Client: _____   Address: _____

Animal name: _____   _____

Client phone: _____   Veterinarian phone: _____

Instructions for aqueous vaccine:

1. Vaccine must be refrigerated.
2. All vaccine is given subcutaneously (under the skin).
3. There will be vaccine left in vials No. 1 and 2. Do not discard.
4. Use 1-ml syringes and 25-gauge, $\frac{1}{2}$-in. needles for injections.

Injection schedule:

Vial No. 1				Vial No. 2				Vial No. 3	
Day	Date	Volume (ml)		Day	Date	Volume (ml)		Day	Date	Volume (ml)
1	_____	0.1		16	_____	0.1		31	_____	0.1
4	_____	0.2		19	_____	0.2		34	_____	0.2
7	_____	0.4		22	_____	0.4		37	_____	0.4
10	_____	0.8		25	_____	0.8		40	_____	0.8
13	_____	1.0		28	_____	1.0		43	_____	1.0
								50	_____	1.0
								57	_____	1.0

Vaccine booster schedule:

Booster injections should be given whenever scratching starts to increase, usually at 1- to 4-week intervals. Please record date and volume of injection on back of this sheet to help to determine the best booster program for your animal.

_____Use Vial No. 3. 1.0 ml/booster

_____Use Vial No. _____ : _____ ml/booster

The vaccine contains the following allergens:

4:3 AQUEOUS HYPOSENSITIZATION INSTRUCTIONS

Injection Procedures

1. Give all injections subcutaneously.
2. Use 1.0-ml syringes and 25-gauge, $1/2$-in. needles.
3. Rotate injection sites each time.

Handling of Vaccine

1. Keep all vaccine refrigerated.
2. Do not discard the vaccine left in vials No. 1 and 2 until the booster vaccine program has been established.

Side Effects of Vaccine

1. At times increased pruritus occurs within 24 hours after giving the injection. If this happens, decrease the dosage to the level given prior to the last injection or the dosage used 3 days before the dosage that caused the reaction.
2. If there is another increase in scratching at the reduced dosage, or if there was no significant decrease in the pruritic reaction, the dog should be re-evaluated to rule out concurrent problems.
3. The dosage or frequency of injections may need to be changed.
4. If necessary, corticosteroids may be administered (short-acting, low-dose) to bring the acute pruritus under control.

Booster Vaccine Schedule

1. Give a booster injection as soon as scratching increases, which may be in 1 week or 1 month. Use 1 ml of Vial No. 3.

4:4 CONTACT DERMATITIS

General Facts

1. Dogs of any age or breed may have symptoms of contact dermatitis.
2. The majority of animals manifest a reaction following irritation of some chemical or solid material in the environment (dyes, floor cleaners, shampoos, topical medications, rug fibers, cotton, wool).
3. An irritant reaction may occur immediately following exposure to the causative agent.
4. An allergic reaction may occur to the same agents (2 above) after months to years of exposure.

Clinical Signs

1. Signs occur only when there is direct contact with the causative agent. Thus, either an intermittent reaction (shampoo) or continuous reaction (rugs) may be observed. Once the reaction occurs, it may persist for a variable period of time after ceasing exposure.
2. Animals with contact reactions to floor coverings usually have red, irritated lesions and scratch the lower abdomen and legs; the top of the body is usually unaffected.
3. If topical medication is the cause, the contact reaction is observed at the site of application.

Diagnosis

1. Isolation (avoidance of contact), followed by re-exposure to the suspected causative agent, is the only satisfactory method of identifying the source of the contact problem.
2. If rugs or bedding are suspected, isolate the animal on hard surfaces. If area rugs are suspected, roll them up and vacuum well. Observe daily for improvement of signs (less scratching and redness). Allow 3 to 5 days for clinical improvement.
3. Do not use any floor cleaners or waxes on the hard surfaces during isolation; wash with water only.
4. If it is impossible to isolate at home, the animal may be removed from the home environment for several days. Hospitalization at the veterinary hospital is often satisfactory.
5. If medications or shampoos are suspected, discontinue their use and treat the animal symptomatically.

Treatment

1. Avoiding exposure is the treatment of choice.
2. If avoidance is not possible, corticosteroids (cortisone) are usually required, preferably a low dose every other day.
3. Try to minimize contact if total avoidance is not possible.
4. Hyposensitization (allergy injections) is not effective for contact dermatitis.

4:5 FOOD ALLERGY

General Facts

1. Food allergies are most commonly caused by an allergic reaction to one or more of the following animal proteins: horse meat, beef, pork, poultry products, milk, eggs, or fish. Food preservatives and dyes have also been reported to cause allergic signs.
2. Symptoms may be seen at any age. A young animal or an older one that has been on the same diet for many years may develop a food allergy.
3. It is not possible to differentiate a food allergy from other types of allergies without diet testing.
4. Many animals with food allergies will not significantly improve by changing commercial diets. All commercial diets (canned, semimoist, dry) contain one or more of the common animal proteins and most contain preservatives.
5. Food allergies are found concurrently with other allergies.

Clinical Signs

1. Clinical signs include scratching and biting, digestive disturbances, or both.
2. Most common digestive signs are excessive gas (flatulence) and loose stool. Occasionally a bloody diarrhea will be observed.
3. Scratching may be mild to severe with either localized or generalized self-trauma.
4. Cats often scratch severely about the head and neck.

Diagnosis

1. Diet testing, followed by provocative exposure (re-exposure) of the suspected foods, is the only definitive method to identify a food allergy.
2. Diet testing procedure
   A. Feed only foods that the dog or cat has had no previous exposure to.
   B. Suggested diets include:
      (1) lamb ($1/3$) and boiled white rice ($2/3$)
      (2) D/D prescription diet
      (3) rabbit or venison ($1/3$) and boiled rice ($2/3$)
   C. Feed the approximate quantity of test diet as regular diet.
   D. Feed the test diet for 14 to 21 days with no other food, treats, or supplements. Observe for less severe symptoms. There may not be complete remission if there are other concurrent problems.
   E. At the end of the test period:
      (1) The animal is re-exposed to one basic component of the regular diet at a time, i.e., one brand and flavor of commercial food or one protein (chicken or hamburger).
      (2) Feed each new addition for one week.
      (3) If symptoms do not become more severe within 7 days, add a second component. This procedure is followed until all of the components of the regular diet have been tested or until a satisfactory balanced diet is obtained.
      (4) If a problem is identified with the provocative testing, revert back to the previous step in the provocative testing in which no problem was observed. Remain at this step until symptoms have subsided and then add another component.

Treatment

1. If the animal reacts to the basic component of the diet, several other brands of commercial diet may be tested to see if one will be tolerated. Avoid all high protein or high meat diets and all scraps and treats.
2. If the dog reacts to several commercial diets, then one must be started from basic ingredients. Start with rice and vegetables, add cottage cheese, and finally meat. Vitamin and mineral supplements should be given if not on a balanced commercial diet.

4:6 FLEA DERMATITIS

General Facts

1. Only the adult flea lives on the dog and cat.
2. Life cycle: flea eggs hatch and form larvae which then develop into adults. This life cycle occurs in the house all year and in the yard mostly from spring through late fall. Fleas can live months without feeding. In climates with warm weather year round there can be a nonseasonal outdoor flea infestation.
3. Indoor flea infestation is usually the result of animals carrying fleas into the house from outdoors.
4. Fleas are commonly found indoors in the carpets, under moldings, and in most areas with moderate temperatures and sufficient moisture.
5. Fleas are on the animals only long enough to feed and then jump off (estimated 15 min/day). Therefore, it is common to find only a few or no fleas on the animal and still have a significant flea problem. Only flea dirt (dried blood) may be found.
6. Dog and cat fleas will infest either species of animal and will bite man, but prefer animals.
7. The sensitivity to fleas varies widely among animals. Often cats tolerate fleas better than dogs.
8. A flea infestation often causes signs of other allergies to become more severe.

Clinical Signs

1. Biting and scratching on the lower back and abdomen are the most common signs of flea infestation.
2. Hot spots often occur secondary to flea infestation.
3. Many dogs and a few cats develop an allergy to flea saliva. If this happens, there is often a disproportionate amount of scratching for the number of fleas observed on the animal.

Flea Control

1. Flea collars vary in efficacy:
   A. Good flea control is generally achieved with flea collars on cats. A few cats are not able to wear collars because of the irritation caused by the collar.
   B. Generally, the larger the dog or the longer the hair of the dog or cat, the poorer the flea control.

2. Most flea sprays, powders, or soaps have a short residual effect and need to be repeated every 2 to 5 days.
3. Flea powders and sprays must reach the skin to be effective. On long-haired animals, an alternative method of continuous flea control should be used.
4. Weekly flea dips (wipe on and let air-dry) are often the most efficient method of flea control for a dog or cat when a collar is not tolerated or efficacious. A bath should be given prior to dipping with the insecticide.
5. Good frequent grooming prevents many flea problems.

Methods for Good Flea Control

This program, if adhered to, should accomplish the following objectives
1. Break the flea life cycle.
2. Maintain relative flea-free animals.
3. Eliminate unnecessary expense in treating flea dermatitis or flea allergy by maintaining constant flea control.
   A. Initial flea control:
      (1) Bathe all dogs and cats, if possible, with flea soap or use an antiseborrheic shampoo if there is a lot of debris and scale on the surface.
      (2) If bathing is impossible, thoroughly dust or spray the animals.
      (3) Fumigate all inside areas the dog or cat has access to, such as house, garage, or shop. Use one or more insect foggers (aerosol bomb) on each floor of the premises. Be sure to read the fogger instructions and follow exactly. It may be more convenient to employ a professional exterminator.
   B. Continuous flea control ;
      (1) Weekly flea baths and dips; or
      (2) Frequent dusting or spraying (every 3 days); or
      (3) Flea collars. Bathing, powders, or sprays may have to be used in conjunction with the collars twice weekly.
   C. Treatment of flea allergy.
      Steps in A and B must be pursued diligently. In addition, corticosteroids may be required to stop the scratching initially.

4:7 DEMODECTIC MANGE

General Facts

1. Demodectic mange is caused by a microscopic mite that lives in the hair follicles of the skin.
2. Most dogs are carriers of the mite, but no clinical signs are observed.
3. Dogs with signs of demodectic mange are believed to (a) have a hereditary predisposition to proliferation of the mites and (b) have a temporary or reversible deficiency in their immune system (resistance).
4. Dogs become infected with the mite at the time of nursing during the first 2 or 3 days of life.
5. The condition is not contagious between infected dogs after the initial prenatal period (2 to 3 days old). It is not contagious to man.
6. The clinical signs are often self-limiting without treatment during the first year of life.
7. There is a higher rate of recurrence associated with females during their heat cycles compared to spayed females.
8. It is recommended not to use the dog for breeding because of the hereditary nature of the disease. Puppies from a symptomatic or recovered female will often have a high percentage of demodectic mange.

Clinical Signs

There are two forms of demodectic mange: localized and generalized.

1. Localized
   A. Usually 1 to 6 small areas of hair loss without inflammation or slight redness are seen, most commonly about the head, neck, and feet. Young dogs, 3 to 12 months of age are most commonly affected.
   B. Frequently, the patches of hair loss become infected, resulting in some scratching and irritation.
2. Generalized
   A. The areas of hair loss become more widespread, often involving several different areas of the body.
   B. Bacterial infection is common. Severe scratching may occur.

Diagnosis

The mites are found on skin scrapings.

Treatment

1. Mild, noninfected, localized cases of demodectic mange are often not treated. A rotenone ointment (Goodwinol) may be applied.
2. Antibiotics must be given if there is a bacterial infection.
3. The most satisfactory treatment is a new medication (Mitaban).
   A. Clip dogs with long hair or dense undercoat prior to starting treatment.
   B. Bathe first and towel dry.
   C. After bathing, wash (sponge on) with the medication diluted according to package instructions. Do not rinse off. Let air-dry.
   D. Repeat the bath and wash every 2 weeks. Usually 3 to 6 treatments are required.
   E. Continue treatment for a minimum of 3 dips or until there are 2 negative scrapings at least 2 weeks apart. Occasionally a second or third series of 6 treatments is necessary.

Prognosis

1. Most dogs will have a good clinical response after 3 to 6 treatments.
2. Up to 25% of the dogs may have a relapse after treatment is stopped. Most problems are related to failure to resolve the bacterial infection or stopping the medication prematurely.

4:8 SEBORRHEA

General Facts

1. Seborrhea is a syndrome characterized by scale (dandruff) or excessively dry or oily skin.
2. In most animals, seborrhea is secondary to some specific disease process such as fleas, mange, fungus (ringworm), allergies, or hormonal abnormalities.
3. In about 10% of the dogs neither internal or external causes can be found. Hereditary factors may predispose these dogs to seborrhea.
4. Many dogs with seborrhea have a bad odor due to a change in the type and number of bacteria on the surface of the skin. This is especially noticeable if the skin is oily.

Diagnosis

1. Identification of the primary cause of the seborrhea requires the "ruling in" or "ruling out" of possible causes based on the history and clinical findings.
2. Tests that may be indicated include skin scrapings, thyroid tests, fungus cultures, diet testing, skin testing, and skin biopsies.

Treatment

1. Specific treatments may include flea control, thyroid hormones, mange dips, or antifungal and allergy medications.
2. Symptomatic treatment for the dandruff and oiliness includes:
   A. Frequent antiseborrheic shampoos (tar, sulfur, selenium).
   B. Oil rinses if there is a dry skin and coat.
   C. Supplementation with a small amount of animal fat and vegetable oil in the diet daily.
   D. Antibiotics if bacterial infection is present.

Index

Numbers in *italics* refer to illustrations; numbers followed by t refer to tables.